Laboratory Animal
and Exotic Pet Medicine
Principles and Procedures

Laboratory Animal
and Exotic Pet Medicine
Principles and Procedures

Second Edition

Margi Sirois, EdD, MS, RVT, LAT

ELSEVIER

ELSEVIER

3251 Riverport Lane
St. Louis, Missouri 63043

Notices

Knowledge and best practice in this field are constantly changing. As new research and experience broaden our understanding, changes in research methods, professional practices, or medical treatment may become necessary.

Practitioners and researchers must always rely on their own experience and knowledge in evaluating and using any information, methods, compounds, or experiments described herein. In using such information or methods they should be mindful of their own safety and the safety of others, including parties for whom they have a professional responsibility.

With respect to any drug or pharmaceutical products identified, readers are advised to check the most current information provided (i) on procedures featured or (ii) by the manufacturer of each product to be administered, to verify the recommended dose or formula, the method and duration of administration, and contraindications. It is the responsibility of practitioners, relying on their own experience and knowledge of their patients, to make diagnoses, to determine dosages and the best treatment for each individual patient, and to take all appropriate safety precautions.

To the fullest extent of the law, neither the Publisher nor the authors, contributors, or editors, assume any liability for any injury and/or damage to persons or property as a matter of products liability, negligence or otherwise, or from any use or operation of any methods, products, instructions, or ideas contained in the material herein.

Library of Congress Cataloging-in-Publication Data

Sirois, Margi.
  Laboratory animal and exotic pet medicine : principles and procedures / Margi Sirois. -- Second edition.
      pages cm.
  Includes index.
  ISBN 978-0-323-17299-8 (paper back)
  1. Veterinary medicine. 2. Laboratory animals--Diseases--Treatment. 3. Exotic animals--Diseases--Treatment.
4. Wild animals as pets. I. Title.
  SF996.5.S57 2016
  636.088'5--dc23
                                                                      2015013301

Content Strategist: Shelly Stringer
Senior Content Development Specialist: Diane Chatman
Publishing Services Manager: Hemamalini Rajendrababu
Project Manager: Maria Bernard
Design Direction: Brian Salisbury

For my family—especially Dan (the-wonder-husband), Jennifer, and Daniel.

Preface

Veterinary technicians and laboratory animal technicians play a vital role in the care of exotic companion animals and animals in biomedical research. Many of the same species found in biomedical research facilities are also seen as pets in the veterinary practice. The diversity in anatomy and physiology of these species poses a particular challenge in their care and treatment. Veterinary technicians and laboratory animal technicians must be well versed in the unique features of these species to render proper care.

This book represents an effort to collect a broad scope of information needed by the student of veterinary technology and laboratory animal technology. A basic knowledge of anatomy and physiology has been assumed throughout the text. Learning objectives at the beginning of each chapter, key points, and chapter review questions are presented to assist in the study of these topics. "Technician notes" throughout each chapter highlight important points and provide helpful tips to improve knowledge and skill. Recommended readings provide additional sources of detailed information on the topics.

The book is organized so that basic principles of laboratory animal medicine are presented early on. Issues related to working with exotic companion animals and their owners in private practice are also discussed. Information on the care and treatment of the common species of laboratory and exotic companion animals follows. The text has been amply illustrated with color photos throughout. Large numbers of tables are used to provide a summary and handy reference for vital information. Common procedures used in diagnosis and treatment of laboratory and exotic companion animals demonstrate how to accomplish complex skills.

As scientific and medical knowledge continues to expand, the need for educated, competent, and compassionate laboratory animal caretakers is increasingly important. The quality and validity of research data are directly related to the quality of animal care provided. It is the veterinary technicians and laboratory animal technicians who provide the daily care on which high-quality science depends. Veterinary technicians are also involved in helping owners of exotic companion animals bond with their pets and maintain the human-animal bond. It is my hope that this book will aid the caretakers of these species (and their owners) in the performance of these crucial responsibilities.

Margi Sirois, EdD, MS, RVT

Acknowledgments

I have been fortunate to have learned from and with many individuals who have helped me nourish my special interest in laboratory animal and exotic companion animal medicine. I am especially grateful to Dr. Bert Lipitz—much of the work of this and the previous edition was envisioned during the time we worked together.

I will always be grateful to my mentors, Harriet Doolittle and Marianne McGurk, and to the many other veterinary technician educators who have encouraged and inspired me. To my friends at Elsevier, especially Shelly Stringer, Penny Rudolph, and Diane Chatman, I thank you all for your attention to detail and focus on excellence. I am forever grateful.

Contents

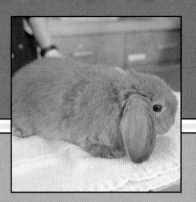

PART ONE

Principles of Laboratory Animal Medicine

Introduction to Exotic and Laboratory Animal Medicine

KEY TERMS

CITES
Dietary factors
Exotic pet
Extralabel use
Extrinsic factors
Intrinsic factors
Institutional animal care
  and use committee
Laboratory animal
Reduction
Refinement
Replacement
Zoonotic disease

LEARNING OBJECTIVES

After studying this chapter, you will be able to:

- Describe what is meant by the term exotic animal.
- Describe what is meant by the term laboratory animal.
- Discuss factors that may predispose an animal to disease.
- Differentiate between intrinsic and extrinsic factors that may predispose an animal to disease.
- List and describe the laws that govern scientific research.
- List the membership and functions of the institutional animal care and use committee.
- Describe the principle of the "three R's" of scientific research.
- Describe legal aspects of exotic animal ownership.
- Discuss laws related to legal aspects of wildlife care.

Exotic and **laboratory animal** medicine encompasses the knowledge and skill required to provide care for exotic pets and laboratory animals. The term **exotic pet** generally refers to any companion animal other than dogs and cats and includes birds, reptiles, amphibians, and a number of small mammals. In the strictest legal terms, an exotic animal is any one that is not native to the area where it is found or housed. Small mammals, sometimes referred to as pocket pets, include rats, mice, hamsters, gerbils, sugar gliders, rabbits, and guinea pigs. The term laboratory animal is used to denote any animal used in research or teaching (Figure 1-1). Animals used in scientific research may also be encountered as production animals in farms and ranches. In many cases; the research being performed is not directly related to the species on which the research is being conducted. The most commonly used laboratory animals are mice and rats. Other animals that may be used in research and teaching include hamsters, guinea pigs, dogs, cats, rabbits, gerbils, and fish. However, nearly any animal or plant may be used in scientific research.

Veterinary practices that treat only exotic pets are fairly common. Some may restrict their practice to just one species, such as avian-only practices. Veterinary practices that treat companion animals including exotic pets are also widespread. A recent survey conducted by the American Veterinary Medical Association indicated that more than 16 million U.S. households have at least one specialty or exotic pet and many had more than one. Survey data is summarized in Table 1-1. Both veterinarians and veterinary technicians receive basic education on handling and care of exotic animal species. However, the in-depth knowledge and skill needed to care for and treat the diverse species likely to be encountered requires additional and continual education.

The entire veterinary health care team has a responsibility to ensure the health and well-being of both pet and research animals. There are numerous legal and ethical issues regarding the care of exotic and laboratory animals. In addition to the many diverse laws involved, there are concerns related to the medications used. Nearly all medications used in exotic and laboratory animal medicine are **extralabel use**. This means that the drugs are used in a manner other than what is specified on the approved label directions. The U.S. Food and Drug Administration publishes specific guidelines under which extralabel use can be legal. Beyond the legal concerns,

administration of these drugs can also be problematic. Most medications are not available in a concentration that allows for the appropriate dose to be measured by conventional means. For example, if 0.5 mL of a medication would be administered to a 20-kg dog, a 400-g chinchilla may need just 0.005 mL. It is not possible to accurately measure this volume in a standard syringe, so the medication would have to be diluted before use.

> **TECHNICIAN NOTE** Many medications used on exotic and laboratory animals must be diluted before use.

DISEASE PREVENTION

Much of the responsibility of a veterinary technician or laboratory animal technician is aimed at preventing disease in the animals for which they provide care. Controlling factors that predispose animals to certain diseases is a primary concern of all members of the veterinary health care team. These predisposing factors can also be considered "stress factors" and may fall into one of several general areas: intrinsic, extrinsic, dietary, and experimental factors (Table 1-2). **Intrinsic factors** include such characteristics as species, age, gender, and heredity. For example, dogs are susceptible to parvovirus while rabbits are not; male cats are at a greater risk of developing feline urologic syndrome than are female cats. **Extrinsic factors** involve specific environmental parameters such as temperature, humidity, lighting, noise, and ventilation. Many species are sensitive to wide fluctuations in these parameters and develop specific diseases when environmental conditions are not appropriate (e.g., ringtail). **Dietary factors** include the quality and quantity of food and water as well as the sanitation of feed and water containers. Experimental factors are those that develop as a function of a specific research protocol in which an animal is involved. They include such parameters as surgery, restraint, and drug effects. Scientific research is designed to minimize the effects of these experimental factors by careful control of all variables in the animal environment.

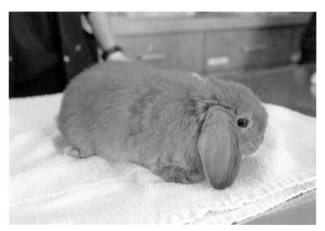

FIGURE 1-1. Rabbits are used in biomedical research and are also commonly encountered in exotic companion animal practice.

TABLE 1-1	Specialty and Exotic Animals	
	HOUSEHOLDS (IN 1000S)	**POPULATION (IN 1000S)**
Fish	7738	57,750
Ferrets	334	748
Rabbits	1408	3210
Hamsters	877	1146
Guinea pigs	847	1362
Gerbils	234	468
Other rodents	391	868
Turtles	1320	2297
Snakes	555	1150
Lizards	726	1119
Other reptiles	365	732
Poultry	1020	12,591
Livestock	661	5045
All others	246	898

From American Veterinary Medical Association, *U.S. Pet Ownership & Demographics Sourcebook (2012),* Schaumburg, IL.

TABLE 1-2	Factors Predisposing Animals to Disease		
INTRINSIC	**EXTRINSIC**	**DIETARY**	**EXPERIMENTAL**
Species variations	Environmental temperature	Quality of food and water	Restraint
Age	Environmental humidity	Availability of sufficient amounts of food and water	Surgical procedures
Sex	Noise	Cleanliness of food and water containers	Medication effects
Genetics	Ventilation		

> **TECHNICIAN NOTE** Control of factors that predispose animals to disease is an important aspect of disease prevention.

LEGAL AND ETHICAL ISSUES

LEGAL ASPECTS OF EXOTIC PET PRACTICE

Exploring the legal aspects of exotic pet ownership is complicated by the fact that the laws may vary considerably in different locations. Federal, state, and local laws may all address some aspect of exotic pet ownership. A species that may be legal to own in one area may be illegal in another or may require a special permit in yet another. Availability of a species in a particular area, even for sale at a pet shop, does not necessarily mean that the species is legal to own. The veterinary team must be familiar with the laws in the local area and be able to properly counsel prospective owners. The veterinarian must also determine whether to treat species that are not legal to own in the local area.

Some of the laws put into place restricting exotic pet ownership are the result of a global effort to minimize illegal trade in animals that could potentially push some species to the brink of extinction in their native habitat. The Convention on International Trade in Endangered Species of Wild Flora and Fauna (**CITES**) was developed to safeguard species from extinction. Currently, 180 countries have agreed to adhere to this international agreement. Approximately 5600 species of animals are protected by CITES. Restrictions are in place that minimize or eliminate the sale of wild caught animals that are protected by CITES. As a result, most common species of exotic animals must be acquired from sources that have bred those animals for the purpose of selling them as pets.

CITES applies only to import and export and not to trade within a country of organisms that were legally imported. Organisms listed under CITES are classified into one of three categories, referred to as Appendix I, II, or III. Appendix I species are those that are currently threatened with extinction, such as the Galapagos turtle. Import or export of these species requires special permits and cannot be for commercial purposes. Permits are issued only under exceptional circumstances. Species listed under CITES Appendix II are not currently threatened with extinction, such as the boa constrictor. Commercial trade is allowed with special permits. Appendix III consists of organisms that are protected in at least one country that has asked for assistance in protecting the species. Certification regarding the country of origin of the species is needed before permission to export is granted.

> **TECHNICIAN NOTE** The Convention on International Trade in Endangered Species of Wild Fauna and Flora is a multinational agreement between governments designed to ensure that international trade in specimens of wild animals and plants does not threaten their survival.

ETHICAL CONCERNS OF EXOTIC PET OWNERSHIP

Owners of exotic pets must ensure that the unique animal husbandry, welfare, and safety requirements of the species are addressed. Many of the common exotic pet species can harbor **zoonotic disease** (diseases that can be transmitted between animals and people). Some of these species can also be dangerous to the community and disruptive to local ecosystems should they escape from their owners. For example, the state of Florida has several species that are not native to the ecosystems where they now live. This includes a large population of Burmese pythons and green iguanas. These species have no natural predators in the areas where they are now present, and their populations have thrived by displacing other species and outcompeting them for resources. Threats to public health do not only include transmission of zoonotic disease. Exotic pets have escaped or been intentionally released and have injured and killed humans and domestic animals. It is important that the veterinary team work closely with owners of exotic pets that they can no longer care for to ensure that the animal is properly placed in another home, a zoo, or animal sanctuary.

LEGAL AND ETHICAL ASPECTS OF WILDLIFE CARE

Federal, state, and local laws exist that protect native wild animals. In most cases, a permit or license is needed to care for or possess native wildlife. Clients may call or bring in native wildlife they believe to be injured or orphaned. The veterinarian may provide emergency care to stabilize the animal but should transfer the animal to a local licensed rehabilitator as soon as possible. Because these orphaned or injured animals have no "owner," the clinic is often not paid for services rendered.

When clients call the practice regarding potentially injured or orphaned animals, it is important to question them regarding the location where the animal was found and why they believe it to be orphaned or injured. In some cases, well-meaning individuals remove animals from nest areas believing that they are abandoned. They may also mistakenly believe that the parents will abandon the baby if it has been touched by a human. In many cases, the client may believe the nest to be abandoned when in fact the parent(s) are sufficiently secretive to not be seen. Many species also visit the nest only one or two times a day so are often not seen by others. The animal in question should be returned to the nest unless it appears weak or has obvious signs of injury (i.e., bleeding, fractures). Clients should also be advised regarding the potential for transmission of diseases such as psittacosis, rabies, and tularemia when handling wildlife.

LEGAL REQUIREMENTS OF LABORATORY ANIMAL USE

Regulation of animal research involves a number of government organizations. In addition, specific guidelines for the use of animals in research are mandated by certain funding agencies. The majority of the regulations were put in place as a result of concern among the general public for the welfare of animals. However, the continued improvement and implementation of those regulations is a welcome responsibility of all individuals working in the field of laboratory animal medicine. Valid scientific research requires excellent animal care.

The Animal Welfare Act

The Animal Welfare Act (AWA) is the principal federal statute governing the sale, handling, transport, and use of animals. The AWA sets standards of care for animals in education, research, or exhibition. The AWA was first passed in 1966 and has been revised several times. It was originally entitled the "Laboratory Animal Welfare Act." The purposes of the original act were to:

- Protect the owners of dogs and cats from theft of such pets
- Prevent the sale or use of dogs and cats that had been stolen
- Insure that animals intended for use in research facilities were provided with humane care and treatment.

> **TECHNICIAN NOTE** The Animal Welfare Act is the principal federal statute governing the sale, handling, transport, and use of animals.

The original act covered nonhuman primates, guinea pigs, hamsters, rabbits, dogs, and cats. In 1970 the original act was amended and renamed the Animal Welfare Act. The 1976 amendments covered broader classes of animals, including all warm-blooded vertebrates, and redefined the regulation of animals during transportation. The current AWA applies to all warm-blooded animals (alive or dead) that are used for research, testing, or teaching, except horses and farm animals used for agricultural research, food, or fiber. The regulations that implement the AWA, commonly referred to as the Animal Welfare Regulations (AWR), are contained in the code of federal regulations Title 9, Chapter 1, subpart A—Animal Welfare. The regulations currently also exempt birds, rats of the genus *Rattus*, and mice of the genus *Mus*. Cold-blooded animals have not been addressed in the AWA.

Later amendments to the AWA included development of standards for exercise for dogs and provisions for improvements of the physical environment of nonhuman primates to promote their psychologic well-being. New limitations were also put in place regarding the performance of multiple survival surgeries. Mandates that the head of the research team (the principal investigator or PI) consult with a veterinarian in the design of experiments that have the potential for causing pain and to ensure the proper use of anesthetics, analgesics, and tranquilizers were added. Requirements for investigation of alternatives to animal use and for the formation of the animal care and use committee were also developed in the later amendments.

The United States Department of Agriculture (USDA) is authorized by law to enforce the animal welfare regulations.

Facilities are required to keep accurate records to show that they are in compliance with legislative requirements. Annual reports are also required (Figure 1-2). Facilities are inspected by an agency of the USDA, the Animal and Plant Health Inspection Service (APHIS). Inspections must occur at least annually. Another agency of the USDA, the Regulatory Enforcement and Animal Care (REAC), has the authority to enforce penalties for violations of the AWA, including closing the facility and fining and suspending individuals and corporations.

Institutional Animal Care and Use Committee

As part of the changes to the Animal Welfare Act of 1985, all animal use in research or teaching done in the United States must be approved by an **Institutional Animal Care and Use Committee** (IACUC), also known as the Animal Care and Use Committee (ACUC). The IACUC is responsible for all aspects of animal use, education, health, and compliance with all laws and regulations. The makeup of the IACUC as required by the AWA includes at least three individuals appointed by the chief executive officer of the institution. One must be a veterinarian with training and experience in laboratory animal medicine and at least one person must have no affiliation with the research facility. Most IACUC's include a nonscientist, or a lay representative, to speak for the general community. Large institutions may have more than one IACUC. The IACUC is an independent entity within the institution or corporation and cannot be overruled by executive action. The IACUC must be qualified to assess the facility's program of veterinary care (Figure 1-3) and review all animal use protocols. Functions of the IACUC are summarized in Box 1-1.

> **TECHNICIAN NOTE** All use of animals in teaching and research must be reviewed and approved by the IACUC.

Animal Use Protocols

Each use of animals in research or teaching must have a specific protocol that describes in detail what is to be done. This includes detailed information regarding the species chosen and number of animals to be used and the rationale for the use of the number of animals of that particular species. Detailed descriptions of all procedures used as well as the individuals involved in each procedure and the qualifications of those individuals are also required. The protocol is also used to allow the IACUC to verify that appropriate pain-relieving medications will be administered for any procedure that causes more than momentary pain or distress to the animals. Animal use protocols also contain results of literature searches to document that the study does not unnecessarily duplicate prior work. Nearly all protocols contain information on euthanasia methods that will be used if needed, even when the procedure is not expected to result in the death of the animal. This helps ensure that appropriate methods are used in the event of unforeseen adverse reactions of an animal.

According to the Paperwork Reduction Act of 1995, an agency may not conduct or sponsor, and a person is not required to respond to, a collection of information unless it displays a valid OMB control number. The valid OMB control number for this information collection is 0579-0036. The time required to complete this information collection is estimated to average 2 hours per response, including the time for reviewing instructions, searching existing data sources, gathering and maintaining the data needed, and completing and reviewing the collection of information.	**OMB APPROVED** 0579-0036

This report is required by law (7 U.S.C. 2143). Failure to report according to the regulations can result in an order to cease and desist and to be subject to penalties as provided for in Section 2150.	Interagency Report Control No. 0180-DOA-AN	Fiscal Year 2013

UNITED STATES DEPARTMENT OF AGRICULTURE
ANIMAL AND PLANT HEALTH INSPECTION SERVICE

1. REGISTRATION NUMBER

2. HEADQUARTERS RESEARCH FACILITY *(Name, address, and telephone number as registered with USDA, include ZIP Code)*

ANNUAL REPORT OF RESEARCH FACILITY
(TYPE OR PRINT)

3. REPORTING FACILITY *(List all locations where animals were housed or used in actual research, testing, teaching, or experimentation, or held for these purposes. Attach additional sheets, if necessary.)*

FACILITY LOCATIONS *(Sites)*

REPORT OF ANIMALS USED BY OR UNDER CONTROL OF RESEARCH FACILITY *(Attach additional sheets, if necessary, or use APHIS FORM 7023A.)*

A. Animals Covered By The Animal Welfare Regulations	B. Number of animals being bred, conditioned, or held for use in teaching, testing, experiments, research, or surgery but not yet used for such purposes.	C. Number of animals upon which teaching, research, experiments, or tests were conducted involving no pain, distress, or use of pain-relieving drugs.	D. Number of animals upon which experiments, teaching, research, surgery, or tests were conducted involving accompanying pain or distress to the animals and for which appropriate anesthetic, analgesic, or tranquilizing drugs were used.	E. Number of animals upon which teaching, experiments, research, surgery, or tests were conducted involving accompanying pain or distress to the animals and for which the use of appropriate anesthetic, analgesic, or tranquilizing drugs would have adversely affected the procedures, results, or interpretation of the teaching, research, experiments, surgery, or tests. *(An explanation of the procedures producing pain or distress on these animals and the reasons such drugs were not used must be attached to this report.)*	F. TOTAL NUMBER OF ANIMALS (Cols. C + D + E)
4. Dogs					0
5. Cats					0
6. Guinea Pigs					0
7. Hamsters					0
8. Rabbits					0
9. Non-human Primates					0
10. Sheep					0
11. Pigs					0
12. Other Farm Animals					
					0
13. Other Animals					
					0
					0
					0

ASSURANCE STATEMENTS

1.) Professionally acceptable standards governing the care, treatment, and use of animals, including appropriate use of anesthetic, analgesic, and tranquilizing drugs, prior to, during, and following actual research, teaching, testing, surgery, or experimentation were followed by this research facility.

2.) Each principal investigator has considered alternatives to painful procedures.

3.) This facility is adhering to the standards and regulations under the Act, and it has required that exceptions to the standards and regulations be specified and explained by the principal investigator and approved by the Institutional Animal Care and Use Committee (IACUC). **A summary of all such exceptions is attached to this annual report.** In addition to identifying the IACUC approved exceptions, this summary includes a brief explanation of the exceptions, as well as the species and number of animals affected.

4.) The attending veterinarian for this research facility has appropriate authority to ensure the provisions of adequate veterinary care and to oversee the adequacy of other aspects of animal care and use.

CERTIFICATION BY HEADQUARTERS RESEARCH FACILITY OFFICIAL
(Chief Executive Officer (C.E.O.) or Legally Responsible Institutional Official (I.O.))
I certify that the above is true, correct, and complete (7 U.S.C. Section 2143).

SIGNATURE OF C.E.O. OR I.O.	NAME AND TITLE OF C.E.O. OR I.O. *(Type or Print)*	DATE SIGNED

APHIS FORM 7023
JUL 2013

FIGURE 1-2. USDA annual report of research facility.

According to the Paperwork Reduction Act of 1995, an agency may not conduct or sponsor, and a person is not required to respond to, a collection of information unless it displays a valid OMB control number. The valid OMB control numbers for these information collections are 0579-0036, 0579-0093, and 0579-0392. The time required to complete these information collections is estimated to average 1 hour per response, including the time for reviewing instructions, searching existing data sources, gathering and maintaining the data needed, and completing and reviewing the collection of information.

OMB Approved
0579-0036
0579-0093
0579-0392

The Animal Welfare Regulations, Title 9, Subchapter A, Part II, Subpart C, Section 2.33 and Subpart D, Section 2.40 require a Program of Veterinary Care.

UNITED STATES DEPARTMENT OF AGRICULTURE
ANIMAL AND PLANT HEALTH INSPECTION SERVICE

ANIMAL CARE

(Program of Veterinary Care for Research Facilities or Exhibitors/Dealers)

OFFICE USE ONLY

DATE RECEIVED:

SECTION I. A PROGRAM OF VETERINARY CARE HAS BEEN ESTABLISHED BETWEEN:

A. LICENSEE/REGISTRANT	B. VETERINARIAN
1. NAME:	1. NAME:
2. BUSINESS NAME:	2. CLINIC NAME:
3. USDA LICENSE/REGISTRATION NUMBER:	3. STATE LICENSE NUMBER:
4. MAILING ADDRESS:	4. BUSINESS ADDRESS:
5. CITY, STATE, AND ZIP CODE:	5. CITY, STATE, AND ZIP CODE:
6. TELEPHONE NUMBER *(Home):* TELEPHONE NUMBER *(Business):*	6. TELEPHONE NUMBER *(Business):*

This is a form that may be used for the Program of Veterinary Care. Also, this form may be used as a guideline for the written Program of Veterinary Care, as required.

The attending veterinarian shall establish, maintain, and supervise programs of disease control and prevention, pest and parasite control, pre-procedural and post-procedural care, nutrition, euthanasia, and adequate veterinary care for all animals on the premises of the licensee/registrant. A written program of adequate veterinary care between the licensee/registrant and the doctor of veterinary medicine shall be established and reviewed on an annual basis. By law, such programs must include regularly scheduled visits to the premises by the veterinarian. Scheduled visits are required to monitor animal health and husbandry.

Pages or blocks which do not apply to the facility should be marked N/A. If the space provided is not adequate for a specific topic, additional sheets may be added. Please indicate Section and Item Number.

I have read and completed this Program of Veterinary Care, and understand my responsibilities.

Regularly scheduled visits by the veterinarian will occur at the following frequency:

_____ *(minimum annual).*

C. SIGNATURE OF LICENSEE/REGISTRANT:	DATE:
D. SIGNATURE OF VETERINARIAN:	DATE:

APHIS 7002
JUN 2011

FIGURE 1-3. USDA form for recording the program of veterinary care.

CHECK IF N/A ☐   **SECTION II. DOGS AND CATS**

A. VACCINATIONS – SPECIFY THE FREQUENCY OF VACCINATION FOR THE FOLLOWING DISEASES:

CANINE			FELINE		
	JUVENILE	ADULT		JUVENILE	ADULT
PARVOVIRUS			PANLEUK		
DISTEMPER			RESP. VIRUSES		
HEPATITIS			RABIES		
LEPTOSPIROSIS			OTHER *(Specify)*		
RABIES					
BORDETELLA					
OTHER *(Specify)*					

B. PARASITE CONTROL PROGRAM – DESCRIBE THE FREQUENCY OF SAMPLING OR TREATMENT FOR THE FOLLOWING:

1. ECTOPARASITES *(Fleas, Ticks, Mites, Lice, Flies)*:

2. BLOOD PARASITES *(Heartworm, Babesia, Ehrlichia, Other)*:

3. INTESTINAL PARASITES *(Fecals, Deworming)*:

C. EMERGENCY CARE – DESCRIBE PROVISIONS FOR EMERGENCY, WEEKEND, AND HOLIDAY CARE:

D. EUTHANASIA

1. SICK, DISEASED, INJURED, OR LAME ANIMALS SHALL BE PROVIDED WITH VETERINARY CARE OR EUTHANIZED. EUTHANASIA WILL BE IN ACCORDANCE WITH THE AMERICAN VETERINARY MEDICAL ASSOCIATION (AVMA) RECOMMENDATIONS AND WILL BE CARRIED OUT BY THE FOLLOWING:

☐ VETERINARIAN   ☐ LICENSEE/REGISTRANT

2. METHOD(S) OF EUTHANASIA:

E. ADDITIONAL PROGRAM TOPICS – THE FOLLOWING TOPICS HAVE BEEN DISCUSSED IN THE FORMULATION OF THE PROGRAM OF VETERINARY CARE:

☐   Congenital Conditions   ☐   Exercise Plan *(Dogs)*

☐   Quarantine Conditions   ☐   Proper Handling of Biologics

☐   Nutrition   ☐   Venereal Diseases

☐   Anthelmintic Alternation   ☐   Pest Control and Product Safety

☐   Other *(Specify)*_____   ☐   Proper Use of Analgesics and Sedatives

FIGURE 1-3, cont'd

Continued

CHECK IF N/A ☐   **SECTION III. WILD AND EXOTIC ANIMALS**

A. VACCINATIONS – LIST THE DISEASES FOR WHICH VACCINATIONS ARE PERFORMED AND THE FREQUENCY OF THE VACCINATIONS *(Enter N/A if not applicable)*:

CARNIVORES:

HOOFED STOCK:

PRIMATES:

ELEPHANTS:

MARINE MAMMALS:

OTHER *(Specify)*:

B. PARASITE CONTROL PROGRAM – DESCRIBE THE FREQUENCY OF SAMPLING OR TREATMENT FOR THE FOLLOWING:

1. ECTOPARASITES *(Fleas, Ticks, Mites, Lice, Flies)*:

2. BLOOD PARASITES:

3. INTESTINAL PARASITES:

C. EMERGENCY CARE

1. DESCRIBE PROVISIONS FOR EMERGENCY, WEEKEND, AND HOLIDAY CARE:

2. DESCRIBE CAPTURE AND RESTRAINT METHOD(S):

D. EUTHANASIA

1. SICK, DISEASED, INJURED, OR LAME ANIMALS SHALL BE PROVIDED WITH VETERINARY CARE OR EUTHANIZED. EUTHANASIA WILL BE IN ACCORDANCE WITH THE AVMA RECOMMENDATIONS AND WILL BE CARRIED OUT BY THE FOLLOWING:

☐ VETERINARIAN   ☐ LICENSEE/REGISTRANT

2. METHOD(S) OF EUTHANASIA:

E. ADDITIONAL PROGRAM TOPICS – THE FOLLOWING TOPICS HAVE BEEN DISCUSSED IN THE FORMULATION OF THE PROGRAM OF VETERINARY CARE:

☐ Pest Control and Product Safety

☐ Quarantine Procedures

☐ Zoonoses

☐ Other *(Specify)* _____

_____

☐ Environment Enhancement *(Primates)*

☐ Water Quality *(Marine Mammals)*

☐ Species-specific Behaviors

☐ Proper Storage and Handling of Drugs and Biologics

☐ Proper Use of Analgesics and Sedatives

F. LIST THE SPECIES SUBJECTED TO TB TESTING, AND THE FREQUENCY OF SUCH TESTS:

FIGURE 1-3, cont'd

CHECK IF N/A ☐ **SECTION IV. OTHER WARMBLOODED ANIMALS**

A. INDICATE SPECIES:

B. VACCINATIONS – LIST THE DISEASES FOR WHICH VACCINATIONS ARE PERFORMED AND THE FREQUENCY OF VACCINATIONS
(Enter N/A if not applicable):

C. PARASITE CONTROL PROGRAM – DESCRIBE THE FREQUENCY OF SAMPLING OR TREATMENT FOR THE FOLLOWING:

1. ECTOPARASITES *(Fleas, Ticks, Mites, Lice, Flies)*:

2. INTERNAL PARASITES *(Helminths, Coccidia, Other)*:

D. EMERGENCY CARE – DESCRIBE PROVISIONS FOR EMERGENCY, WEEKEND, AND HOLIDAY CARE:

E. EUTHANASIA

1. SICK, DISEASED, INJURED, OR LAME ANIMALS SHALL BE PROVIDED WITH VETERINARY CARE OR EUTHANIZED, EUTHANASIA WILL BE IN ACCORDANCE WITH THE AVMA RECOMMENDATIONS AND WILL BE CARRIED OUT BY THE FOLLOWING:

☐ VETERINARIAN   ☐ LICENSEE/REGISTRANT

2. METHOD(S) OF EUTHANASIA:

F. ADDITIONAL PROGRAM TOPICS – THE FOLLOWING TOPICS HAVE BEEN DISCUSSED IN THE FORMULATION OF THE PROGRAM OF VETERINARY CARE:

☐ Pasteurellosis   ☐ Species Separation

☐ Pododermatitis   ☐ Malocclusion/Overgrown Incisors

☐ Cannibalism   ☐ Pest Control and Product Safety

☐ Wet Tail   ☐ Handling

☐ Other *(Specify)*_____

FIGURE 1-3, cont'd

BOX 1-1	Functions and Responsibilities of the IACUC

- The facility should be inspected and the program of veterinary care should be reviewed at least every 6 months
- Protocols involving the use of live animals should be reviewed
- Complaints involving the care and use of animals should be investigated
- Evaluation reports should be prepared every 6 months
- Recommendations to the institutional official should be made
- Suspending an activity involving animals should be authorized
- Proposed activities should meet the following requirements:
  - Discomfort, distress, and pain to the animals will be avoided or minimized
  - Alternatives to procedures that may cause more than momentary or slight pain or distress to the animals have been considered
  - No unnecessary duplication of previous experiments will be done
  - Procedures that may cause more than momentary or slight pain or distress to the animals will be performed with appropriate sedatives, analgesics, or anesthetics
  - The PI will consult with attending veterinarians when planning procedures
  - Procedures will not include the use of paralytics without anesthesia
  - Animals that would otherwise experience severe or chronic pain or distress that cannot be relieved will be painlessly euthanized at the end of the procedure
  - Animals' living conditions will be appropriate
  - Personnel conducting procedures on the species being maintained or studied will be appropriately qualified and trained in those procedures
  - Medical care will be provided by a qualified veterinarian
  - Activities that involve surgery will include appropriate provision for preoperative and postoperative care of the animals according to established veterinary and nursing practices
  - All survival surgeries will be performed with aseptic procedures, including surgical gloves, masks, sterile instruments, and aseptic techniques
  - Major operative procedures on nonrodents will be conducted only in facilities intended for that purpose, which will be operated and maintained under aseptic conditions
  - Nonmajor operative procedures and all surgeries on rodents that do not require a dedicated facility will be performed with aseptic procedures
  - No animal will be used in more than one major operative procedure from which it is allowed to recover, unless:
    - Justified for scientific reasons by the PI in writing
    - Required as routine veterinary procedure or to protect the health or well-being of the animal as determined by the attending veterinarian, or
    - In other special circumstances as determined by the administrator with written request and supporting data sent to the administrator, APHIS, and USDA

Guide for the Care and Use of Laboratory Animals

The Guide for the Care and Use of Laboratory Animals (referred to simply as the "Guide") is the primary reference on animal care and use (Figure 1-4). The Guide is written under the direction of the Institute for Laboratory Animal Research (ILAR) of the National Academy of Sciences and is used throughout the world to guide the care of research animals. ILAR provides advisory and educational services both to the biomedical industry and the public.

The Guide contains recommendations based on published data, scientific principles, expert opinion, and experience with methods and practices that are consistent with high-quality, humane animal care and use. The Guide contains detailed information on all aspects of biomedical research facilities, including methods for monitoring animal care and use, provisions for veterinary care, qualifications and training of personnel, and the establishment of an occupational health and safety program. Additional information includes standards for the animal environment, animal husbandry and management, veterinary care, and design and construction of animal facilities.

Research facilities that receive funding from the Public Health Service (PHS) are required to utilize the Guide in

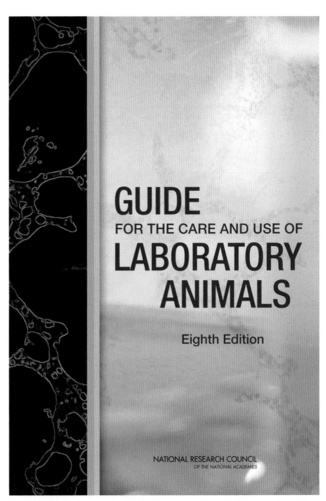

FIGURE 1-4. Guide for the Care and Use of Laboratory Animals.

the development and implementation of an animal care and use program. One significant consequence of that requirement is that the Guide covers all aspects of the facility, not just the animals. Species that are excluded from the Animal Welfare Act regulations are in fact covered by the regulations contained in the Guide. Box 1-2 contains the major areas addressed in the Guide. A related publication, the Guide for the Care and Use of Agricultural Animals in Research and Teaching (the Ag Guide) applies to the use of farm animals in nonbiomedical research protocols (e.g., agricultural research and teaching).

> **TECHNICIAN NOTE** Research facilities that receive funding from the Public Health Service must meet the standards in the Guide for the Care and Use of Laboratory Animals.

BOX 1-2	Standards Contained in the Guide for the Care and Use of Laboratory Animals

1. Qualifications and credentials of personnel
2. Occupational safety and health
3. Veterinary care
4. Animal environment (housing and care)
5. Animal procurement and transportation
6. Surgical and postsurgical care
7. Pain relief
8. Euthanasia techniques
9. Physical plant design

PHS Policy on Humane Care and Use of Laboratory Animals

The Public Health Services is one of many agencies within the United States Department of Health and Human Services. PHS has specific policies on the utilization and care of vertebrate animals in research and education. The PHS Policy is based on the nine U.S. Government Principles adopted by the Office of Science and Technology Policy in 1985. The nine specific principles are listed in Box 1-3.

The PHS Policy also requires that when euthanasia of research animals is necessary, it be conducted in a manner that relieves pain and suffering of the animals. A committee of the American Veterinary Medical Association publishes the *AVMA Guidelines for the Euthanasia of Animals*. The AVMA Report discusses only methods and agents for euthanasia supported by data from scientific studies. It emphasizes professional judgment, technical proficiency, and humane handling of the animals. Deviations from the Report are permitted by the PHS Policy only if the IACUC determines that they are justified for scientific reasons.

The Office of Research Integrity (ORI) is focused on promoting integrity in biomedical and behavioral research funded by PHS. ORI oversees institutional investigations into research misconduct and promotes the responsible conduct of research through educational, preventive, and regulatory activities.

Good Laboratory Practices

Facilities that receive funding from the Food and Drug Administration (FDA) or the Environmental Protection Agency (EPA) must adhere to the Good Laboratory Practice

BOX 1-3	U.S. Government Principles for the Utilization and Care of Vertebrate Animals Used in Testing, Research, and Training

I. The transportation, care, and use of animals should be in accordance with the AWA (7 U.S.C. 2131 et. seq.) and other applicable federal laws, guidelines, and policies.

II. Procedures involving animals should be designed and performed with due consideration of their relevance to human or animal health, the advancement of knowledge, or the good of society.

III. The animals selected for a procedure should be of an appropriate species and quality and the minimum number required to obtain valid results. Methods such as mathematical models, computer simulation, and in vitro biologic systems should be considered.

IV. Proper use of animals, including the avoidance or minimization of discomfort, distress, and pain when consistent with sound scientific practices, is imperative. Unless the contrary is established, investigators should consider that procedures that cause pain or distress in human beings may cause pain or distress in other animals.

V. Procedures with animals that may cause more than momentary or slight pain or distress should be performed with appropriate sedation, analgesia, or anesthesia. Surgical or other painful procedures should not be performed on unanesthetized animals paralyzed by chemical agents.

VI. Animals that would otherwise suffer severe or chronic pain or distress that cannot be relieved should be painlessly killed at the end of the procedure or, if appropriate, during the procedure.

VII. The living conditions of animals should be appropriate for their species and contribute to their health and comfort. Normally, the housing, feeding, and care of all animals used for biomedical purposes must be directed by a veterinarian or other scientist trained and experienced in the proper care, handling, and use of the species being maintained or studied. In any case, veterinary care shall be provided as indicated.

VIII. Investigators and other personnel shall be appropriately qualified and experienced for conducting procedures on living animals. Adequate arrangements shall be made for their in-service training, including the proper and humane care and use of laboratory animals.

IX. Where exceptions are required in relation to the provisions of these principles, the decisions should not rest with the investigators directly concerned but should be made, with due regard to principle II, by an appropriate review group such as an institutional animal care and use committee. Such exceptions should not be made solely for the purposes of teaching or demonstration.

(GLP) regulations, even when the funding is for research not involving animals. The FDA enforces a number of laws designed to protect the health and safety of the general public, such as the Food, Drug, and Cosmetic Act. The Food, Drug, and Cosmetic Act mandates that manufacturers of products provide documentation that their products are safe when used in their customary way. While the FDA does not specifically mandate that items such as cosmetics or other consumer products undergo animal testing, they do require documentation that the product or its ingredients are safe. Many manufacturers mislead the public into thinking that a product was not tested when in fact they might be using safety data on the ingredients that was performed previously or by another company. The FDA does allow for and encourage manufacturers to utilize nonanimal alternatives to document product safety, but it also requires that such alternatives are scientifically valid. The EPA is a federal government agency that administers laws that protect human health and the environment. One of these laws, the Toxic Substances Control Act, requires that chemicals made, used, or imported into the United States do not pose a risk to human health or the environment. The EPA may request specific animal safety testing and can remove products from the market or restrict their use if the safety of the product cannot be adequately determined.

The GLP regulations apply to both animal and nonanimal studies funded by either the FDA or EPA and have specific mandates for personnel training, record keeping, and quality assurance. Development and adherence to Standard Operating Procedures (SOPs) is also mandated by the GLP regulations. SOPs are step-by-step descriptions of all scientific and husbandry procedures performed in a facility. The SOPs cover everything from cleaning of the floors to procedures used in preparing patients for surgery.

> **TECHNICIAN NOTE** Facilities that receive funding from the Food and Drug Administration or the Environmental Protection Agency must adhere to the Good Laboratory Practice regulations.

National Institutes of Health (NIH)

NIH is another of the agencies of the Public Health Services. The primary focus of NIH is to support and conduct biomedical research. NIH comprises both an extramural research program and an intramural research program. The intramural program encompasses projects that are conducted in one of NIH's own laboratories. The extramural program provides grants and contracts to support research and training in thousands of universities, medical schools, and other research and research training institutions both nationally and internationally.

Scientists submit grant proposals to NIH, which then undergo an extensive peer review process. The process involves a panel of experts that evaluate the scientific merit of the proposal as well as its priority in providing information relevant to the mission of NIH.

Institutions that receive funding from NIH must comply with PHS policies and submit an annual report to the Office of Laboratory Welfare (OLAW). The report must include details on any changes to the institution's program of animal care, changes in the membership of the IACUC, dates of IACUC evaluations and facility inspections, and summaries of any minority opinions expressed by IACUC members. The chief executive officer of the institution and the IACUC chairperson must sign the report.

NIH Research Laboratories

NIH scientists conduct their research in NIH laboratories. NIH facilities include a research hospital where clinical trials are conducted. NIH facilities also include the National Library of Medicine. The Library produces and publishes indexes of scientific literature published throughout the world as well as housing a large medical bibliographic database. The NIH Institute of Environmental Sciences is concerned with the study of environmental hazards on human health. NIH institutes and centers are listed in Box 1-4. The USDA, FDA, and NIH have a formal cooperative arrangement to facilitate implementation of, and foster institutional compliance with, the Animal Welfare Regulations and the PHS Policy.

Association for Assessment and Accreditation of Laboratory Animal Care (AAALAC)

AAALAC is a private nonprofit organization that promotes the humane treatment of animals in science through a voluntary accreditation program. AAALAC does not promulgate its own regulations. Accreditation standards rely on widely accepted guidelines, such as the *Guide for the Care and Use of Laboratory Animals*. AALAC publishes position statements on certain issues, such as the use of farm animals, occupational health and safety, or adequate veterinary care.

AAALAC evaluates all aspects of an animal care and use program, including the organization's procedures and overall performance in the area of animal care and use in research, education, testing, or breeding. Detailed evaluations include institutional policies, animal husbandry, veterinary care, and the physical plant. Programs using nontraditional research animals, such as farm animals, fish, or birds, are eligible to seek accreditation and must meet rigorous standards even though these species are exempt from federal regulations.

> **TECHNICIAN NOTE** AAALAC administers a voluntary accreditation program.

Research institutions seek AAALAC accreditation because it signifies a commitment to excellence. The accreditation process encourages rigorous assessment of the institution's policies and procedures with a focus on continual improvement. Some private biomedical funding organizations strongly recommend that grantees using animals in their studies be part of an AAALAC-accredited program. The AAALAC standards for animal care, facilities, and staff of this association are the highest for the industry. Institutions that are AAALAC accredited have little trouble meeting other standards.

BOX 1-4	NIH INSTITUTES AND CENTERS

- Center for Information Technology (CIT)
- Center for Scientific Review (CSR)
- Eunice Kennedy Shriver National Institute of Child Health and Human Development (NICHD)
- Fogarty International Center (FIC)
- National Cancer Institute (NCI)
- National Center for Advancing Translational Sciences (NCATS)
- National Center for Complementary and Alternative Medicine (NCCAM)
- National Center for Research Resources (NCRR)—(April 13, 1962–December 23, 2011)
- National Eye Institute (NEI)
- National Heart, Lung, and Blood Institute (NHLBI)
- National Human Genome Research Institute (NHGRI)
- National Institute of Allergy and Infectious Diseases (NIAID)
- National Institute of Arthritis and Musculoskeletal and Skin Diseases (NIAMS)
- National Institute of Biomedical Imaging and Bioengineering (NIBIB)
- National Institute of Dental and Craniofacial Research (NIDCR)
- National Institute of Diabetes and Digestive and Kidney Diseases (NIDDK)
- National Institute of Environmental Health Sciences (NIEHS)
- National Institute of General Medical Sciences (NIGMS)
- National Institute of Mental Health (NIMH)
- National Institute of Neurological Disorders and Stroke (NINDS)
- National Institute of Nursing Research (NINR)
- National Institute on Aging (NIA)
- National Institute on Alcohol Abuse and Alcoholism (NIAAA)
- National Institute on Deafness and Other Communication Disorders (NIDCD)
- National Institute on Drug Abuse (NIDA)
- National Institute on Minority Health and Health Disparities (NIMHD)
- National Library of Medicine (NLM)
- NIH Clinical Center (CC)

THE THREE R'S: REDUCTION, REFINEMENT, AND REPLACEMENT

All biomedical research workers feel compassion for the lives of the animals that may be sacrificed in the quest for scientific progress. We demand, at least, that when animal research is done that it conform to strict guidelines and principles. It is in this light that researchers formulated and abide by the principles of the "3 R's."

REDUCTION

The goal of **reduction** is to use the absolute least number of animals that will achieve the research goals. In considering the number of animals needed for an experimental plan, a number of factors must be considered. Statistical analysis requires that a certain minimum number of test subjects be used for results to be statistically significant.

For research designed to develop a new surgical technique, a sufficient number of animals must be used to establish surgical competency and consistent results. There also must be enough subjects to take individual variations into account. When submitting an experimental protocol for review by funding agencies or the IACUC, the PI must provide a rationale for the number of animals requested. The funding agency and the IACUC are then responsible for determining if the number of animals requested is reasonable or excessive.

REFINEMENT

The concept of **refinement** refers to several basic principles. A focus on refinement requires that an experimental procedure be chosen that causes the least amount of stress, pain, anxiety, and disturbance of normal life to the animal and still meets the experimental goals. If the least amount of pain and distress cannot be achieved because of experimental design and goals, pain and distress must be alleviated with medications. In addition, refinement also refers to the education and skill level of the scientists and research technicians involved in performing the procedures. Procedures must be performed only by properly trained personnel. Refinement also requires that the research be of great value to mankind. All of the above basic principles are reviewed by the funding agency and IACUC prior to approval of any research protocol.

The highest refinement is achieved when the most skilled investigator uses procedures that cause the least discomfort to the animal to achieve a result that is of maximum benefit to mankind.

REPLACEMENT

Replacement refers to research that utilizes lower forms of life, computer models, or other artificial means whenever possible. Replacement substitutes a nonliving model for a living animal if possible to achieve the scientific results needed. Tissue cultures are often used to replace the actual live animal. Artificial models and computer models can sometimes simulate conditions that exist in live animals.

The substitution of rodents for primates, dogs, and cats is constantly taking place. Plants can also be used for some studies. Scientists must search for the lowest form of life available to satisfy the scientific need. Research into development of more nonanimal research subjects is ongoing. The goal to do more research on inanimate objects is the challenge of the future.

> *TECHNICIAN NOTE* Researchers adhere to the principles of the "three R's": Reduction, Refinement, and Replacement.

THE MORALS AND ETHICS OF ANIMAL RESEARCH

In an effort to understand all the moral and ethical issues concerning animal research, sociologists have devised different ways of classifying people. One way of categorizing people is to look at the organized groups that are formed for people of like interests and beliefs. These are "special-interest" groups. Special-interest groups have always banded together to try to influence others into believing as they do. For example, state and national veterinary and veterinary technician associations tend to speak for the profession on most matters concerning animals. We want the public to understand our concerns and agree with our opinions. We ask our associations to convey the message to the general public and to our legislators, who develop regulations that affect the practice of veterinary medicine. The same basic concept is used by any of the special interest groups we may consider.

If we attempt to classify all Americans into groups on the basis of how they would answer the question, "What are the rights of animals?" we find that there are six basic groups of organizations. They can be classified as:

1. Animal exploitation groups
2. Animal use groups
3. Animal control groups
4. Animal welfare groups
5. Animal rights groups
6. Animal liberation groups

The classification is based on an examination of the official doctrine of each group. Many individuals may feel differently from the official doctrine on certain points. Also individuals and groups may fall into more than one category on different issues.

ANIMAL EXPLOITATION GROUPS

Individuals in these groups generally believe that animals were put on earth for use by humans. They believe that animals are our absolute property. They cannot conceive of animals feeling pain as we do, and even if they did, it should not be of any concern to them. Individuals in this group are often advocates of bull fighting, cock fighting, etc. They tend to have no sense of suffering of animals; it means nothing to them.

Fortunately, almost all the activities advocated by these groups are illegal in our country. That doesn't mean that some of it doesn't go on in certain parts of the United States despite being against the law. As recently as 100 years ago we see that this type of behavior was not considered unusual or bad. As man has progressed morally and socially, this behavior has become less accepted.

ANIMAL USE GROUPS

Individuals in these groups believe that animals are here for use of humans but that we must be responsible about that use. This responsibility includes sparing an animal pain and discomfort if it is at all possible. Most individuals that work in laboratory animal facilities are included in this group. Others included in this classification are people who eat meat and wear leather, hunting and fishing groups, breeders of purebred dogs, cats, and livestock, circuses, zoos, horse and dog racing. In general, individuals in this group see nothing wrong with using animals to better mankind and animals, as long as the use is not abusive to the animals.

ANIMAL CONTROL GROUPS

Animal control group members believe that governments should write laws that express the sentiments of most of the population and that these laws should be carried out to the letter regardless of pressure from groups who would have them believe that the laws are unfair. They answer that if the law is unfair, change the law. Government organizations, such as the USDA is an animal control group. Veterinary organizations, such as the AVMA, and therefore all their members, believe in animal control. Animal control varies from place to place and from one year to the next. All the changes are being made in one direction: to improve the quality of care and welfare of animals. Veterinarians, as a group, advocate the continued improvement of the health and well-being of animals. Individuals in the animal control group believe that the current law represents the will of the people. They are not against change if done legally, but will enforce the law as presently written.

ANIMAL WELFARE GROUPS

Animal welfare organizations, such as the SPCA, believe that people should treat each animal as kindly as possible and that they should be required by law to do so. If an animal is mistreated or neglected for whatever reason, this group believes we have a duty to relieve their suffering. This can include euthanasia to relieve or prevent animal suffering. Organizations in this group actively pursue legislation to promote animal welfare. Many animal shelters fall into this group. This group does not oppose well-controlled animal research that does not cause pain or distress and is of important scientific value, but it does not believe that unwanted animals should be used for research.

Many research-related laws are based on suggestions from animal welfare organizations. Biomedical research workers and animal welfare advocates may disagree on certain points, but generally coexist very well and support many of the same causes.

ANIMAL RIGHTS GROUPS

Supporters of animal rights believe that animals have intrinsic rights that should be guaranteed just the way human rights are guaranteed. This would include not being killed, eaten, used for sport or research, or abused in any way. Organizations in this group include the National Anti-Vivisection Society and noneuthanasia animal shelters. They will not consider euthanasia under any circumstance. Individuals in this group strongly believe that animal research for whatever purpose or value should never be done because it violates the basic rights of animals.

TECHNICIAN NOTE Animal rights groups will not consider euthanasia under any circumstance and are opposed to the use of any animals in research.

ANIMAL LIBERATION GROUPS

Individuals and organizations in this group believe that animals should not be forced to work or produce for our benefit in any way. Although it is sometimes difficult to separate the ideals of Animal Rights and Animal Liberation, the most extreme advocates of Animal Liberation feel that a person owning a pet is a form of enslavement. Some in this group are activists who may condone and encourage illegal methods such as civil disobedience and break-ins in an effort to garner public support for their positions. Despite their radical views, this group has grown in popularity by appealing to common feelings that many people have toward animals, especially welfare-minded individuals. Important groups in this category are: People for the Ethical Treatment of Animals (PETA) and the Animal Liberation Front (ALF).

PETA, the largest of the animal liberation groups, was founded in 1980 by Ingrid Newkirk and Alex Pacheco. Although radical in approach, this group has served to expose neglected and inadequate areas in animal research. Ingrid Newkirk once published an article containing a statement of her belief of the equality of all life. Individuals and organizations in the animal liberation groups believe that all life is equal and that if we are not willing to do research on our children and ourselves, we should not do it on animals.

Animal rights advocates and animal liberationists imply that all animal research is wrong and cruel to animals. Additionally they believe that animal research is unnecessary, unproductive, and could be replaced by other forms of research. Animal experimentation is portrayed as always being painful, unnecessary, and of no major benefit to anyone. Research scientists are said to be sadistic murderers who are interested only in money. No one can argue with the moral convictions of people who feel in their heart that animals should not be used for the benefit of humans under any circumstance. But their argument that says that animal research is worthless, abusive, out of control, unproductive, and could easily be replaced must be answered. Activists continue spreading false information to the public in order to attract support to stop animal research. Manufacturers and product distributors that market consumer products with the labels "cruelty-free" contribute to the misinformation by implying that no animal testing has been performed on the products.

Some years ago the laboratory animal community realized that although abuses within their ranks were rare, any abuse at all had to be eliminated. People in research are also pet owners and caring human beings. They know that their work is important and necessary, and they have accepted the 3 "R's" principles of Replacement, Reduction, and Refinement, which acts as a guideline for all their thinking. The development of the field of laboratory animal science and the development of the skilled, caring technician is a result of progress and change. Legislation and policy has continually moved toward more welfare and better care and accountability as demanded by the general public.

BENEFITS OF ANIMAL RESEARCH

Medical advances that occurred as a direct result of animal research include such things as human immunizations (polio, diphtheria, measles, etc.), development of antibiotics, insulin to treat diabetic patients, chemotherapy for cancer, and development of pharmaceuticals to treat hypertension and mental illness. Surgical advances have also resulted from animal research, including hip replacement surgery, organ transplants, cardiac bypass, and many others (Table 1-3). Humans are living longer and maintaining a higher quality of life because of many of these advances. Many of the medical advances have also provided information to allow improvements in the care of pet and farm animals. In spite of these facts, some activists refuse to believe that the research has provided any benefits at all. Their belief that research persists because it is easy, inexpensive, and quick is not supported by the evidence. Animal research is, in fact, quite expensive. This accounts for part of the reason why animal researchers are also developing additional adjunctive techniques for research. There are significant incentives to developing techniques such as cell and tissue cultures and mathematical and computer models. Those adjunctive techniques are now routinely used and have replaced animal use in the early stages of research projects. These nonanimal methods have been eagerly adopted by the scientific community whenever possible. This has significantly reduced the numbers of animals used in research and has increased the speed of development of new medical therapies. In addition, many of the tests used on animals have been refined so that the animals do not suffer significant pain or distress. For example, the LD-50 and Draize tests have been significantly improved and now use far fewer animal subjects than when they were first developed while still providing valid data.

Some animal liberationists also fail to focus on the fact that some animal research is required by law. Before laws such as the Food, Drug, and Cosmetic Act were enacted, untested products were given to humans, often with tragic results. For example, when sulfa-based antimicrobials were first used, there was no requirement for manufacturers to prove product safety. The medication was contained in ethylene glycol (a component of antifreeze) because it was not soluble in water. Over 100 people were killed after taking the drug in that form. The Food, Drug, and Cosmetic Act requires extensive safety documentation before any new drugs are given to humans. The current requirements result in approximately 10 to 12 years of laboratory study and animal and human clinical trials before a medication can be released for human use.

TABLE 1-3	Some Major Scientific Advances Resulting from Animal Research	
YEAR	**ANIMAL MODEL(S)**	**SCIENTIFIC ADVANCE**
2008	Rat	Spinal cord regeneration techniques advanced
2007	Mouse	Principles for introducing specific gene modifications in mice by the use of embryonic stem cells discovered
2006	Nematode	RNA interference, or gene silencing, by double-stranded RNA discovered
2005	Gerbil	Discovery of the bacterium *Helicobacter pylori* and its role in gastritis and peptic ulcer disease
2004	Mouse	Odorant receptors and the organization of the olfactory system discovered
2003	Clam, mouse, dog, rat, pig, rabbit, frog	Noninvasive imaging methods (MRI) for medical diagnosis developed
2002	Nematode	Mechanism of cell death discovered
2000	Mouse, rat, sea slug	Brain signal transduction discovered
1998	Rabbit	Nitric oxide as signaling molecule in regulation of blood pressure discovered
1997	Mouse, hamster	Prions discovered and characterized
1995	Mouse, nonhuman primate	Gene transfer for cystic fibrosis developed
1992	Pig	Laparoscopic surgical techniques advanced
1990	Dog, sheep, cow, pig	1990 organ transplantation techniques advanced
1984	Mouse	Monoclonal antibodies developed
1982	Armadillo	Treatment for leprosy developed
1975	Monkey, horse, chicken, mouse	Interaction between tumor viruses and genetic material discovered
1973	Bee, fish, bird	Animal social and behavior patterns discovered
1971	Pig	Development of computer-assisted tomography (CAT scan)
1970	Rat, guinea pig	Lithium approved
1968	Monkey	Rubella vaccine developed
1964	Rat	Regulation of cholesterol discovered
1956	Dog	Open heart surgery and cardiac pacemakers developed
1954	Mouse, monkey	Polio vaccine developed
1952	Guinea pig	Discovery of streptomycin
1951	Mouse, monkey	Development of yellow fever vaccine
1945	Mouse	Penicillin tested
1943	Rat, dog, chick, mouse	Functions of vitamin K discovered
1942	Monkey	The Rh factor discovered
1936	Cat	Anticoagulants developed
1933	Horse	Vaccine for tetanus developed
1932	Cat, dog	Function of neurons discovered
1929	Chicken	Discovery of antineuritic and growth-stimulating vitamins
1928	Monkey, guinea pig, rat, mouse	Pathogenesis of typhus discovered
1921	Dog, rabbit, fish	Discovery of insulin and mechanism of diabetes
1919	Guinea pig, horse, rabbit	Mechanisms of immunity discovered
1905	Cow, sheep	Pathogenesis of tuberculosis discovered
1902	Pigeon	Malarial life cycle described
1901	Guinea pig	Development of diphtheria antiserum
1885	Dog, rabbit	Vaccine for rabies developed
1881	Sheep	Vaccine for anthrax developed
1756	Cow	Vaccine for smallpox developed

KEY POINTS

- Exotic pets other than dogs and cats are companion animals and include birds, reptiles, amphibians, rats, mice, hamsters, gerbils, sugar gliders, rabbits, and guinea pigs.

- Laboratory animals are any species used in research or teaching.
- The most commonly used laboratory animals are mice and rats.
- Treatment of exotic and laboratory animals often involves extralabel use of medications.

- Factors that may predispose an animal to disease include intrinsic, extrinsic, dietary, and experimental factors.
- The Convention on International Trade in Endangered Species of Wild Flora and Fauna is a multinational agreement focused on safeguarding species from extinction.
- A variety of federal, state, and local laws exist related to exotic pets and wildlife.
- The Animal Welfare Act sets standards of care for laboratory animals and is implemented through the Animal Welfare Regulations.
- All use of animals in research and teaching must be reviewed and approved by the institutional animal care and use committee.
- Research facilities that receive funding from the Public Health Service must meet the standards in the Guide for the Care and Use of Laboratory Animals.
- Facilities that receive funding from the Food and Drug Administration (FDA) or the Environmental Protection Agency (EPA) must adhere to the Good Laboratory Practice (GLP) regulations.
- AAALAC administers a voluntary accreditation program for research facilities.
- Researchers adhere to the principles of the "three R's": Reduction, Refinement, and Replacement.

REVIEW QUESTIONS

1. The term _____ _____ generally refers to any companion animal other than dogs and cats.

2. Any animal used in research or teaching is referred to as a _____ _____.

3. Nearly all medications used in exotic and laboratory animal medicine are considered _____ use.

4. Predisposing factors such as species, age, gender, and heredity are considered _____ factors.

5. Name the organization formed to safeguard species from extinction.

6. The government agency that oversees the use of animals in an educational or research institution is the _____.

7. The _____ _____ _____ is the principle federal statute governing the sale, handling, transport, and use of animals.

8. The Guide for the Care and Use of Laboratory Animals was written under the direction of the _____.

9. The _____ oversees institutional investigations into research misconduct and promotes the responsible conduct of research through educational, preventive, and regulatory activities.

10. The institutional group charged with evaluation of animal use and inspection of facilities is _____.

11. The group that provides voluntary accreditation of biomedical research facilities is _____.

12. The use of procedures that causes the least amount of stress, pain, anxiety, and disturbance of normal life to the animal is an example of _____.

13. List the three R's of research and briefly explain each.

14. Name the minimum membership of an IACUC.

15. Name the two most active animal liberation groups in the United States.

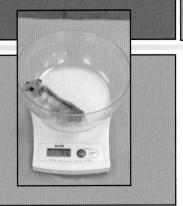

Exotic and Research Animal Facilities

OUTLINE

LEARNING OBJECTIVES

After studying this chapter, you will be able to:

- Describe unique aspects of clinic management for exotic pet practice.
- List unique equipment and supplies needed for exotic pet practice.
- Describe the principles of scientific research.
- Describe basic considerations in experimental design.
- List the members of the research team and describe the role of each.
- Describe considerations in design and construction of a research facility.
- Describe different types and modes of caging.
- List advantages and disadvantages of different types and modes of caging.
- Describe environmental concerns in laboratory animal facilities.
- Differentiate between microenvironments and macroenvironments.
- Describe feeding and watering devices used for laboratory animals.
- Describe basic administrative responsibilities in a laboratory animal facility.
- List and describe types and sources of animals for research.

EXOTIC ANIMAL PRACTICE

The decision to treat exotic animals requires that veterinarians not only take responsibility for the knowledge and skill required to treat the diverse species that may enter the clinic but also ensure that staff members are properly trained in handling, restraint, and clinical procedures needed. Although veterinarians and veterinary technicians receive basic information in these areas while studying to earn their credentials, the in-depth knowledge and skill required to treat them on a regular basis will require advanced education.

The veterinary clinic staff will also have to consider other unique aspects of the behavior of these species to avoid undue stress on the animals as well as other clients. Not all clients will appreciate sharing a waiting area with a large snake. Similarly, some small exotic animals, such as mice, are prey species that will be unduly stressed by the presence of predators such as domestic cats. The veterinary hospital policies and procedures will need to be modified to consider these issues.

While some supplies and equipment are the same as those used when examining and treating dogs and cats, others are more specialized. For example, it is important to obtain an accurate weight on these animals, but the scales used to weigh dogs and cats are rarely capable of providing an accurate weight on small mammals such as mice and hamsters. A special scale is needed that can measure weight in grams and also contain the animal while it is being weighed (Figure 2-1). Some of the more common items needed to treat exotic companion animals are summarized in Box 2-1.

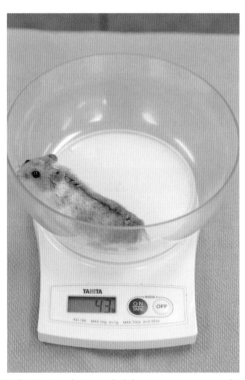

FIGURE 2-1. A scale is needed that can measure weight in grams and also contain the animal while it is being weighed.

BOX 2-1	Supplies Needed for Exotic Pet Practice

3 to 5 French red rubber catheters
2- to 5-mm uncuffed endotracheal tubes
Gram scale
Heat lamps
Incubators
Nasolacrimal cannulas
Perches
Stainless steel feeding needles
Magnification loupe

It is also necessary to arrange an area within the practice where exotic animals can be examined and hospitalized without exposure to domestic species. While some exotic animals can be maintained in dog and cat cages with small modifications, others will require specialized caging to keep them from escaping.

BIOMEDICAL RESEARCH

Scientific research is carried out by scientists and veterinary professionals with the goal of improving mankind's knowledge of anatomy, physiology, disease processes, and methods to control and treat diseases. Three basic types of research are performed: **basic research**, **applied research**, and **clinical research**.

> *TECHNICIAN NOTE* The three basic types of research are basic research, applied research, and clinical research.

BASIC RESEARCH

Basic research is primarily concerned with advancing fundamental knowledge of physical, chemical, and functional mechanisms of life processes and diseases. Such research is often performed using computer models or plants. The knowledge gained from basic research often provides guidance in developing applied or clinical research endeavors.

APPLIED RESEARCH

Applied research involves the use of existing knowledge toward solving a specific biomedical problem and is often directed toward detailed objectives, such as development of new vaccines or surgical procedures. This type of research may be performed on computer or mathematical models, cell or tissue cultures, or live animals. The choice of a specific biomedical research model is based on the ability of the model to mimic or predict responses in another species. When a live animal is selected as an applied research subject, it is referred to as an **animal model**. The choice of a particular species of animal model helps direct the research plan. It is common to develop multiple research plans utilizing more than one species of animal model. This helps to minimize concern over differences (e.g., anatomy, physiology) in the animal models and the species for which the research is designed.

CLINICAL RESEARCH

Clinical research is designed to build on the knowledge gained in basic and applied research. Clinical research is always conducted on live animals, including humans. The United States Food and Drug Administration (FDA) requires that certain products, particularly new medications, undergo clinical trials using small groups of human volunteers. This allows the FDA to verify that the research performed on non-human animal models is applicable to humans. The FDA also requires that all research (basic, applied, and clinical) funded or reviewed by its agency be conducted in accordance with the Good Laboratory Practices (GLPs). The GLPs vary depending on the type of research and purpose of the study. More information on GLPs is located in Chapter 1.

Research Design

In all types of research, the design of the research protocol is guided by the initial question to be answered or problem to be solved. Once a researcher has identified this specific question or problem, a detailed search of the scientific literature is conducted to identify whether the question or problem has been addressed by other researchers. If the literature search yields no answers or solutions, the scientist develops a **hypothesis**. The hypothesis is simply a theory based on current knowledge that could answer the question or provide the solution. From that point, the scientist works with additional research team members to develop the experimental design. The design incorporates the detailed description of methods to be used, standard operating procedures (SOPs) for the research, choice of biomedical model, personnel needed, and a budget showing anticipated costs for the project. The research may be funded by the institution for which the scientist works or by independent or government agencies such as the American Cancer Society or National Institutes of Health (NIH).

> *TECHNICIAN NOTE* Research is designed to test just one variable.

Experiments are usually designed so that just one variable is tested. The variable is the one characteristic, condition, or factor being studied or treatment being applied. Most experiments have several test groups. The experimental group(s) is the one for which the variable is being manipulated. The control group(s) is similar in composition (e.g., species, gender, age) but receives no manipulation of the variable. Animals are randomly assigned to one or the other group and strict adherence to SOPs is used to ensure that the groups differ only in the manipulated variable. The data collected from the control and experimental groups are then compared. Statistical analysis is performed to determine the effect, if any, of the manipulated variable.

If the research utilizes animals, the experimental design must then be submitted to the Institutional Animal Care and Use Committee (IACUC) for review and approval prior to undertaking the experiment. The composition and responsibilities of the IACUC are mandated by federal law and discussed in more detail in Chapter 1.

THE RESEARCH TEAM

The research team may comprise a number of members, depending on the type of experiment and the available resources. The scientist that developed the hypothesis and planned the experimental design is known as the **principal investigator (PI)**. This individual often has an advanced degree (e.g., PhD) in a specific field, such as neurology or cardiology. In addition to planning and coordinating the experiment, the PI also compiles and interprets the data collected and reports the research findings to the scientific community.

Laboratory animal technicians (LAT), laboratory animal technologists (LATG), and assistant laboratory animal technologists (ALAT) are also vital members of the research team. The criteria to obtain certification as an LAT, LATG, or ALAT are determined by the American Association of Laboratory Animal Science (AALAS). This organization was formed in 1950 and is composed of individuals from all aspects of the study and care of laboratory animals. A group of AALAS members, the Certification and Registry Board (CRB), is charged with developing standards of education and performance for LATs, LATGs, and ALATs and for developing and administering the certification examination for each of the three classifications. The current standards for certification are summarized in Table 2-1. Certification by AALAS is often a requirement of participation on the research team. The ALAT, LAT, and LATG are usually involved in the daily care of the animals in the experimental and control groups and have the primary responsibility for ensuring that all environmental variables are properly controlled. The LAT or LATG may also function as research technicians and perform the specific treatment needed for the experimental

TABLE 2-1	Eligibility Requirements for AALAS Certification	
EDUCATION	**WORK EXPERIENCE**
ALAT Examination	
No high school diploma or GED	+2 years
High school diploma or GED	+1 year
Any college degree of 2 years or more	+0.5 year
LAT Examination	
High school diploma or GED	+3 years
Any 2-year associate's degree	+2 years
Any 4-year bachelor's degree or higher	+1 year
ALAT certification plus high school diploma, GED, or college degree	+0.5 year after receiving ALAT certification
ALAT certification	+2 years after receiving ALAT certification
LATG Examination	
High school diploma or GED	+5 years
Any 2-year associate's degree	+4 years
Any 4-year bachelor's degree or higher	+3 years
LAT certification plus high school diploma, GED, or college degree	+0.5 year after receiving LAT certification

group, as well as collect and process data from the experimental and control groups.

> **TECHNICIAN NOTE** AALAS administers the certification examinations for laboratory animal technicians, laboratory animal technologists, and assistant laboratory animal technicians.

A laboratory animal veterinarian is also part of the research team. The veterinarian is usually one that has a special interest in laboratory animals and is a member of the American Society of Laboratory Animal Practitioners (ASLAP) or certified as a laboratory animal veterinarian by the American College of Laboratory Animal Medicine (ACLAM). ASLAP is a professional organization composed of veterinarians with a special interest in laboratory animal medicine. ACLAM provides standards of training and experience for laboratory animal veterinarians and develops and administers the certifying examination for laboratory animal veterinarians. As part of the research team, the laboratory animal veterinarian is responsible for overseeing all aspects of animal health and for advising the PI and other research team members on the proper handling and treatment of the animals and compliance with regulations related to animal care and use.

The administrator of the laboratory animal facility also plays a crucial role in biomedical research. The administrator is responsible for all aspects of the operation of the facility, including supervision of staff and ensuring that appropriate records are maintained.

FACILITY DESIGN

The quality of research data is directly connected to the quality of animal care. Appropriate housing and care of animals are essential to the health and safety of both the animals and the personnel. The specific design needs of a research facility vary with the nature of the work performed. Animal facilities are planned with a focus on minimizing the spread of disease from one part of the facility to another. Biomedical research facilities that are part of a larger institution are usually isolated from the rest of the institution. Facility managers make every effort to maintain a constant and controlled environment. Most biomedical research facilities contain the following areas: animal rooms, surgical suite, cage-washing area, offices, storage areas, necropsy laboratory, clinical laboratory, and personnel shower and lounge areas.

> **TECHNICIAN NOTE** Animal facilities are designed to minimize the spread of disease from one part of the facility to another.

Materials used in construction of laboratory animal facilities are waterproof and seamless. Special attention is paid to interfaces between walls, doors, floors, and windows. These areas must be readily cleaned and not damaged by regular use. Movement of items such as large pieces of equipment and racks of cages has the potential to damage the facility. Materials must be chosen that are capable of withstanding such use. Windows and doors also require special consideration. Exterior windows are not usually present in animal facilities. Doors in animal rooms are usually designed to open inward. Windows may be present in the doors of animal rooms to allow for observation of the room without entering the room.

ANIMAL ROOMS

The number of animal rooms depends on the total number of animals as well as the number of different species maintained at the facility. Different species are housed in different areas. This is particularly important when the facility maintains species that have normal flora that are pathogenic to other species also housed in the facility.

All animal rooms are designed so they can be maintained with consistent environmental parameters. This is a crucial consideration. Any variables in environment could compromise the validity of research being performed. Animal rooms must be easy to clean, with waterproof walls, floors, and electrical sources. Drains that can be opened and flushed are also important.

SURGICAL SUITE

Areas used for preparation of animals, performance of surgical procedures, and surgical or anesthetic recovery are commonly found. Surgical procedures performed on laboratory animals must be accomplished with aseptic technique. Many of the procedures performed on laboratory animals also require special instrumentation and equipment because of the wide variety of anatomic and physiologic variations among different species.

CAGE-WASHING ROOMS

Separate areas for use in washing cages and other supplies (e.g., food bowls, water containers) are important to minimize the spread of disease in the facility (see Figure 2-2). Cage-washing areas are also separated from animal rooms because the washing procedure creates a significant amount of noise that may be a significant source of stress for laboratory animals. There are usually "clean" and "dirty" sides to most cage-washing areas. Ventilation is always important, as is noise control. Workers in this area may wear ear plugs or protective clothing if hazardous substances are present. Cage-washing areas should be away from animal rooms but accessible through corridors.

> **TECHNICIAN NOTE** Cage-washing areas are separated from animal rooms to minimize exposure of the animals to the noise of the washing equipment.

Several types of cage and bottle washers may be used in biomedical research facilities. This equipment is designed to standardize washing procedures. Washers can be walk-through types, cabinet types, or tunnel types (Figure 2-3). All are able to bring water to temperatures capable of sanitizing equipment. Proper attention to safety protocols is vital when working with this equipment.

LABORATORIES

All procedures performed on animals are done outside the animal rooms so that the other animals are not alarmed. An assortment of different laboratory areas is usually present for this purpose. These include radiography, diagnostic, necropsy, and treatment areas.

PERSONNEL AREAS

Aside from office spaces and record-keeping areas, there are special rooms for eating and employee breaks. Changing and shower rooms are also important. Most facilities require their employees to change into special protective clothing when working inside the animal complex. In some cases workers must shower before dressing in the protective clothing.

RECEIVING AND STORAGE AREAS

Different areas are needed for receiving and storing medications, supplies, animal feed, and equipment. These rooms tend to be rather noisy and should be separated from animal room areas. Feed storage rooms must be kept free of vermin and excessive moisture. There is typically no water source in feed storage rooms. The temperature and humidity are usually kept low to protect against spoilage and mildew. Shelves or pallets that contain animal feed or bedding material must be kept at least 20 cm off the floor and away from the wall (Figure 2-4).

> **TECHNICIAN NOTE**   Animal food and bedding must be stored off the floor and away from the wall.

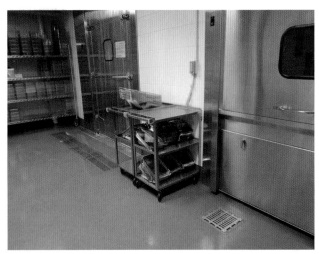

FIGURE 2-2. Cage washer room. A separate area is maintained for sanitation of cages and other supplies to minimize spread of disease and prevent excessive noise in animal areas.

TYPES OF FACILITIES

CONVENTIONAL FACILITY

Conventional facilities consist of animal rooms and support areas that have single doors opening onto a central corridor. This design is common in small facilities and requires some special considerations to minimize disease spread. In most cases, animal cages are cleaned within the room and the dirty cages and materials immediately taken to the washing area. Dirty cages and supplies cannot be left in the corridor because the potential for contamination of other areas is great. Technicians usually make an effort to keep the movement of dirty cages in one direction to minimize potential contamination of other areas.

DOUBLE-CORRIDOR FACILITY

This type of facility, sometimes referred to as a clean/dirty facility, consists of animal rooms and support areas that have two doors: one door opens onto the "clean" corridor and the other opens onto the "dirty" corridor (Figure 2-5). Traffic in all areas is unidirectional, with only clean cages and supplies entering the clean corridor and only dirty supplies and cages entering the dirty corridor. Personnel cannot leave by the clean corridor door.

> **TECHNICIAN NOTE**   Double-corridor facilities are the most commonly encountered type of research facility.

BARRIER FACILITY

Barrier facilities are similar in design to the double-corridor facility except that personnel must shower before entering the animal rooms. They are often required to dress in disposable

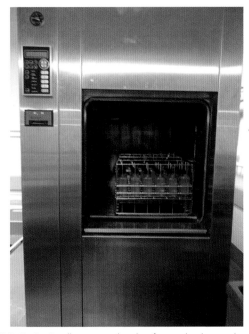

FIGURE 2-3. Small cages and racks of water bottles can be cleaned in this industrial washer.

clothing. Entry areas for barrier facilities typically have an airlock, and all materials must be autoclaved before being moved in to the animal rooms. Ultraviolet light may be used within the airlock to sterilize equipment and supplies. Air pressure in animal rooms is also carefully monitored. Barrier facilities are generally used to house germ-free animals.

CONTAINMENT FACILITIES

Design and use concerns for containment facilities are similar to those required in barrier facilities. In addition, personnel are usually required to shower when leaving the facility. Disposable clothing and all materials and supplies used in the animal rooms are autoclaved before being passed out of the facility through a special waste portal. This type of facility is normally used for housing animals with infectious or zoonotic diseases. The air passing out of the facility is also treated, either with filtration or heating, to remove any infectious organisms. The type of filtration needed for this purpose is referred to as high efficiency particulate air (HEPA) filtration. HEPA filters are capable of removing particles as small as 0.3 μm.

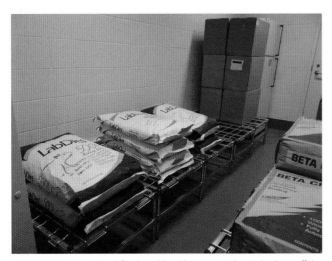

FIGURE 2-4. Animal feed and bedding material must be kept off the floor and away from the wall

ENVIRONMENTAL CONCERNS

Animals must be housed in an environment that maintains constant conditions of temperature, humidity, lighting, and ventilation. The facility will have a system to monitor the environmental parameters for the animal rooms (Figure 2-6). All components of the environment with the animal rooms comprise the **macroenvironment** of the animal housing areas. The optimal level for each of those factors varies depending on the species and, in some cases, on the specific use of the animals (e.g., breeding). The macroenvironment is often quite different from the **microenvironment**. Microenvironment refers to those same environmental factors specifically within the primary enclosure of the animals. The primary enclosure is the cage, run, pen, or other individual housing of a specific animal. The microenvironment is affected by the macroenvironment. However, because a specific animal room may not have constant environmental factors in all parts of the room, there may be some variation in the microenvironment within individual cages. For example, the cages located in the bottom of a rack of cages may have somewhat lower temperatures than those housed higher on the rack.

TEMPERATURE AND HUMIDITY

Variation in temperature and humidity can affect the metabolism and behavior of animals. Variations introduce variables into an experimental design that may render data invalid. Temperature requirements vary depending on the species. For example, rodents tend to have higher temperature requirements than rabbits (Table 2-2). Species that are from tropical areas, such as primates, tend to have higher temperature requirements. Animal rooms are maintained in a temperature that is within the **thermoneutral zone** (TNZ) for the species. TNZ is defined as the range of temperature where an animal does not need physical or chemical mechanisms to control heat production or heat loss. When the TNZ is exceeded, the animal must find ways to create heat loss. In the case of rodents, this is difficult because they do not have the ability to

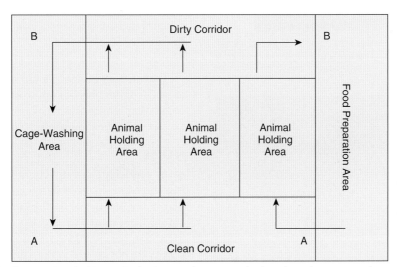

FIGURE 2-5. The flow of traffic through a double-corridor facility. **A,** Clean cages, food, and supplies are moved into animal rooms through the clean corridor. **B,** Dirty cages, food, and water bowls are moved out of animal rooms through the dirty corridor and into the cage-washing area.

sweat (except for pads of feet) and they do not pant. In most cases, the optimal temperature for development, comfort, reactivity, and adaptability is slightly below the TNZ.

Humidity requirements also vary depending on the species. Most animal rooms can be maintained at 45% to 55% relative humidity. Rodents require relative humidity of 40% to 70%, whereas dogs, cats, and primates are best maintained at 30% to 70% humidity.

> *TECHNICIAN NOTE* Most animal rooms can be maintained at 45% to 55% relative humidity.

VENTILATION REQUIREMENTS

Proper ventilation in animal housing units supplies oxygen to the animals and removes noxious odors and contaminants from the air. Ammonia, which is a byproduct of the breakdown of metabolic waste products (urine and feces), can build up to toxic levels if not removed through proper

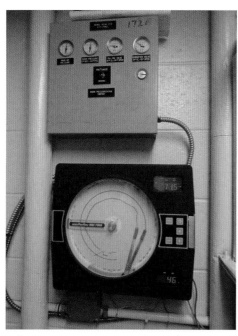

FIGURE 2-6. A monitoring station that tracks temperature, humidity, and air pressure and records temperature and humidity in an animal room.

TABLE 2-2	Recommended Environmental Temperatures and Humidity Levels for Common Laboratory Animals		
	°C	°F	RELATIVE HUMIDITY (%)
Rodents	18-26	64-79	40-60
Rabbits	16-22	61-72	30-70
Dogs, cats, primates	18-29	64-84	30-70
Livestock, poultry	16-27	61-81	30-60

Adapted from *The Guide for the Care and Use of Laboratory Animals,* Washington, DC, 1996, National Academy Press.

air circulation. Air circulation also allows for removal of thermal loads caused by animal respiration, lights, and equipment.

Animal rooms must have between 10 and 15 complete air changes each hour. These air changes affect the macroenvironment of the room. Microenvironments must be designed so that the same concerns (removal of ammonia, thermal load, etc.) are addressed. Air changes that occur too rapidly may result in drafts within the animal cage. Recirculation of air is discouraged. When room air must be recirculated, it must first be passed through filters and decontaminated. HEPA filters are routinely used for this purpose.

AIR PRESSURE CONCERNS

The air pressure in an animal room may be considered positive or negative. When a room is under positive pressure, air flows from the room to the outside when the door is opened. When the door of a negatively pressurized room is opened, air flows from the hall into the room. The pressure in a given room is determined by the purpose or specific use of the room. For example, an animal ward used for quarantine of infectious patients is maintained with negative air pressure so that the infectious agent is not likely to enter the hall area when the door is opened. Surgical suites are usually maintained under positive pressure so that contaminants from outside the surgical suite do not enter the room when the door is opened.

ILLUMINATION

There is usually no natural light from windows in most animal rooms because animals react differently to seasonal light changes, which would be considered a variable. Whenever possible a **diurnal illumination** system is used in which room lights are left on for 12 hours and then turned off for 12 hours. Certain experimental protocols may require variations in the light/dark ratio. Breeding animals of certain species have special requirements.

> *TECHNICIAN NOTE* Research animals are usually maintained using a diurnal illumination system.

The intensity of light should be sufficient for technicians to work comfortably but not so excessive as to harm the animals. Albino mice and rats can incur retinal damage from excessive illumination levels.

NOISE

Many species are sensitive to noise. Rats, for example, may stop breeding in excessively noisy surroundings. Rabbits may injure themselves. Both gerbils and rats can go into seizures when exposed to excessive noise. In most cases special fire and emergency alarms are used in animal facilities. These alarms are not as loud as the usual alarms in the frequencies that animals hear best and may combine other warning signs such as a flashing light to cut down on noise.

Animals that are sensitive to noise should be housed away from cage-washing equipment, elevators, personnel areas, and loud species such as dogs and nonhuman primates.

Many rooms that produce excessive noise require the operator or technician to wear ear plugs or other protective devices.

SOCIAL ENVIRONMENT

The social environment of an animal refers primarily to physical contact and visual, auditory, and olfactory communication with members of the same species. Animal species whose behavior is social should be housed in pairs or social groups when not prohibited by experimental design. For example, dogs and primates develop social hierarchies when maintained in groups. These social groupings may in fact be necessary to the proper development of the individuals in some species. Cages used for housing cats must have resting boards or ledges placed above the floor level to accommodate the cat's normal behavior.

> **TECHNICIAN NOTE** Cages for housing cats must contain a resting board or ledge above floor level.

An understanding of a species' normal social behavior is essential when planning for group housing. Territorial or communal concepts must be considered. With many species, especially primates, social rank, age, and sex enter into housing considerations.

The length of confinement may in some cases determine the type of primary enclosure.

The animal environment should also consider the species' activity patterns. Many laboratory animal species have typical activity patterns that include such behaviors as play and foraging. If not strictly prohibited by an experimental protocol, animals should be housed to allow these normal behaviors.

PRIMARY ENCLOSURES

All laboratory animals must be contained in some way. The primary enclosure of a research animal can be considered as the outer limit within which that the animal can move without assistance from human beings. This could be a shoebox cage for a rodent, a fenced-in field for a goat, or a glass tank for a frog. Primary enclosures must be capable of containing the animal without using unnecessary restraint. The enclosure must protect the animal from hazards and environmental extremes and provide for the well-being of the animal. Proper feeding and watering equipment must be available. Overcrowding and indiscriminate mixing of animals may result in fighting, cannibalism, or barbering. The primary enclosure must also allow for observation of the animals without disturbing their normal physiologic and behavioral functions.

CAGING MATERIALS

A wide variety of materials can be used to construct primary enclosures. These include stainless steel, aluminum, and plastics.

Each type of material has specific advantages and disadvantages. Stainless steel is the strongest of all caging materials and is smooth, rust free, and resistant to most cleaning chemicals. Disadvantages include its relatively high cost when compared with other materials. Stainless steel cages may also produce microenvironments with significantly lower temperatures than may be desired. Aluminum is a lightweight material that has a relatively low cost. It tends to be less durable than stainless steel. Although cages may also be made from galvanized metals, these are not desirable because they are usually easily damaged by cleaning chemicals and can develop rust.

Plastics used for construction of primary enclosures include polycarbonate, polypropylene, and polystyrene. Plastic cages are less expensive than metal cages. Polycarbonate cages have high impact strength, high heat resistance, and high chemical resistance. They are the most expensive of the plastics. Polycarbonate cages are transparent, allowing for ready observation of the animals in the cage. Polypropylene cages are somewhat less heat resistant with slightly less impact strength. Cages made of polypropylene are opaque so animals cannot be directly observed. Polystyrene cages have low impact strength and are the least heat and chemical resistant of the plastics. Polystyrene is primarily used for disposable cages.

> **TECHNICIAN NOTE** Because polycarbonate cages are transparent, observation of the animals in the cage can be accomplished without handling the animals or opening the cage lid or door.

TYPES OF CAGING

The choice of specific cage types and arrangements used in housing of laboratory animals depends on the species being housed and the experimental design.

Shoebox Cages

Shoebox cages are solid-bottomed cages usually composed of plastic. The cage top is usually composed of a grid of stainless steel and may incorporate a feeding station (Figure 2-7). Filter tops are a common feature of this type and may be either a bonnet type of filter or a flat filter held in place with a specially designed filter holder. The filter serves to control the microenvironment of the cage. These cages may be easily stacked or placed on shelves (Figure 2-8).

> **TECHNICIAN NOTE** Rats, mice, and other small rodents are commonly housed in shoebox cages.

Suspended Caging

Suspended caging refers to racks that hold a series of mesh-bottomed cages that slide in and out of the rack on rails. The cages may be composed of plastic or stainless steel and have a wire mesh or plastic grid floor. Depending on the specific design, the cage may provide access to the animals only from

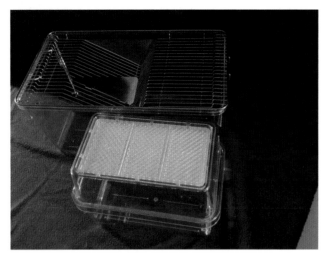

FIGURE 2-7. A shoebox cage showing the V-trough area for food and water *(top)* and the microisolator top *(bottom)*.

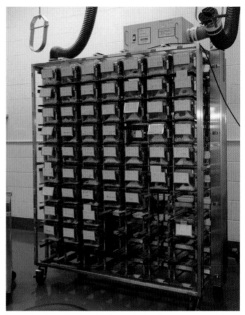

FIGURE 2-8. Rack of shoebox cages for small rodent housing.

the top of the cage, or they may have front access doors. This system provides excellent ventilation through the cages but poor control of microenvironment.

Metabolism Cages

Metabolism cages are used to collect urine and feces in such a way that the total volume can be measured and analyzed. Food and water sources are usually located outside the cage so that they do not add to the volume of waste collected.

Gang Cages

This type of cage is used for housing of social groupings of animals. The exact cage configuration varies depending on the species being housed. All gang housing has multiple sites for food and water distributed throughout the cage to discourage domination by a few animals in the group.

> TECHNICIAN NOTE   Multiple sites for food and water must be distributed throughout the cage when multiple animals are housed in the same enclosure.

Transportation Cages

Cages on wheels are used to move an animal from one area of a facility to another. Some transportation cages incorporate other systems within such as primate squeeze cages. Squeeze cages have a device that moves one wall of the cage inward to immobilize the animal. Because animals only stay in transportation cages for short periods, food and water sources are not required. Special cages that provide food, water, and adequate space are required when animals are to be transported long distances by truck, plane, or rail.

Pens and Runs

Large pens or runs are primarily used to house dogs, sheep, goats, and other farm animals. If outdoors, special measures must be used to maintain safety and keep other animals out

of the enclosure. The use of an outdoor area, such as a pasture, may allow easier accommodation of an animal's social and behavioral needs. However, some loss of control over the animal's nutritional needs is possible, and health care and direct surveillance of individual animals may become more complicated. Consideration of adequate shelter must also be addressed. Animals must be provided either a natural or constructed shelter from weather extremes. Ground or base surfaces of outdoor facilities can be covered with dirt, absorbent bedding, sand, gravel, grass, or any other material that can be removed for cleaning or replaced when needed. Animals must also be acclimated to outdoor housing in advance of any seasonal changes. Pens or runs may be located indoors to improve environmental control.

Activity Cages

This type of cage is used to provide exercise areas for animals. The exact cage configuration varies depending on the species being housed. Dog runs can be considered activity cages. Primates may have jungle gyms or swings; rodent activity cages often have exercise wheels.

Inhalation Cages

This cage type is an enclosed chamber for use when strict control of environmental parameters is needed. They are routinely used for studies requiring inhalation of vaccine or antibiotic. Inhalation cages allow the substances to be applied directly into the cage without contaminating the room air.

Recovery Cages

Similar to intensive care cages in a veterinary hospital, these cages provide strict control of temperature, humidity, oxygen pressure, and so forth (Figure 2-9). Intravenous lines, catheter access ports, and monitoring devices may also be incorporated.

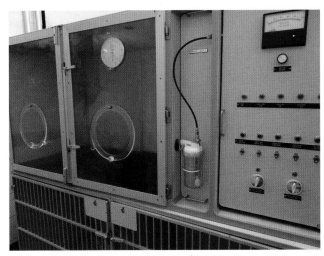

FIGURE 2-9. An oxygen cage used for recovery.

TABLE 2-3	Floor Space Requirements for Common Laboratory Animals	
SPECIES	**WEIGHT (G)**	**FLOOR AREA (IN²)/ANIMAL**
Mice	<10	6
	Up to 15	8
	Up to 25	12
	>25	>15
Rats	<100	17
	Up to 200	23
	Up to 300	29
	Up to 400	40
	Up to 500	60
	>500	>70
Hamsters	<60	10
	Up to 80	13
	Up to 100	16
	>100	>19
Guinea pigs	<350	60
	>350	>101
Rabbits	<2	1.5
	Up to 4	3.0
	Up to 5.4	4.0
	>5.4	>5.0
Cats	<4	3.0
	>4	>4.0
Dogs	<15	8.0
	Up to 30	12.0
	>30	>24.0

SPACE REQUIREMENTS

Calculating the space required of a primary enclosure requires consideration of a large number of factors. The cage must be large enough to allow normal postural movements and also provide an enriched environment that allows normal behavioral function. Floor space requirements are calculated on the basis of the animal's body weight or body surface area. Determination of adequate space may be based on such factors as animal health, reproduction, growth, behavior, and activity. Animals involved in long-term research studies may need greater space and, at minimum, need to have space considerations reassessed on a regular basis. In addition, animals housed in pairs or groups may require more or less than the calculated floor space. Some primates, for example, may require greater cage space when group housed to minimize aggression among individuals. Small rodents often huddle close together when group housed and do not necessarily require greatly increased space. The minimum floor space for selected species of laboratory animals is located in Table 2-3.

ENVIRONMENTAL ENRICHMENT

When planning for housing of animals, consideration of floor space alone may be inadequate. Some species make extensive use of vertical space. Other species may not require a large space if the enclosure is sufficiently complex. For example, cats, dogs, and primates often benefit from the inclusion of raised resting ledges. A number of research studies have demonstrated that certain forms of enrichment have a significant impact on an animal's health and development. Studies have confirmed that experimental results may be compromised when animals are not provided with suitable enrichment activities appropriate for their species. Rabbits, for example, respond poorly to conditions where sudden noises occur. An enrichment program in this case might include playing soft music during part of the day to acclimate the animals to some regular noise level.

TECHNICIAN NOTE Experimental results may be compromised when animals are not provided with suitable, appropriate enrichment activities.

Additional methods that are used for enrichment of laboratory animal environments include cage modifications, such as containers for burrowing or hiding (Figure 2-10) and resting ledges, enrichment devices, such as chew toys and climbing ropes, pair or group housing, and human interaction. Encouraging normal foraging behavior is also a type of enrichment. For example, seeds, fruits, or other small treats can be hidden within the cage bedding materials to encourage this behavior in species that have foraging instincts.

Activity cages, jungle gyms, running wheels, and simple tubes in which animals can hide are all used as enrichment devices (Figure 2-11).

The choice of a specific enrichment method must consider the normal behavior of a species as well as the experimental protocol. The goal of an enrichment program is to provide a mechanism for the animal to express an innate behavior that results in positive effects on its health and well-being. Some innate behaviors (e.g., predator/prey behaviors) may cause excess stress in the animals and are not considered appropriate enrichment. Forced exercise should never be used as an enrichment method. Similarly, some species, particularly rats,

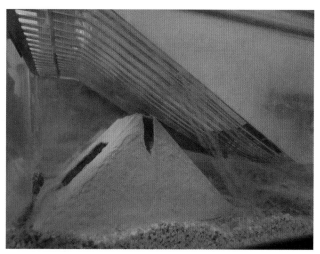

FIGURE 2-10. A simple cardboard enrichment device.

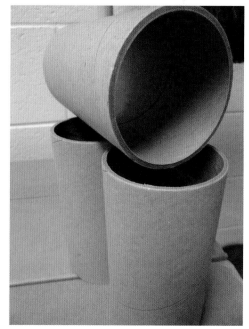

FIGURE 2-11. Cardboard tubes used as enrichment devices.

may respond poorly to handling when housed in a highly enriched environment. It is important that animals be acclimated to human handling in advance of their use in a research protocol and introduction of enrichment devices.

EXERCISE PROGRAMS

The Animal Welfare Act requires that dogs housed in U.S. Department of Agriculture (USDA)–licensed breeding or research facilities be provided with appropriate exercise. The exercise plan must be in writing and developed in conjunction with the veterinarian in charge of animal care for the facility. Dogs older than 12 weeks that are kept in primary enclosures providing less than twice the minimum floor space required for their size must be provided with regular exercise. When dogs are housed in groups, the specific requirement for exercise does not apply if the minimal floor space is at least equal to that which would have been required had each dog been housed individually. Only the attending veterinarian for the facility can make exceptions to the requirement. Acceptable exceptions include bitches with litters, animals that are overly aggressive, or any other situation in which the health or well-being of the dogs or group of dogs would be adversely affected. Dogs that cannot be provided with direct physical contact with other dogs must be provided with regular human interaction.

FEEDING AND WATERING DEVICES

Feeding and watering devices vary with the type of food (e.g., pelleted, powdered), the type of cage, and the species of animals present. Feeding devices must be placed so that food is readily available but not allowed to become contaminated with feces or urine. Feeding devices are normally composed of stainless steel or plastic because of the durability and ease of cleaning those materials. Special considerations are needed for animals in group or outdoor housing to ensure that all animals are able to gain access to the food. Experimental designs may also call for specific types of feeds and feeding containers.

> **TECHNICIAN NOTE** Feeding devices are normally composed of stainless steel or plastic.

V-shaped feeders are components of many rodent cages. The cage lid contains a preformed V-shaped area into which food pellets can be placed. Animals take the food through the bars. There is usually space for a water bottle within the same area. J-shaped feeders are also used for pelleted feed. The feeder hangs inside the cage but off the cage bottom and uses gravity to allow the feed to enter the accessible area at the bottom of the feeder. Rabbits and guinea pigs are commonly fed by J-shaped feeders (Figure 2-12). Slotted feeders also hang inside cages and are routinely used for feeding pelleted food to rodents.

> **TECHNICIAN NOTE** Feeding devices placed on the cage floor must be cleaned frequently.

A variety of glass or stainless steel bowls or crocks may also be used as feeding devices. Dogs, cats, and primates are commonly fed with bowls. Powdered rodent diets are often provided in bowls. The bowl may be placed on the cage floor, but contamination of food must be addressed by frequent cleaning of the food bowl. Some bowls incorporate a screen to minimize this problem. Feed bowls may also be attached by a bracket to the wall or cage door.

Unless specifically prohibited by an experimental design, clean, fresh water must be available to all animals at all times. Water may be supplied in a bottle that fits within the V-shaped trough of a rodent cage or by a sipper tube that is placed through the cage bars (Figure 2-13). Bottles

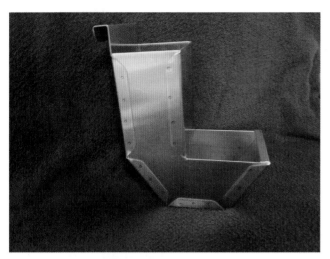

FIGURE 2-12. J-shaped feeder.

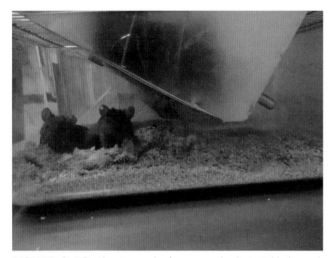

FIGURE 2-13. The sipper tube for a water bottle is visible beneath the V-trough of this shoebox cage.

that are suspended within the cage should be made of glass so that the animals cannot damage them by gnawing or scratching.

Bottles placed outside the cage may be made of plastic; these are most often polycarbonate. Sipper tubes must be examined daily to ensure proper operation.

Some sipper tubes contain a ball bearing that allows water to move through the tube only when the animal contacts it. If the ball bearing or tube is damaged, water often empties freely from the bottle, resulting in a wet cage and an animal with no water. Water bottles also require regular cleaning and refilling with fresh water (Figure 2-14).

AUTOMATIC WATERING SYSTEMS

Automatic watering systems have become very popular in large institutions. Although these systems eliminate the need for constant refilling and washing of bottles, they may be expensive, and all require routine care and maintenance. Automatic watering systems contain built-in pressure-reducing stations to reduce the water pressure in

the source line to a level that is appropriate for delivery to the animal. The system must be flushed regularly to remove the potential for the buildup of bacteria in the water lines. Filtering systems are often included to remove any particulates from the source water. The automatic watering system terminates at the drinking valve placed either inside or outside the animal cage (Figure 2-15). Disadvantages of automatic watering systems include the inability to determine the water consumption of an individual animal. In addition, the drinking valves must be regularly checked for evidence of leaks or clogging within the lines or valves. Some animals may be unfamiliar with the operation of the systems and may need to be trained to use them effectively.

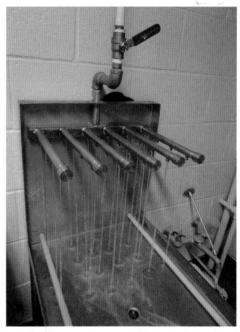

FIGURE 2-14. Devices are available to fill many water bottles at once when manual filling is needed.

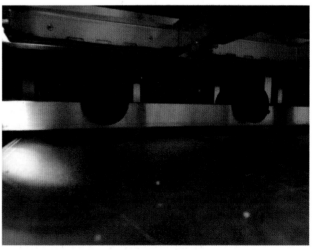

FIGURE 2-15. Cage rack showing individual valves for an automatic watering system.

FACILITY ADMINISTRATION

Although the veterinary technician or laboratory animal technician may not have direct responsibility for management of the animal facility, numerous administrative responsibilities may apply. Record-keeping requirements for animal facilities are specified in the Animal Welfare Act, the Guide for the Care and Use of Laboratory Animals, and Public Health Services policies as well as other federal, state, and local guidelines. The technician may also be involved in calculating costs related to experimental design. In many cases, the principal investigator must provide a portion of any grant money received to the animal care facility, referred to as the **per diem cost**. This refers to the total costs per day for housing of the animals. In addition to costs of feeding, watering, bedding, cleaning, waste disposal, veterinary care, and other basic animal care requirements, the costs related to operation of the housing facility (e.g., electricity, equipment depreciation) are also included when per diem costs are calculated. The technician may also be responsible for inventory control related to supplies, animal feeds, equipment, and acquisition of animals.

ANIMAL ACQUISITION

Federal laws require that animals used in research and teaching be acquired only from USDA-licensed dealers. Animal dealers must be licensed by the USDA and must adhere to Animal Welfare Act standards of care. Dealers must comply with detailed record-keeping and waiting period requirements. For example, any animal not bred by the animal dealer must undergo a 5- to 10-day waiting period to verify the origin of the animal before the animal can be transferred to another dealer or sold to a research facility. The USDA conducts unannounced inspections of dealers to ensure compliance. Animals bred specifically for research purposes are referred to as purpose bred. **Purpose-bred** animals are usually purchased from USDA class A dealers. Nearly half the dogs and cats needed for research are bred for that purpose. The USDA also licenses class B dealers. These dealers are permitted to obtain animals from a variety of sources, including animal shelters. These animals are referred to as **random source**. Some research protocols may not allow the use of random source animals because the genetic makeup and health status of the animal is usually unknown. In some cases, state laws and local policies may prevent animal dealers from obtaining shelter animals for research.

Regardless of the source, all animals acquired by the facility should be quarantined before being introduced into the animal colony. This will help ensure that the animals are not harboring disease that may infect the animals already present in the facility. The quarantine period also allows the animals to recover from the stress of transportation. Quarantine periods vary with different species at different facilities and are affected by the research protocol for which the animals are intended. Minimum 48-hour quarantine periods are common. Animal records are reviewed and diagnostic tests are usually performed on animals during the quarantine period. These include physical examination and fecal and blood tests. Once the quarantine period has passed, animals may then require a period to acclimate to the specific conditions in the facility (e.g., outdoor housing, group housing) and may also receive additional medical treatments to ensure optimal health before being used in any research protocol.

Gnotobiology

The study of animals with completely known flora and fauna is referred to as **gnotobiology**. The development of gnotobiology in the 1950s represented a significant conceptual and technologic advance in the commercial breeding of animals for research.

In biomedical research, the use of animals with defined flora and fauna minimizes the variables associated with normal variations among individuals of the same species. In addition, defined flora animals may be required when specific procedures are performed. For example, many animals harbor normal microorganisms that can overgrow when an animal is immunosuppressed. If immunology studies are being performed, this overgrowth may invalidate test results or lead to ambiguous results. When animals have undefined or unknown microflora, they are referred to as conventional. Defined flora animals may be of several types: axenic, **gnotobiotic**, **specific pathogen free**, cesarean derived, and **barrier sustained**.

> **TECHNICIAN NOTE** Variables are minimized when animals with defined flora and fauna are used in biomedical research.

Axenic Animals

The term *axenic* literally means "without strangers." These animals are also referred to as germ free. **Axenic animals** have no evidence of microorganisms except those that pass to the animal through the placenta before birth. Axenic animals remain germ free as long as they are maintained in barrier facilities under strict conditions of sterility. Food and water must be sterilized before being given to these animals. This results in the need for heavy supplementation of dietary vitamins and minerals because sterilization usually destroys these substances. Axenic animals have some unique anatomic features, including a thinner-walled intestine with a larger lumen. Axenic animals tend to grow more quickly, absorb fats better, and have a longer lifespan.

Gnotobiotic

Animals that are considered gnotobiotic have a well-defined microflora. These animals have been demonstrated to have specific microorganisms, and only those microorganisms specified are present.

Specific Pathogen Free

Specific pathogen–free (SPF) animals are those that have been demonstrated to be free of certain pathogens. SPF animals may not be free of pathogens other than those specified. Other than the pathogen specified, SPF animals have undefined microflora.

Cesarean Derived

Animals delivered surgically by removal of the uterus (hysterectomy) of the mother with delivery of the fetuses in a sterile isolation chamber are referred to as **cesarean derived**. Usually, the entire uterus is removed and passed through a disinfectant before being aseptically placed in the sterile isolator. The uterus is then incised and the fetuses removed.

Barrier Sustained

Animals derived by cesarean section may then be maintained in sterile, controlled environments. These animals are referred to as barrier sustained or barrier reared. The barrier may be a single microisolator cage, a barrier room, or an entire barrier facility. All supplies, food, water, and equipment used with these animals are sterilized before being introduced to the barrier environment. Personnel involved in animal care must also adhere to strict procedures to keep the animals from becoming contaminated by pathogens.

QUALITY ASSURANCE

Monitoring of the health of the animals in a facility is vital to ensuring that the animals are not introducing variables into an experiment. Programs of veterinary care are in place in all facilities and are aimed at preventing disease and identifying the presence of any pathogens. Although the animals are observed daily, it is not usually feasible to perform diagnostic testing on every animal in the facility on a regular basis. A well-defined program of periodic physical examination and laboratory evaluations of animals is an essential component of animal care. A morbidity and mortality reporting system will also allow early identification of potential problems. A quality assurance program should be designed for each of the species maintained at the facility. One method that can be used for monitoring animal health is the use of **sentinel animals**. Sentinel animals are those that are susceptible to particular pathogens. These animals are located in various animal rooms and experimental areas. Periodically, serologic testing, fecal analysis, and fecal and blood cultures are taken from these sentinel animals to identify the presence of any microorganisms in the animal colonies.

> **TECHNICIAN NOTE** Sentinel animals are used to monitor for the presence of any microorganisms in the animal colonies.

FACILITY SECURITY

The welfare of the animals, safety of personnel, and protection of the reliability of research require that animal housing facilities have a focus on security. This is necessary because of the potential for sabotage by animal rights or liberation activists. In addition, animal care and research protocols

can be compromised simply when an unauthorized individual from within the facility accidentally wanders into a controlled environment. The security system should control access to the facility as a whole as well as individual rooms within the facility. Common security systems include keyed entry and coded keyless entry systems. The facility manager must determine which personnel are authorized to enter controlled areas and issue appropriate access keys or numbers. Keys and codes should be changed on a regular basis, particularly when there is a change in personnel. Coded security systems can also be used to restrict the ability to modify environmental parameters (e.g., lighting, temperature) to authorized personnel.

Security system alarms are often integrated with alarm systems for fire and other emergency situations. Because alarms within animal rooms must be silent, monitoring of alarms should be handled at a central monitoring area.

OCCUPATIONAL SAFETY AND HEALTH

The Occupational Safety and Health Administration (OSHA) is a division of the U.S. Department of Labor. OSHA is responsible for enforcing laws that protect workers from workplace hazards. Federal OSHA regulations allow states to adopt their own regulations. Some of the state OSHA regulations are identical to the federal ones. OSHA standards call for the employer to post certain notices and maintain written safety plans. Employers must make protective equipment available to workers. OSHA requirements are summarized in Box 2-2.

The OSHA "Right to Know" law requires that personnel be informed about any potential chemical exposure on the job. The law also requires the use of appropriate safety equipment that is prescribed by the chemical manufacturer when handling a chemical. The safety equipment must be provided by the employer at no cost to employees. Use of personal protective equipment is not optional; personnel must wear what is prescribed.

Another component of the Right to Know law is the hazardous materials plan. This plan describes the details of the Material Safety Data Sheet (MSDS) filing system and the secondary container labeling system for the facility. The plan also lists the person responsible for ensuring that all employees have received the necessary safety training. All employees have a right to review any of these materials. The plan must also contain an up-to-date list of chemicals known to

BOX 2-2	OSHA Requirements

- Display job safety and health protection posters
- Record occupational injuries and illnesses
- Display warning and identification signs
- Provide written plans for job safety and health
- Provide protective equipment for employees
- Train employees in proper procedures and use of protective equipment
- Document all training received by personnel

be on the premises. Before using any chemicals, employees should review the MSDS and learn the procedures to follow for cleaning up a spill. When cleaning up any spill, employees must always wear disposable gloves and any other protective equipment specified on the MSDS. Unless prohibited by the instructions on the MSDS, the spill site and any contaminated equipment must be washed with a detergent soap and water.

The Centers for Disease Control and Prevention (CDC), National Institutes of Health (NIH), and the Public Health Service also promulgate regulations that require an occupational health and safety program as part of an animal care and use program. The specific program depends on the facility, types of research protocols, and animal species maintained at the facility. The National Research Council publication *Occupational Health and Safety in the Care and Use of Research Animals* contains guidelines and references for establishing and maintaining an effective, comprehensive program.

Identifying Hazards

Potential hazards in animal care facilities include animal bites, exposure to caustic chemical cleaning agents, allergens, and zoonoses. Laboratory and veterinary technicians must be aware of these potential hazards and provided with training and equipment to minimize injury to themselves and to the animals in their care. The degree of knowledge and training required of individuals in a specific occupational health and safety program is determined by the level of potential risk given their normal responsibilities. The intensity, duration, and frequency of any exposure to hazards and the susceptibility of the personnel to the hazard are also considered when identifying which personnel are at risk of exposure to specific hazards.

All personnel involved in animal care must be trained regarding zoonoses, handling of waste materials, chemical safety, and microbiologic, anesthetic, and radiation hazards. The potential for allergic responses of personnel to animals and to any unusual events or agents that might be part of experimental procedures must also be addressed. A high standard of personal cleanliness is essential for personnel involved in animal care. Facilities for washing and showering as well as disposable clothing may be required.

The safety of both animals and personnel depends on training and rigorous adherence to safety procedures. Written policies regarding procedures for working with hazardous biologic, chemical, and physical agents are essential. Methods to monitor and ensure compliance with safety policies should also be instituted. Special facilities and safety equipment are needed to protect personnel, the public, animals, and the environment from exposure to hazardous biologic, chemical, and physical agents used in animal experimentation.

The CDC and NIH publication *Biosafety in Microbiological and Biomedical Laboratories* defines specific procedures for working with hazardous materials.

Facilities used for animal experimentation with hazardous agents should be separate from other animal housing and support areas and research and clinical laboratories.

Areas where animals are involved in protocols requiring the use of hazardous agents should be clearly identified and access to them should be limited to authorized personnel.

Floor drains should always contain liquid or be sealed by other means. Hazardous agents must be contained within the experimental area. Control of airflow is vital to minimize escape of contaminants. Features such as airlocks, negative air pressure, and HEPA air filters provide additional barriers against release of contaminants in the work area or the outside environment.

Biosafety Hazard Considerations

Special considerations must be given to hazards that are unique to the biomedical industry. Biohazards are biologic substances such as used hypodermic needles and patient samples containing infectious agents that pose a threat to human health. It can also include substances harmful to animals. Containers that contain biohazardous material are marked with a specific symbol (Figure 2-16). The Centers for Disease Control and Prevention (CDC) is a U.S. government agency that has established specific guidelines for the safe handling and management of infectious agents in the biomedical industry. **Biosafety levels** are graded as I, II, III, and IV; the higher the number; the greater the risk. The following is a brief summary of the precautions for each biosafety level. It should be noted that the requirements for each level increase and that requirements for lower levels are automatically included in higher levels.

Biosafety Level I. The agents in biosafety level I are those that ordinarily do not cause disease in humans. It should be noted, however, that these otherwise harmless substances may affect individuals with immune deficiency.

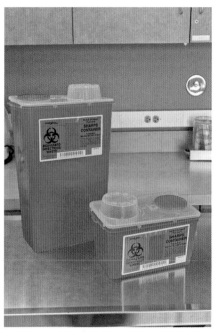

FIGURE 2-16. A biohazard container for handling of hazardous materials and sharps.

Examples of products and organisms found in biosafety level I include most soaps and cleaning agents, vaccines administered to animals, and infectious diseases that are species specific, such as canine infectious hepatitis virus.

There are no specific requirements for the handling or disposal of biosafety level I materials other than the normal sanitation that would be used in a home kitchen. This always includes complete washing of counters, equipment, and hands.

Biosafety Level II. The agents in biosafety level II are those that have the potential to cause human disease if handled incorrectly. At this level, specific precautions are taken to avoid problems. The hazards in this level include mucous membrane exposure, possible oral ingestion, and puncture of the skin. Examples of organisms in this level are the bacterial agents that cause toxoplasmosis and salmonellosis. Generally, substances in this group have a low potential for aerosol contamination.

Although precautions will vary with the specific substances, these are the general requirements for biosafety level II.
- Limited access to the area, including signs that warn of biohazards
- Wearing of gloves, laboratory coats, gowns, face shields, and use of Class I or Class II biosafety cabinets to protect against splash potential or aerosol contamination
- Appropriate use of sharps containers
- Specific instruction for the disposal and/or decontamination of equipment and potentially dangerous materials, including monitoring and reporting of contamination problems
- Physical containment devices and autoclaved, if needed

Biosafety Level III. Agents in biosafety level III are substances that can cause serious and potentially lethal disease. The potential for aerosol respiratory transmission is high. An example of an organism in this category is *Mycobacterium tuberculosis*. At this level, primary and secondary barriers are required to protect personnel. General requirements at this level are as follows:
- Controlled access
- Decontamination of waste
- Decontamination of cages, clothing, and other equipment
- Testing of personnel to evaluate possible exposure
- Use of Class I or Class II biosafety cabinets or other physical containment devices during all procedures
- Use of personal protective gear for all personnel

Biosafety Level IV. It is unlikely that persons with limited experience in handing biohazards will ever encounter substances that are included in biosafety level IV. Agents found in this category pose a high risk of causing life-threatening diseases. Included in this level are Ebola and Marburg viruses and other dangerous and exotic agents. Facilities that handle these substances exercise maximum containment. Personnel shower-in and shower-out and dress in full body suits equipped with a positive air supply. Individuals who plan to work in these facilities will undergo extensive training to ensure safety.

Personnel Health

Animal care workers must participate in a program of medical evaluation and preventive medicine. New employees should have a thorough health screening to identify any potential risks to the employee or the animals for which that employee may provide care. Regular medical check-ups are also advisable for employees who work with pathogenic organisms or with species known to be carriers of zoonotic diseases. In some cases, employees may require immunization against certain diseases for the protection of both employees and the animals in the facility. Common vaccines administered to animal care personnel include tetanus, rabies, and hepatitis B virus. Whenever a research protocol involves specific pathogenic organisms for which vaccines are available, vaccinations are recommended. Biosafety in Microbiological and Biomedical Laboratories contains recommendations for vaccination of personnel. All animal care personnel should be vigilant in reporting accidents, bites, scratches, and allergic reactions.

Many diseases of nonhuman primates are zoonotic and can represent serious hazards. Screening for tuberculosis is required for technicians, investigators, maintenance workers, security personnel, and any others who may come in contact with nonhuman primates. Certain species of nonhuman primates are susceptible to tuberculosis and may be asymptomatic carriers of the herpes simplex B virus. Personnel who are bitten or scratched by a carrier of herpes B virus can develop fatal meningitis. The facility must have a program for reporting and treating any animal bites or scratches.

KEY POINTS

- Specialized equipment and caging may be needed to care for exotic companioon animals in the private veterinary clinic.
- Veterinary practices that decide to treat exotic animal patients must provide for the advanced training needed to properly care for these animals.
- The three basic types of research are basic research, applied research, and clinical research.
- AALAS administers the certification examinations for laboratory animal technicians, laboratory animal technologists, and assistant laboratory animal technicians.
- The quality of research data is directly related to the standards of animal care.
- Animal facilities are desiged to minimize the spread of disease from one part of the facility to another.
- Facilities used for biomedical research may be designed with single corridors or with separate clean/dirty corridor systems.
- Barrier facilities are used to house germ-free animals.
- Environmental conditions (e.g., temperature, lighting, ventilation) are carefully controlled in facilities that house animals.

- Macroenvironment refers to the environmental conditions within a room used to house animals.
- Microenvironment refers to the environmental conditions within an individual animal cage.
- The temperature ranges used for housing of animals is within the thermoneutral zone for each species.
- Air pressure within animal rooms is maintained as positive or negative pressure based on the specific use of the room.
- Animals are housed in social groupings whenever possible.
- A variety of materials can be used for construction of primary enclosures.
- Cage types include shoebox cages, suspended cages, and special use cages.
- Determinations of minimum space requirements for animals are based on factors such as animal health, reproduction, growth, behavior, and activity.
- Adequate food and water must be provided in a device that the animal is capable of using.
- Automatic watering systems are commonly used in larger animal housing facilities.
- Animal acquisition is governed by federal, state, and local regulations.
- Gnotobiology refers to the study of animals with completely known flora and fauna.

REVIEW QUESTIONS

1. Research directed toward specific objectives, such as development of new drugs, is referred to as _____ _____.

2. The use of computer models or plants in research is an example of _____ _____.

3. Veterinarians who have reached the highest degree of proficiency in laboratory animal medicine are board certified by _____.

4. Name the organization that determines the criteria for certification for ALAT, LAT, and LATG.

5. The level of certification that requires a minimum of a GED or high school diploma and at least 3 years of experience is the _____.

6. A biomedical facility designed for housing of germ-free animals is referred to as a _____ facility.

7. Define *microenvironment*.

8. Define *thermoneutral zone*.

9. Animal rooms must have a minimum of _____ room air changes per hour.

10. Which type of room should be under negative air pressure?

11. A diurnal lighting system is one that uses ___ hours of light followed by ___ hours of darkness.

12. A type of plastic used for cages that is transparent and has high impact strength and resistance to high heat and chemicals is _____.

13. The study of animals with completely known flora and fauna is referred to as _____.

14. Animals that are known to be free of certain pathogens are referred to as _____ _____ _____.

15. Animals kept in animal rooms and experimental areas that undergo periodic testing to identify the presence of any microorganisms in the animal colonies are referred to as _____ _____.

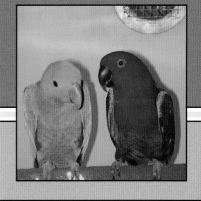

3 Birds

KEY TERMS

Anisodactyl
Apteria
Choana
Cloaca
Coverts
Crop
Gizzard
Heterophil
Passerines
Pododermatitis
Proventriculus
Psittacines
Pterylae
Remiges
Sexually dimorphic
Syrinx
Urates
Uropygial gland
Zygodactyl

LEARNING OBJECTIVES

After studying this chapter, you will be able to:
- Describe the unique features of the anatomy of birds
- Discuss the basic behavior of birds.
- Discuss the basics of client education, husbandry, and nutrition for avian species.
- Describe how to obtain a complete and thorough history of the avian patient.
- Explain the different capture and restraint techniques used for birds.
- Identify methods of sample collection for laboratory analysis.
- Describe how to obtain high-quality diagnostic images of avian patients.
- Discuss nursing care and supportive therapy techniques for the avian patient.
- Identify and discuss some of the common diseases and presentations of the avian patient to the veterinary clinic.
- List the common infectious diseases, noninfectious diseases, and zoonoses found in the avian patient.
- Describe the routine clinical procedures performed on avian species.
- Explain the unique aspects of avian anesthesia and surgery.

The taxonomic class Aves contains more than two dozen orders or birds. Some variation exists in classification of different species of birds. Most species encountered in exotic companion animal practice are members of the orders Passeriformes (**passerines**) or Psittaciformes (**psittacines**). Avian species that may be encountered in biomedical research are primarily in the order Galliformes (fowl) (Box 3-1).

Passeriformes
- Canary
- Finch

Columbiformes
- Dove
- Pigeon

Psittaciformes
- Cockatoo
- Macaw
- Parrot
- Conure
- Budgerigar
- Lovebird
- Cockatiel
- Parakeet
- Lorikeet

Galliformes
- Turkey
- Chicken
- Duck

In biomedical research, chickens, turkeys, and ducks serve as animal models for studies of atherosclerosis, hypertension, and muscular dystrophy. There are numerous additional diseases, including glaucoma, cataracts, and human neural tube defects, that have utilized chicken embryos. Studies related to vaccine development and a variety of pharmacokinetic studies have also involved avian species.

UNIQUE ANATOMIC FEATURES

Because of the large number of taxonomic families in the class Aves, there is some diversity in anatomic features among different families of birds. However, some generalizations can be made. A review of external features may aid in further study as well as handling and examination of these animals (Figure 3-1). A full discussion of all anatomic and physiologic features unique to birds is beyond the scope of this text. The following sections provide an overview of some of those unique features.

INTEGUMENT

The integument comprises the skin, beak, claws, feathers, and associated structures. The skin is very thin and delicate with a dry, wrinkled appearance. It may have a reddish appearance in some areas due to visibility of some underlying muscle and blood vessels. The feet and legs are covered with scales composed of raised areas of highly keratinized epidermis separated by a fold.

The psittacines are known as hookbills due to their curved upper beak. Their second and third digits point anteriorly while digits I and IV are oriented posteriorly (known as

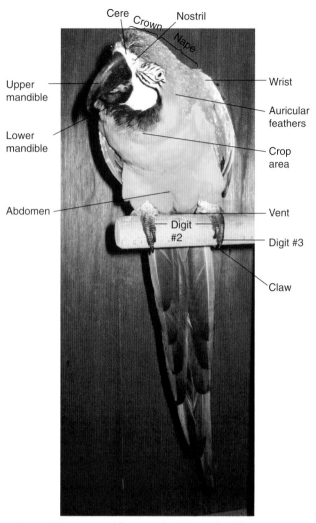

FIGURE 3-1. External features of a blue and gold macaw *(Propyrhura maracana)*. (From Colville TP, Bassert JM: *Clinical anatomy and physiology for veterinary technicians*, ed 2, St. Louis, Mosby, 2008.)

zygodactyl). Passerines have a pointed or slightly curved beak. Their first digit points posteriorly while digits II–IV point anteriorly (known as **anisodactyl**).

Birds do not have sweat glands. They will dissipate heat by increasing their respiratory rate and holding the wings away from the body. Hyperthermia is usually characterized by open-mouth breathing and panting. Birds that are hypothermic will have fluffed feathers. Most birds do possess a **uropygial gland**, also referred to as the preen gland. This is a bilobed gland with one duct opening that empties into a lone papilla, found dorsally at the base of the tail (Figure 3-2). The gland secretes a lipoid sebaceous material that is spread over feathers during preening to help with waterproofing. This gland is absent in the ostrich, emu, cassowaries, bustards, frogmouth, many pigeons, woodpeckers, and Amazon parrots.

> **TECHNICIAN NOTE** The uropygial gland secretes a lipoid sebaceous material that is spread over feathers during preening.

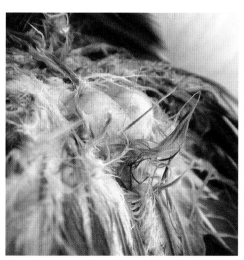

FIGURE 3-2. Uropygial gland of a Meyers parrot located at the base of the tail dorsal to the pygostyle. (From Sirois M: *Principles and practice of veterinary technology*, ed 3, St. Louis, Mosby, 2011.)

Feathers

Feathers are necessary for flight, to protect the skin from trauma and exposure, and to aid in thermoregulation, camouflage, and communication. Birds spend several hours a day preening, or rearranging and conditioning their feathers. Feathers' follicles are located in specific tracts over the surface of the body called **pterylae**. These tracts are separated by nonfeathered areas of skin called **apteria**. The tracts overlap each other to give the bird a fully feathered look.

Birds have several types of feathers (Figure 3-3). The contour feathers cover the body and wings and are identified as flight feathers or body feathers. The large, primary flight feathers (**remiges**) are found on the outer end of the wing. The secondary flight feathers are located on the wing between the body and the primaries. Body feathers, also known as **coverts**, provide surface coverage over most of the rest of the bird. Down feathers insulate the bird and have a soft, fluffy appearance. Cockatoos, cockatiels, and African greys have

powder down, which breaks down to produce a white, dusty powder. A healthy bird of these species will have a fine layer of this powder over most of its body and most noticeably on the beak. Molting occurs in all species and results in periodic replacement of old feathers. Developing feathers have a vascular supply that regresses as the feather grows. The shafts of these "blood feathers" appear dark and bleed profusely if cut or damaged, possibly leading to the death of the bird.

> *TECHNICIAN NOTE* Birds have several types of feathers: contour, semiplume, down, filoplume, and bristle.

MUSCULOSKELETAL SYSTEM

The avian musculoskeletal system contains many adaptations that enable flight. The avian skeleton is lightweight in comparison to that of a similarly sized mammal due in part to the presence of many pneumatized bones. These pneumatic bones are linked with air sacs and filled with air. They are located in the skull, vertebrae, pelvis, sternum, ribs, humerus, and sometimes the femur. The remaining bones are medullary bones and have thin walls that contain high levels of calcium as compared to bones of mammals. Many avian bones are also fused, which decreases the overall weight of the bird and improves strength. The skull bones are fused, which strengthens the beak structure. The atlas (first cervical vertebrae) has a single condyle, giving the neck great range of motion. The large sternum supports the pectoral muscles, which are needed for flight, and may contain a bony ridge, the keel, to which the muscles attach. A large portion of the caudal vertebrae is fused to form the synsacrum, which stabilizes the back during flight and can withstand the pressures related to perching and landing after flight.

The largest muscles in the body are the pectorals, which account for approximately 20% of the bird's weight. Because of their mass, they are used to determine the body condition of the bird and are ideal for intramuscular injections. Wings have paired muscle groups responsible for raising or

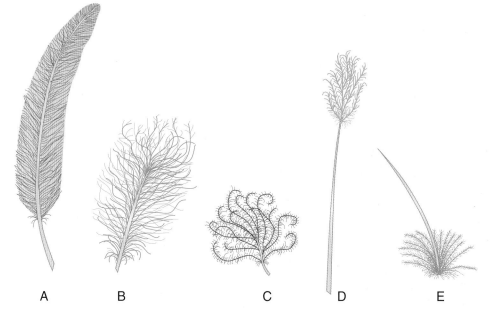

A   B   C   D   E

FIGURE 3-3. Types of feathers. **A,** Contour. **B,** Semiplume. **C,** Down. **D,** Filoplume. **E,** Bristle. (Courtesy Avid Systems). (From Colville TP, Bassert JM: *Clinical anatomy and physiology for veterinary technicians*, ed 2, St. Louis, Mosby, 2008.)

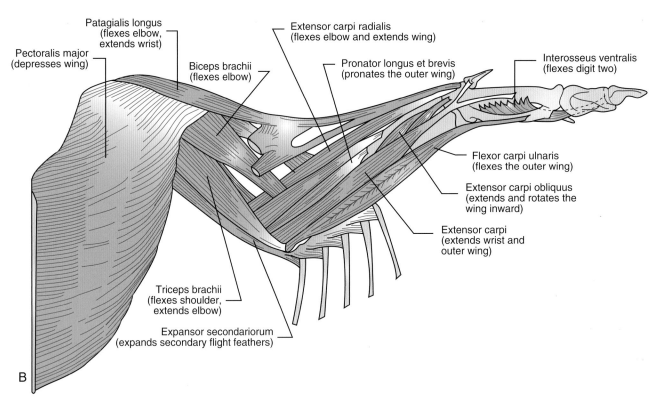

FIGURE 3-4. Wing muscles and their function. **A,** Dorsal view. **B,** Ventral view. (From Colville TP, Bassert JM: *Clinical anatomy and physiology for veterinary technicians,* ed 2, St. Louis, Mosby, 2008.)

depressing the leading edge of the wing, pulling the wing forward or backward, extending, or flexing the wing (Figure 3-4).

RESPIRATORY SYSTEM

Birds possess a highly specialized and efficient respiratory system. Air enters the respiratory system through the nares and

continues over an operculum, which is a cornified flap of tissue located immediately behind the nares in the nasal cavity. Air then travels through the many sinuses in the head and then enters the oral cavity through the slitlike opening in the roof of the mouth known as the **choana**. The choana is a V-shaped notch in the roof of the mouth that directs air from the mouth and nasal cavities to the glottis. The choana closes during swallowing. This structure should be surrounded by many sharp papillae. If the papillae are blunted or absent, this may be indicative of disease or malnutrition. Birds lack an epiglottis, so air travels through the glottis at the base of the tongue and down the trachea. At the caudal portion of the trachea lies the **syrinx** and is the voice box of birds. Birds produce vocalizations by forcing air over the syrinx and vibrating membranes during the expiratory phase of respiration. The complexity of a bird's vocalizations depends on the number of muscles in the syrinx. The air continues into the small lungs located dorsal near the spine, where gas exchange takes place. There are no lobes or alveoli and therefore the lungs do not inflate. Inspiration of air occurs by extension of the intracostal joints drawing in inspired air with a bellowslike action into the caudal air sacs. Both inspiration and expiration require active muscle contraction. Air flows into the air sacs, which are thin-walled hollow spaces that have lightly vascularized membranes and are found throughout the body. There are a total of nine air sacs—four paired air sacs and one unpaired. The paired air sacs are cranial thoracic, caudal thoracic, cervical, and abdominal. The one unpaired air sac is the interclavicular air sac, which is located in the thoracic inlet between the clavicles. From the caudal air sac the volume of air is pushed into the lungs so that airflow within the lung tissue is predominantly unidirectional, caudal to cranial.

Normal respiratory effort in the bird should not be noticeable, and the beak should remain closed. In some cases there may be increased head and tail movement and increased abdominal effort after exercise. The bird should return to normal within a few minutes.

> **TECHNICIAN NOTE** The choana is a V-shaped notch in the roof of the mouth that directs air from the mouth and nasal cavities to the glottis.

DIGESTIVE SYSTEM

The high metabolism of birds requires ingestion of large amounts of food. The beaks will vary with the diet and foraging strategies. Generally the beak is used to grasp food and crush it with the aid of the tongue. Birds do not have teeth. The mouth consists of a hard upper palate, a soft lower palate, a distinctive tongue, scattered taste buds, and salivary glands. The mouth is relatively dry because little saliva is produced.

When food is swallowed, it travels through the esophagus to the stomach. In several species the esophagus expands in the interclavicular space to create a **crop**. The crop anatomy varies between species and can be a dilation of the esophagus, a single pouch, or a double pouch (Figure 3-5).

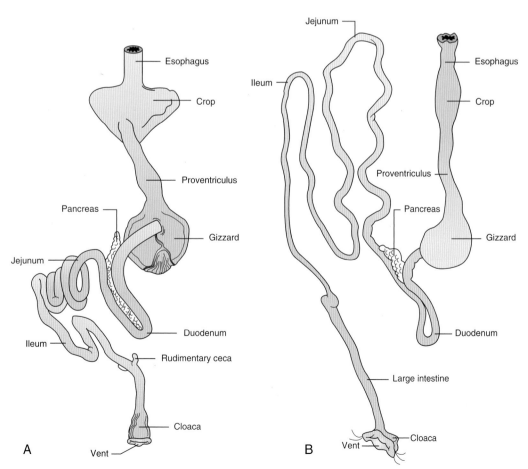

FIGURE 3-5. General diagram of avian digestive system. **A,** Rock dove. **B,** Hawk. (From Colville TP, Bassert JM: *Clinical anatomy and physiology for veterinary technicians,* ed 2, St. Louis, Mosby, 2008.)

It softens food and allows continuous passage of small amounts of food to the **proventriculus**, or true stomach. The proventriculus is unique to birds; however, it is very similar to the stomach of mammals, containing digestive acid and enzymes.

> TECHNICIAN NOTE The crop serves to soften food and allows continuous passage of small amounts of food to the proventriculus.

The food next passes into the ventriculus, or **gizzard**. This is a thickly muscled organ that grinds food into smaller particles. The intestinal tract is very similar to that of mammals. Birds have a pancreas that is a relatively large gland and rests in the loop of the duodenum. The gallbladder is absent in most parrots but is found in many other avian species. The large intestine terminates at the **cloaca**. The cloaca is the common terminal chamber of the gastrointestinal, urinary, and reproductive systems. The cloaca is divided into three compartments, the coprodeum, urodeum, and the proctodeum. The coprodeum is the cranial portion of the cloaca that receives feces from the rectum. The urodeum is the middle part of the cloaca into which the ureters enter dorsolaterally on both sides. In males the ductus deferens enters near the ureters, while in females a single oviduct enters the urodeum dorsolaterally on the left side. The proctodeum is the caudal part of the cloaca. If a phallus is present, it would be located on the floor of the proctodeum. Psittacines do not have a phallus, but it is found in many other avian species.

The external opening of the cloaca is called the vent, from which the droppings are passed. In most species the vent is horizontally flattened rather than circumferential as in mammals. Normal bird droppings have three distinct components: liquid urine, semisolid white or cream **urates**, and feces. The droppings will vary in consistency, depending on the diet.

UROGENITAL SYSTEM

The paired kidneys of birds are closely attached to the vertebrae. They empty into the ureters, which carry the liquid urine and semisolid urates to the cloaca. Urine is not concentrated in the kidneys; rather it moves retrograde into the coprodeum and rectum, where resorption of water, sodium, and chloride takes place. Urates are the major excretion product in birds and comprise the white portion of the droppings. Birds do not have a urinary bladder.

> TECHNICIAN NOTE Urates are the major excretion product in birds.

In the female bird, only the left side of the reproductive tract develops fully. As in mammals, an ovary, oviduct, and vagina are present. Various regions of the oviduct produce the egg white and eggshell. The entire process from ovulation to egg laying takes approximately 15 hours. The female lays eggs even if no male is present.

The male bird has paired testes located internally near the kidneys. During periods of active breeding, they enlarge dramatically. Sperm cells travel to the cloaca through the epididymis and then the ductus deferens. Most birds do not have a penis or phallus, and mating takes place when the vents of the male and female birds come in contact.

CIRCULATORY SYSTEM

The heart of birds closely resembles that of mammals, but it is proportionally about one and one half times larger. Heart rates range from 250 to 350 beats per minute in large parrots and up to 1400 beats per minute in the very small species. Blood pressure in birds is typically higher than in mammals.

The red blood cells of birds are oval and contain a nucleus. Birds do not have lymph nodes, and the lymphatic system is less extensive.

SPECIAL SENSES

The nervous system centers that receive and process stimuli from the senses are similar to those of mammals with a couple of exceptions. The brains of birds are large in proportion to body size. The control centers for vision and hearing are larger than those for taste, touch, and smell. Vision is highly developed in the avian species. The eyes of birds are relatively large, and a significant part of the avian skull is devoted to housing and protecting the eyes. The shape of the eyes is determined by the orbits. Bird eyes can be round, flat, or tubular, depending on the species (Figure 3-6). Diurnal birds (birds that forage or hunt in the daytime) have round or relatively flat eyes, whereas nocturnal species (those that forage and hunt at night) have tubular eyes. Tubular eyes have a pupil with a larger diameter than the retina, allowing more light into the eye.

The lens and anterior chamber of the avian eye are similar to those of mammals with the exception of the presence of a highly vascular, ribbonlike structure called the pectin

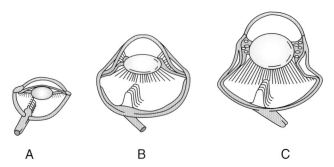

A   B   C

FIGURE 3-6. Shapes of the avian eye. **A,** Flat. **B,** Round. **C,** Tubular. (From Colville TP, Bassert JM: *Clinical anatomy and physiology for veterinary technicians,* ed 2, St. Louis, Mosby, 2008.)

oculi. The pectin oculi provides environmental stabilization of the fluid within the eye. Bird vision is very acute, and they can perceive color. Birds often look closely at something with one eye, tilting their head for a better view. In many species, the color of the iris is often darker in young birds. The iris contains striated muscles that allow voluntary control over the size of the pupils. Thus, pupillary light response is not a good diagnostic indicator in birds. Blinking is done using the nictitating membrane, or third eyelid. This structure is mostly transparent. Most birds completely close their eyes when they sleep.

> **TECHNICIAN NOTE** Birds have voluntary control over the size of the pupils.

The avian ear is simpler than that of mammals, but has exceptional acoustical ability. Located on the sides of the head and slightly below the eyes, the ears of birds are hidden from view by feathers that protect the ear during flight and yet allow sound to pass through. The external auditory canal funnels sound to the middle ear and tympanic membrane. There is a single bone in the middle ear in contrast to the three bones in mammals. It is called the columella and connects to the inner ear. The inner ear is similar to that in mammals and consists of a membranous labyrinth that helps to maintain balance and equilibrium and converts sounds into nerve impulses that are sent to the brain.

Birds have fewer taste buds than most mammals. Taste buds are located on the roof of the mouth and scattered over the soft palate. The sense of smell varies greatly in birds. In a few species such as the turkey vulture, the sense of smell is highly developed for locating food, but in the average companion species it is thought that the sense of smell is poorly developed.

The sense of touch is an important sense in many species for finding food and for defense. The skin of birds contains sensory nerve endings that respond to pain, heat, cold, and touch. Some are very responsive to the slightest feather movement, and some birds will respond when the tips of the feathers are touched.

AVIAN BEHAVIOR

Most birds have a higher than average intelligence resulting in a patient that is both entertaining and challenging to alter behaviors. Many of the behaviors that owners wish to modify are the result of instinctive avian reactions or related to the stresses of captivity. Knowledge of normal avian behavior is needed to have an understanding of the problem behaviors that birds exhibit in captivity.

Many parrots use their agile feet to hold food while they eat or manipulate objects they are interested in exploring (Figure 3-7). They tend to be good climbers, often moving around their cage using a combination of beak and feet. Birds will wag their tail back and forth when happy and relaxed. Birds grind their beak when they are comfortable and ready to fall asleep. Some birds will regurgitate food for those that they are closely bonded to, whether it is the owner or another bird. The typical behavior that indicates defecation in a calm bird is a slight wiggle of the tail, followed by a squat and an uplifted tail. Birds defecate frequently and more often when afraid or stressed.

> **TECHNICIAN NOTE** Many avian behaviors that owners wish to modify are the result of instinctive avian reactions or related to the stresses of captivity.

Fear is a common behavior in pet birds, and personnel should be aware of this and take appropriate measures to reduce the stress involved with clinic visits. When a bird is frightened, it may fling itself about the cage, struggle violently, flap its wings, scream loudly, or take flight in response to sudden movements or unfamiliar sights or sounds. Clients often seek help with such problems as biting, chewing, excessive vocalization, or destructive feather behavior.

CHEWING

Mouthing is a term used to describe a juvenile parrot using the tongue to explore surfaces. Juvenile parrots pass through an innocent "beaking" phase, in which they attempt to taste or chew almost anything, somewhat like what is commonly seen in puppies. Unlike puppies, birds do not grow out of this behavior (Figure 3-8). Clients should be counseled to supervise the parrot when out of its cage and provide the pet with well-designed safe toys to destroy. Toys that are safe to destroy such as paper-based manufactured or homemade or natural wood toys embedded with nuts provide much-needed enrichment for these intelligent confined creatures.

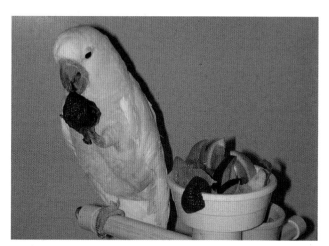

FIGURE 3-7. Birds are very agile and use their feet as utensils for eating. (From Sirois M: *Principles and practice of veterinary technology,* ed 3, St. Louis, Mosby, 2011.)

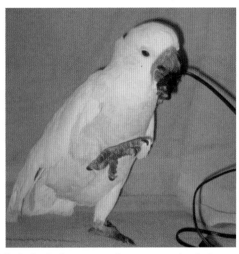

FIGURE 3-8. Birds are naturally curious and will chew on almost anything. (From Sirois M: *Principles and practice of veterinary technology,* ed 3, St. Louis, Mosby, 2011.)

BITING

Birds bite to exhibit dominance, express fear, exhibit jealousy, or as a result of hormonal fluctuations during puberty or the breeding season. Biting may not be an instinctual behavior but rather one that captive birds have developed in this confined world created for our companion birds. In the wild, most birds generally fly away rather than using their beak as a weapon. Some protective birds may bite the owner in an effort to communicate with the person to move away from perceived danger. It is important for the owner to realize that the bird must not be allowed to bite as a way of controlling any situation. Mature parrots are more likely to bite during handling as a method of defense. Larger psittacines, such as macaws, can exert up to 300 pounds of pressure per square inch, inflicting deep bruises and lacerations. Birds such as cockatiels and budgies have the potential to draw blood with their bites. Biting is a common behavior problem and identifying why the bird is biting is the first step to a resolution.

DOMINANCE

Psittacines may attempt to become dominant over their flock, and in the captive companion bird world this is their human family. It is important that the owner and other household members use certain techniques to maintain the dominant position in the home. Birds should be taught to consistently step up on or down from the owner's hand when asked. Clipping the bird's wings to limit its flying ability can diminish dominance behaviors, such as flying down from a curtain rod to attack members of the household. When holding the bird, keep it at mid-chest level. Never allowing it to sit on the head or shoulders keeps it from attaining the highest perch, a position of great power. Situating the cage or perches so that the bird is below eye level also discourages dominant behavior.

VOCALIZATION

Parrots are naturally loud creatures and vocalize for many reasons: communication, entertainment, exercise, and in response to discomfort or restraint. Birds tend to be very noisy at dawn and dusk and feeding time. Noise levels vary between species, and parrots can scream loud enough to damage human hearing, so hearing protection is recommended when working with these species. Some birds have the ability to repeat what they hear. Vocalizations may become a problem in some insecure or dependent birds that call constantly to their owner. Some species are relatively quiet, but all birds make a certain amount of noise. Owners may actually encourage the bird to make more noise by responding to the loud calls with anger or shouting in an effort to quiet the bird.

SELF-MUTILATION

Feather-destructive behavior, also called feather picking or plucking, is a well known but poorly understood condition. The bird uses its beak to chew on and pull out any feathers that are accessible, including any that start to grow back. Some birds remove all but the feathers on their heads, and some may damage skin as well as muscle (Figure 3-9). Some affected birds may have an underlying medical condition that initiates plucking, but some healthy birds respond to stress with self-mutilation. Stresses can be in the form of separation anxiety from their owner, from a change in the cage location, or the addition of a new pet or family member. This is a difficult problem to solve and may become a chronic condition. It is most common in cockatoo species and African greys. The most important first step in correcting this behavior is a thorough medical workup to rule out any underlying pathologic conditions. Once a medical condition has been ruled out or treated, the behavior modification and training can be implemented. Once feather-destructive behavior has been established, behavior

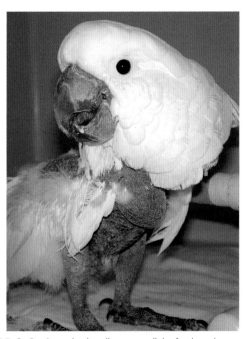

FIGURE 3-9. Some birds will remove all the feathers they can reach, which produces an image such as this cockatoo with a featherless body and fully feathered head. (From Sirois M: *Principles and practice of veterinary technology,* ed 3, St. Louis, Mosby, 2011.)

modification and training may decrease the severity of the disorder but will rarely stop the habit completely.

INAPPROPRIATE BONDING

Some owners will unintentionally allow a parrot to form a sexual bond with them by inappropriate petting. Petting the bird repeatedly over its back and tail sends a message to that bird that is similar to the courtship behaviors performed in the wild. Cuddling and feeding the bird warm foods by hand or mouth can have similar inappropriate bonding results. Panting and masturbation may follow and should be avoided, especially in cockatoos. Chronic masturbation can lead to a chronic prolapsing cloaca and a dilated vent that may require a corrective surgery. This is a difficult situation for the owner to correct, since it involves disrupting the owner's tight bond with the bird with behavior modification.

Correction of behavior problems takes time, an understanding of the underlying cause, and judicious use of behavior modification. Prolonged physical or mental isolation of the bird, withholding food or water, and physical punishment are totally unacceptable methods of dealing with these problems. All may result in permanent emotional or physical damage to the bird.

HUSBANDRY

Many birds that present to the veterinary clinic for the first time will have medical problems related to improper diet and husbandry. Client education needs to be available for a vast range of topics including proper cages and perch dimensions, substrate, safe transport, nutrition, and disease prevention.

HOUSING

Enclosures for birds come in many shapes and sizes that are designed to appeal to the client but may fail to address the needs of the bird. The enclosure should be spacious, and the minimum size would allow the bird to spread its wings without touching the sides of the cage. The cage should be wider than it is tall. It should be easy to clean and disinfect regularly and be constructed of a durable, nontoxic, lead-free material. Galvanized metal contains zinc and could be toxic if the bird pecks at it. Stainless steel cages are preferred. Cage bars must have appropriate spacing to ensure that the bird cannot squeeze through the bars or get caught in the bars (Table 3-1). Newspapers or paper towels are inexpensive and are very safe substrates for birds and don't promote the growth of pathogens as do other organic substrates such as wood shavings and corncob bedding. Some of the later substrates can also be ingested and create a gastrointestinal foreign body with the possibility of obstruction. The position of the enclosure should be in a draft-free area, out of direct sunlight, and in an area of the house where the family routinely congregates. The cage should not be placed close to the kitchen area. Fumes from self-cleaning ovens, non-stick cooking pans, cleaning products, and burnt food can be toxic to birds. The environmental temperature should range between 61° and 81° F with humidity levels in the range of

TABLE 3-1	Recommended Cage Bar Spacing for Companion Psittacine Species
BIRD	**CAGE BAR SPACING (IN INCHES)**
Large macaws and cockatoos	¾-1½
Large parrots, Amazon parrots, African grey parrots	¾-1
Cockatiels and small conures	½-¾
Budgies and lovebirds	⅜

(From Mitchell M, Tully T: *manual of exotic pet practice*, St. Louis, WB Saunders Company, 2009.)

30% to 70%. Wide fluctuations in temperature and humidity can predispose birds to illness. Very young birds may require an external heat source.

> **TECHNICIAN NOTE** The primary bird enclosure must be large enough for the bird to spread its wings, should be wider than they are tall, and maintained in a draft-free area.

Perches should be made from branches of clean, nontoxic hardwood trees and shrubs free of pesticides, mold, or wood rot. Birds need varying sizes, textures, and irregularly shaped perches to decrease the pressure placed on any one point of the foot and decrease the potential for pododermatitis. Food dishes, toys, mirrors, and other accessories should be provided without overcrowding the bird. If there is insufficient room for the bird to move about, the bird may not exercise appropriately and may become entrapped in parts of the accessories or toys and be injured. Toys should be made of nontoxic substances and of appropriate size for the bird so as not to allow for ingestion of the pieces.

NUTRITION

Different species of birds have different nutritional requirements. Nutritional deficiencies are common in companion birds. Comprehensive research on the specific nutritional requirements of different species is not readily available. Fresh water should be provided at all times. Food and water containers should not be placed below any perches to decrease the possibility of fecal contamination. Birds should be offered fresh food on a daily basis. For most companion birds, pellets should comprise approximately 70% of the diet and a variety of fresh fruits and vegetables approximately 30%. A calcium source such as cuttlefish bones or calcium blocks should also be available. Grit is not essential for captive psittacine species, and some birds may become impacted if provided with grit. However, in captive poultry and pigeons, studies suggest that it may increase the digestibility of feed by as much as 10%.

Feeding the bird at the dinner table and from the client's mouth should be discouraged since some human foods are too high in salts and sugars and some can be toxic to the bird such as chocolate and avocado. Health problems due to deficiencies and imbalances associated with all-seed diets are common. Conversion from seeds to pellets is encouraged.

IDENTIFICATION

Individual birds may be identified with leg bands or with microchips. Leg bands may contain radio frequency identification chips. The microchip is a tiny computer chip that has an identification number programmed into it and is encapsulated within a biocompatible material. The whole device is small enough to fit inside a hypodermic needle and can be simply injected intramuscularly, where it will stay for the life of the bird. This provides a permanent, positive identification that cannot be lost, altered, or intentionally removed. The microchip devices are sold as a disposable syringe and large needle unit for one-time use. The bird should be anesthetized for the procedure because the microchip is injected into the pectoral muscle via a 15-gauge needle and can be a very painful and stressful procedure. The site should be aseptically prepared. After the chip has been inserted, scan the bird to verify that it is functioning correctly (Figure 3-10).

RESTRAINT AND HANDLING

Restraint is required for the safety of the patient and the personnel working with the bird. Capturing a bird needs to be done in a room that can be sealed and has no escape route or hiding places for the bird to get to. Close and lock the door and remove any cage accessories. Darkening the room may help reduce the stress of capture. Smaller birds may try to fly around in their cages to avoid capture. A terry cloth towel is often useful when capturing and restraining birds ranging in size from the cockatiels or conures to the largest parrots (Figure 3-11). Place the towel over the patient, gain control of the head, pin the wings to the body, and pick the patient up. Paper towels are sometimes used when restraining budgies, cockatiels, or conures. The bird should be allowed to chew on the towel if it wishes, which keeps its beak busy and makes it less likely for the holder to be bitten. The use of a towel to capture a bird helps keep the birds from developing a fear of hands. The use of gloves is discouraged because this too will create a fear of hands. Gloves also reduce the handler's tactile sensation and ability to feel subtle movements and reactions to the stress of restraint.

> **TECHNICIAN NOTE** A terry cloth towel is used when capturing and restraining birds.

Larger parrots may be caught in the cage, in the carrier, on the floor, or from a table top. Never capture a bird from the owner's shoulder. This is dangerous because the

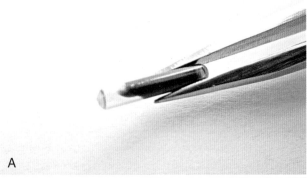

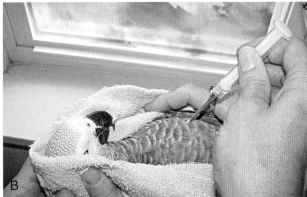

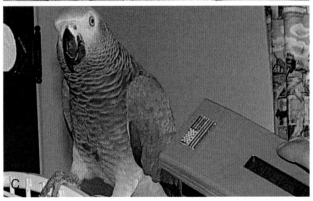

FIGURE 3-10. A, AVID microchip. B, Inserting the microchip into the pectoral muscle of an African grey parrot. C, Avian microchip reader. (Courtesy AVID ID Systems.)

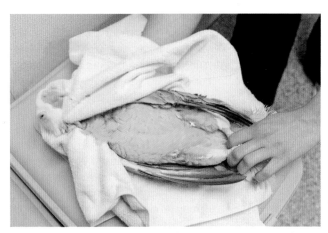

FIGURE 3-11. A towel is often useful in capture and restraint of birds.

bird may bite the owner. As with small birds, a slow and deliberate approach works best. A quiet, soothing tone of voice should be used when approaching the bird. In most cases a towel is used during capture to avoid injury to the bird or technician. Once the bird is captured the towel can be wrapped around the bird to control the wings and the legs. With or without a towel the body of the bird can be tucked under your arm once you have control of the head. This will aid in restraint of the wings. As with all methods of restraint you must monitor carefully for stress, hypoxia, and hyperthermia.

In some practices a restraint board is used for procedures that require the awake (not anesthetized) bird to remain completely still, such as for radiographs or implantation of microchips for identification or in other situations when both hands may be needed to perform complicated tasks (Figure 3-12). However, manual restraint allows for better

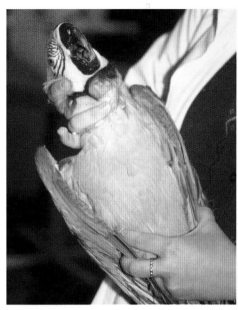

FIGURE 3-13. Securing a psittacine, using an Elizabethan grip. (From Sirois M: *Principles and practice of veterinary technology*, ed 3, St. Louis, Mosby, 2011.)

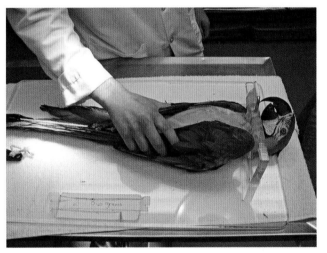

FIGURE 3-12. The avian restraint board is an effective method of restraining a pet bird. (From Mitchell M, Thomas T: *Manual of exotic pet practice*, St. Louis, WB Saunders Company, 2009.)

observation of the bird's condition and a faster reaction time to return the bird to its cage or carrier if the patient is becoming too stressed during restraint. Larger birds can be restrained with an Elizabethan hold. The bird is gripped around the cervical region while extending the neck. This prevents the bird from dropping its head down and biting your fingers. This looks like a chokehold, but it is a great way to restrain macaws or other birds that have fragile facial skin that bruises easily with traditional restraint methods. With the other hand, keep the wings pinned to the sides of the body (Figure 3-13).

Restraint can be a very stressful experience for a bird. It is not unusual for the bird to show signs of extreme distress when released. The bird will typically pant and exhibit open beak breathing, have hot feet, hold its wings away from its body, and fluff the feathers in a manner to allow air to cool the skin. Birds with featherless areas on their faces, such as African greys and macaws, may blush.

CLINICAL PROCEDURES

PHYSICAL EXAMINATION

For pet birds the physical examination begins by obtaining a detailed history (Figure 3-14). Husbandry-related problems are very common findings with the first visit to an avian practitioner. Many medical conditions can be directly related to poor diet and husbandry. Once the history has been completed, the patient should be observed from a distance.

Evaluate the bird's ability to recover from the stress of transport to the clinic. The respiratory rate should be smooth and regular, and a healthy bird should show no signs of increased effort. Observe the bird's perching/walking ability, posture, and feather condition. If the bird is exhibiting a tail bob, forward movement of the head, or open-beak breathing, this could be a sign of respiratory distress and may need immediate attention. Evaluate the mentation and stance. If the bird is trying to sleep, is droopy eyed, wobbling, or barely hanging on to the perch, immediate medical attention may be necessary.

Prior to proceeding to the hands-on examination, evaluate the droppings in the cage. When a bird is stressed or excited, the droppings may be mostly urine. Seedeaters will have drier droppings than those with a diet supplemented with fruits. If the bird is anorexic, the droppings will be fewer in number. Look for blood, parasites, or undigested seeds because these findings may be indicative of disease. The feces may be green or light brown and may vary in consistency between species and diet. The color of the droppings can be affected by the color of the food consumed. The urine should be clear and the urates can appear white to a pale tan (Figure 3-15). Aside from disease considerations, water intake, diet, and the species in question all influence the appearance of droppings. It is important to obtain an accurate weight of the patient. Some birds will sit on the scale while others may require that you place them in box or small cage in order to weigh them (Figure 3-16).

> **TECHNICIAN NOTE** The physical examination includes observation from a distance and may also include a systematic hands-on examination.

Table 3-2 contains some physiologic data for common avian species. The physical examination should proceed systematically. A typical physical examination routine is as follows: Examine the eyes, ears, nares, beak, and oral cavity. Palpate the crop and esophagus, neck, pectoral region, coelom and pelvic region, wings, legs, feet, and back. Evaluate the feather quality and check the preen gland. Auscultate the heart, air sacs, lungs, and sinuses. Examine the cloaca and evert the mucosa to examine for lesions.

Eyes should be clear and bright, bilaterally symmetrical, and free of discharge. Evaluate the eyes with a focal light source and note the patient's pupillary light response.

AVIAN HISTORY FORM

General History

Bird's name _____ Sex: M _____ F _____ UNK _____

How was bird sexed?   Blood test _____   Surgical? _____

Any specific identification? (i.e.: tattoo, band, microchip) _____

If bird is female, has she produced eggs in the past? (if yes, please describe) _____

Bird is a: Pet _____ Breeder _____

How did you acquire the bird?   Store _____ Breeder _____ Other (describe) _____

Date acquired? _____

Do you have any other pets? Y _____ N _____

If yes, please specify, including ages and when acquired _____

Housing

Is this bird kept: Indoors _____ Outdoors _____ Both _____ (if both, please specify % time in each)

_____

Is the bird housed alone? Y _____ N _____ If no, describe _____

If bird is caged, what type of cage? _____

What do use on the bottom of the cage? _____

How often is the cage cleaned? _____

Method/frequency of cleaning food/water dishes _____

Any toys in the cage? Y _____ N _____ If yes, describe _____

Has the bird's environment changed recently? Y _____ N _____ If yes, describe _____

At night, do you cover the bird? Y _____ N _____

How many hours of darkness does the bird have each day? _____

Diet

What foods are offered to your bird/in what total percentages? (i.e.: 50% seed, etc.) _____

What percentages of these foods do you remove from the cage at night? _____

Any supplements offered? Brand name? _____

Any treats offered? Type? How often? _____

Any recent diet changes or new foods? Y _____ N _____ If yes, describe _____

How is water offered? (i.e.: sipper bottle, bowl) _____

Reason for Today's Visit

What signs have you noticed that prompted today's visit? _____

How long have you noticed the problem? _____

Has your bird been sick previously? _____

Has the bird ever been seen by any other veterinarian? Y _____ N _____ If yes, when/why?

_____

Have any tests been performed previously on your bird? Please circle all that apply:

Psittacosis; CBC; Psittacine beak and feather disease; Polyoma disease; Parasites; Other bloodwork;

Other (please describe) _____

Additional comments (your comments regarding the reason for this visit):

FIGURE 3-14. Avian history form filled out by clients annually or as needed. (From Sirois M: *Principles and practice of veterinary technology*, ed 3, St. Louis, Mosby, 2011.)

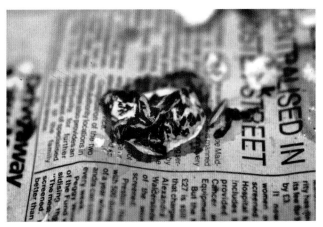

FIGURE 3-15. Normal parrot dropping, showing white urate, dark faecal material and some liquid urine. (From Tully TM, Dorrestein GM, Jones AK: *Handbook of avian medicine*, ed 2, Edinburg, WB Saunders, 2009.)

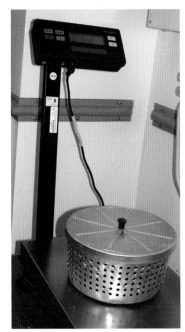

FIGURE 3-16. Weighing the patient is a vital part of monitoring health status. The scale should be able to read to ±1 gram. (From Sirois M: *Principles and practice of veterinary technology*, ed 3, St. Louis, Mosby, 2011.)

Periophthalmic swelling or conjunctivitis can be indicative of ocular or sinus abnormalities. The ears are located on the sides of the head, behind and slightly below its eyes, and appear as a hole in the head (Figure 3-17). Note the presence of any debris.

The head should be examined for symmetry, feather condition, swellings, and any evidence of trauma. Nares should be smooth, evenly colored, and symmetric. Birds have a keratinized plate inside the nostril called an operculum. The beak should be smooth and shiny and free of dry, flaky regions. In some species such as cockatoos a fine powder layer on the beak is a normal finding and if absent this may be a sign of disease. *Knemidokoptes* spp. infections are presented as proliferate growths on the beak and feet (Figure 3-18). In any species a beak that is malformed, growing excessively, or is in poor condition may be signs of disease and require additional testing. Healthy birds should not need regular beak trimmings.

With the bird in an upright position expose the oral cavity by using gauze or tape strips to gently fatigue the powerful muscles controlling the beak (Figure 3-19). In smaller birds, a hemostat or paper clips or small tape strips can be used for this purpose. Observe the color, texture,

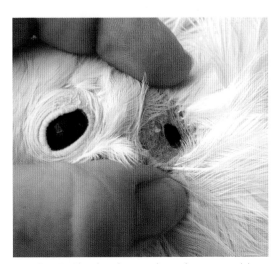

FIGURE 3-17. The short horizontal canal is protected by contour feathers that can be gently swept forward to expose the ear for examination. (From Sirois M: *Principles and practice of veterinary technology*, ed 3, St. Louis, Mosby, 2011.)

TABLE 3-2	Physiologic Data for Common Avian Species				
BIRD	**AVG WT**	**HEART RATE bpm**	**RESP RATE bpm**	**SEXUAL MATURITY**	**AVG CAPTIVE LIFE SPAN**
Budgerigars	30 g	500-600	60-70	6 months	6 years
Lovebirds	38-56 g	400-600	60-80	8-12 months	4 years
Cockatiels	75-125 g	400-500	40-50	6-12 months	6 years
Conures	80-100 g	500-600	60-70	1-3 years	10 years
Lories	100-300 g	300-500	35-50	2-3 years	3 years
Cockatoos	300-1100 g	150-350	20-30	1-6 years (species dependent)	15 years
Eclectus parrots	380-450 g	160-300	20-30	3-6 years	8 years
Amazon parrots	350-1000 g	160-300	20-30	4-6 years	15 years
Macaws	200-1500 g	120-300	15-32	4-7 years (species dependent)	15 years
African greys	400-550 g	200-350	25-30	4-6 years	15 years

(From Sirois M: *Principles and practice of veterinary technology*, ed 3, St. Louis, Mosby, 2011.)

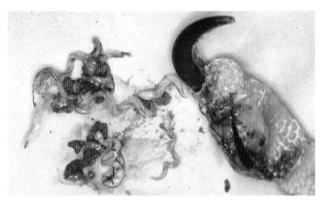

FIGURE 3-18. Cockatiel with *Knemidokoptes pili* mite infestation, known as the scaly leg and face mite (side view). (From Hnilica, KA: *Small animal dermatology: a color atlas and therapeutic guide*, ed 3, St. Louis, Elsevier, 2011.)

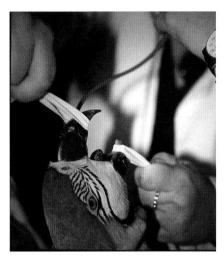

FIGURE 3-19. Oral examination method. (From Sirois M: *Principles and practice of veterinary technology*, ed 3, St. Louis, Mosby, 2011.)

and moisture in the oral cavity. Evaluate for the presence of swelling, ulceration, erosions, or plaques. Closely examine the choanal slit and its papillae. The papillae should be sharp. If they are absent or blunted, this could be a sign of disease and will require a further workup. Assess the hydration status while looking in the mouth. In a dehydrated patient, the eyes may appear dull, dry, and sunken and the skin around them may appear withered and wrinkled. Skin around the eye and covering the keel, when moved to the side, will be slow to shift back into position. The oral and cloacal mucosa will also be tacky or dry in appearance in a dehydrated bird.

Palpate all areas of the bird for masses and swellings, evidence of trauma or self-mutilation, or any other abnormalities. Use a transilluminator to shine through the crop and evaluate the general thickness of the mucosa. Evaluate the air sacs for air sac mites (in passerines). Palpate the pectoral mass. The pectoral muscles should be solid, well formed, and rounded. The ratio of muscle mass to sternum is measured on a scale from 1 (very thin) to 9 (obese). The pectoral muscles should be checked for evidence of a microchip.

Evaluation of the abdomen is very limited or impossible in small birds. In larger birds, abdominal palpation is used to detect organs that feel hard or unusually shaped. The abdomen or coelom should be concave or flat. In all birds, the vent should be clean and covered by dry feathers. Palpate the pelvic region and extremities for symmetry and masses.

Both wings should be gently examined, with care taken to curve the wing in the direction of the body at all times. Some birds are very sensitive and struggle when their wings are manipulated. If a stressed bird is struggling too much, release the wing and start again when the struggling ceases.

Examine skin and feather quality. The delicate skin is usually white and underlying structures, such as muscle or blood vessels, are somewhat visible. Birds are prone to pressure sores, calluses, and secondary infections on their feet and legs. These most commonly occur on the interdigital pad or the plantar surface of the intertarsal joint. Walking or perching on rough or hard substrates, obesity, restricted exercise, and diets low in vitamin A are predisposing factors. Evaluate the feet and legs for any lesions or masses and **pododermatitis** (Figure 3-20).

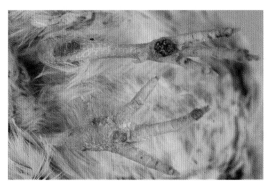

FIGURE 3-20. Pododermatitis. (From Tully TM, Dorrestein GM, Jones AK: *Handbook of avain medicine*, ed 2, Edinburg, Saunders, 2009.)

The feathers should be clean, symmetric, smooth, and structurally sound. Evidence of blood feathers (i.e., growing feathers) should be noted. The presence of the powder down, which is produced by cockatoos, cockatiels, and African greys, should be evaluated. The nails and skin on the legs should be inspected for condition and any abnormal growth. Feather condition is a good indicator of overall health. Stress bars are sometimes found, and these represent a period of malnutrition or stress while the feathers were being developed. These bars are symmetrical and segmental malformations in the barbs and barbules (Figure 3-21).

Examine the uropygial gland. It should be smooth and evenly colored and excrete a creamy material.

To auscultate the avian patient best, use a pediatric or neonatal stethoscope. Auscultate the heart from the ventral midline along the keel. Heart rates vary with excitation and species but range from 100 to 600 bpm. Auscultate dorsal midline between the shoulder blades to evaluate the lungs, which are located dorsal near the spine in the coelomic cavity. If the heart cannot be auscultated in the region, this may be a sign of lung pathology. Listen to the top of the bird's

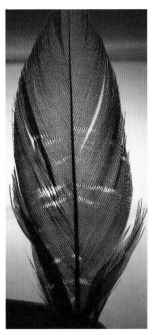

FIGURE 3-21. Stress bars and feather discolorations are signs of potential stressors during feather development, such as malnutrition. Stress bars are normally perpendicular to the feather shaft. (From Sirois M: *Principles and practice of veterinary technology*, ed 3, St. Louis, Mosby, 2011.)

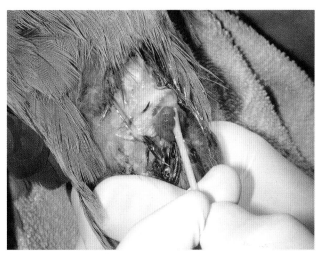

FIGURE 3-22. Everting the cloaca with a cotton-tipped applicator. (From Sirois M: *Principles and practice of veterinary technology*, ed 3, St. Louis, Mosby, 2011.)

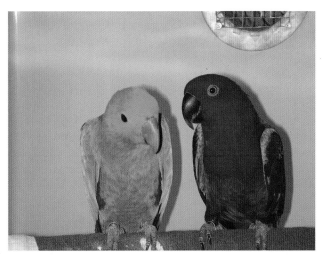

FIGURE 3-23. Eclectus parrots are sexually dimorphic. The male is green and the female is red. (From Sirois M: *Principles and practice of veterinary technology*, ed 3, St. Louis, Mosby, 2011.)

head. Any sound evident with auscultation of the head can be an indicator of possible sinus problems.

Examine the cloaca for any lesions or masses. Tissue should not protrude from the cloaca. The tissue in this area may be distended if the bird is developing an egg, is constipated, or has a cloacal mass.

In order to examine the cloacal mucosa properly it must be everted. To evert the cloaca, place the bird in dorsal recumbency and gently insert a slightly moistened cotton-tipped applicator into the cloaca. Slowly remove the applicator, angling the tip ventrally and everting a small sampling of mucosa for examination (Figure 3-22). Do this procedure in all four quadrants of the cloaca as if you were looking at a clock: 12 o'clock, 3 o'clock, 6 o'clock and 9 o'clock. Examine the cloacal tissue closely for evidence of papillomatous growths. Applying 5% acetic acid (apple cider vinegar) will cause papillomas to blanche. This is not definitive because other abnormalities can blanche as well. The only way to truly diagnose papillomatosis is by tissue biopsy.

DETERMINING GENDER

In some species of birds, the species are **sexually dimorphic**, meaning the male and female differ in appearance (Figure 3-23). However, for the majority of species of pet birds, the males and females look identical. The gender of a bird can be determined by endoscopy; however, DNA sexing is a safer alternative to the surgical approach and is available through some labs around the country. With a very small amount of whole blood, the gender of a bird can be determined in a few days. DNA sexing uses the polymerase chain reaction (PCR) to analyze the DNA from the sex chromosomes of the bird.

GROOMING

Beak, nail, and wing trimming are common procedures performed on pet birds. Healthy birds should not need regular beak trimming. Overgrowth of the beak may result from malocclusion resulting in insufficient wear on the beak. Patients presented for overgrowth of the beak should be evaluated to determine the cause.

> **TECHNICIAN NOTE** Beak, nail, and wing trimming are common procedures performed on pet birds.

Reducing the length and grooming the beak can be done with a Dremel Motor Tool (Dremel, Inc., Racine, Wisconsin). Cone-shaped aluminum oxide grinding stones work well on beaks. To prevent the spread of disease, it is best to have a separate grinding stone per patient, which the owner can bring to each visit. To perform this procedure the restrainer holds the bird in an upright position. The person performing the trim holds the beak closed with one hand and applies the Dremel with the other. Care should be taken not to cover the nares as you hold the beak shut (Figure 3-24). Monitor the patient closely for hypoxia and hyperthermia. Once you have achieved the desired length or shape, a small amount of mineral oil can be applied to remove the dust and make the beak aesthetically pleasing.

Trimming a bird's wings is one method to decrease the bird's ability to fly. This is done by selectively trimming some of the primary and secondary feathers. The flight feathers are numbered from the inside out, 1 through 10. There is a natural break in the direction of the feathers with the feathers of the manus (primaries—P-1 to P-10) angled out, and the feathers on the brachium and antibrachium (secondaries—S-1 to S-10) angled in. Instruments used to perform a wing trimming are varied and include suture scissors, cat nail trimmers, wire cutters, and sharp-sharp scissors. Prevent the spread of disease by sterilizing the trimmers between each bird.

It is very important to discuss with the client to determine how much flight is needed and how aesthetically pleasing they want it. A nice, aesthetically pleasing trim leaves the distal two primary feathers and trims only four to eight feathers on each wing. The recommendation is to trim both wings evenly for balance. The general rule of wing trim is that the heavier bodied a bird is, the fewer feathers are removed.

The trim is done up high under the coverts, so that the jagged edges of the cut feathers are not showing (Figure 3-25). Evaluate the feather to be trimmed and ensure that it is not a blood feather. These should be avoided, and if one is located the mature feather on either side should be left as support. Flying ability should be tested in the clinic prior to the bird being sent home. Flight distance should be limited to less than 25 feet, and lift to under 2 feet. Additional feathers can be trimmed after a flight test if necessary.

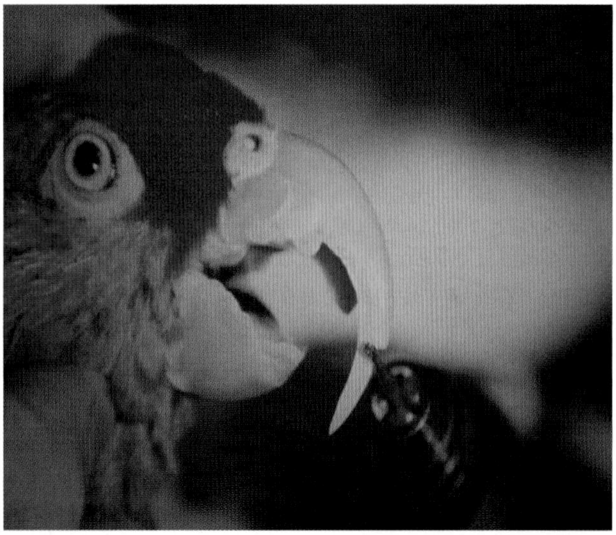

Nail trimming is an important preventive care procedure. Excessive nail length can result in improper perching and the nail could be traumatically avulsed. An overgrown nail could get caught in the grate commonly found in the bottom of most birdcages or on the carpet as the bird wanders around the house. Untrimmed nails can grow into the pad of the foot causing cellulitis or abscess formation. The size and temperament of the bird determines the number of people required to perform the trim. Towel restraint is commonly used.

Birds with light-colored nails have easily visible blood vessels, improving the chances of a nail trim without any bleeding. In birds with black nails, an understanding of the structure of the nail is important. However, even with extreme care it is not unusual to cut the quick of at least one nail, causing bleeding. Owners should be warned that this might happen. Any blood loss in birds should be considered serious. In very small birds, loss of what appears to be a minute amount of blood is potentially fatal. When bleeding is noticed, a hemostatic powder must be pressed immediately onto the nail.

The most common tools used for nail trims include Resco trimmers, the Dremel (motorized) tool, files, nail scissors, fingernail trimmers, and cautery instruments. These should be disinfected or sterilized after using to help prevent the spread of disease between birds (Figure 3-26). The Dremel tool, typically used on large birds, uses a grinding tip to blunt the tips of the nails. This hand-held motorized tool is noisy and can overheat nail tissues if applied too long. Flat or rounded fine-tooth files are preferred by some for nail trims of birds of any size. This method slowly blunts the nail tips, causing some birds to become impatient and struggle. Clients can be trained to do this at home if both pet and owner are willing. Some veterinarians use electrocautery instruments to trim nails and prevent bleeding at the same time. Many birds exhibit pain reactions, presumably related to the high heat of the instrument. This method of nail trimming should be done primarily on anesthetized animals.

FIGURE 3-24. Trimming a beak with the Dremel. (From Sirois M: *Principles and practice of veterinary technology*, ed 3, St. Louis, Mosby, 2011.)

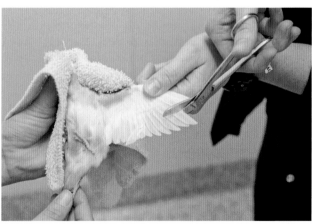

FIGURE 3-25. Wing trim procedure.

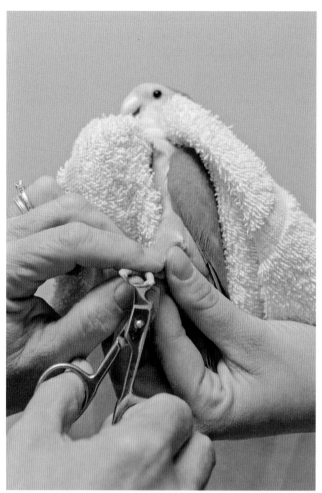

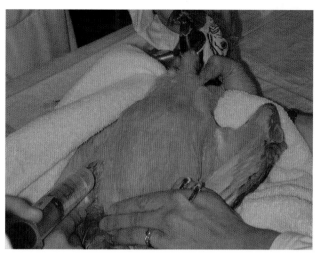

FIGURE 3-27. A blue and gold macaw is receiving a dose of subcutaneous fluids in the right inguinal region. (From Sirois M: *Principles and practice of veterinary technology*, ed 3, St. Louis, Mosby, 2011.)

FIGURE 3-26. Grasp one toe at a time, keeping the other toes safely away from the trimmer so that the other toes or toenails will not be cut by mistake.

INJECTIONS AND BLOOD COLLECTION
Subcutaneous Injection

Subcutaneous sites are found in the inguinal, axillary, and dorsal regions. The inguinal region is the preferred site to administer subcutaneous fluids and medications (Figure 3-27). With the patient restrained in dorsal recumbency, pull the legs straight down and apply a small amount of alcohol to the medial side of the most proximal portion of the leg, parting the feathers. Using a small-gauge needle, preferably 23-26 gauge, insert the needle just under the skin. Administer 5 to 10 mL/kg/site. Use only isotonic fluids that have been warmed to body temperature. Similar administration techniques are used for the axillary and dorsal regions; however, you cannot get as much fluid into these areas.

> *TECHNICIAN NOTE* The inguinal region is the preferred site to administer subcutaneous fluids and medications.

Intramuscular Injections

For intramuscular injections the pectoral muscles are most commonly used. These represent the largest muscle mass on

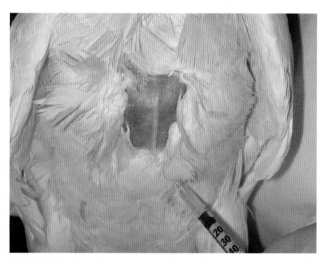

FIGURE 3-28. The pectoral muscles are the optimal injection site for IM injections in birds. (From Sirois M: *Principles and practice of veterinary technology*, ed 3, St. Louis, Mosby, 2011.)

the bird and are found on both sides of the keel (Figure 3-28). Always use a small-gauge needle (26-25 gauge) to reduce the amount of muscle damage and don't use the same area of muscle every time. Palpate the keel and don't mistake the crop or abdominal region for the pectoral muscles. Have the patient in an upright position, then wet the feathers slightly so you can visualize the skin. A maximum of 0.2 to 0.3 mL can be administered in one site for a large bird. If you need to administer a large volume via this route, use multiple sites and alternate these sites each treatment time to decrease the chances of muscle necrosis. Birds have a renal portal system, so drugs administered in the caudal third of the body may go through the kidneys before reaching the rest of the body. Keep this in mind when administering potentially nephrotoxic drugs.

Intravenous Catheter Placement

Intravenous (IV) catheters are normally placed for anesthetic procedures but not routinely for daily venous access. In the anesthetized patient IV catheters are fairly easy to secure with tissue glue or suture, but once the patient is recovered, it is very difficult to maintain a patent catheter. The avian patient is apt to chew out the IV catheter within seconds of placing the patient back into its cage. If the patient is extremely debilitated, it is possible to secure the catheter well enough for a few days. Aseptic catheter care must be performed on a daily basis with all catheters placed for long-term medication administration.

Intraosseous Catheter Placement

Intraosseous catheters (IO) can be used in the same manner as an IV catheter to administer CRI fluid therapy, blood, antibiotics, and other medications. IO catheters can be placed in any bone that has a marrow cavity such as the distal ulna and proximal tibia. Pneumatic bones such as the humerus and femur cannot be used, since these communicate with the respiratory system. The distal ulna is fairly well tolerated and easier to maintain in debilitated birds, more so than the proximal tibia. Depending on the size of the patient, 20- to 22-gauge spinal needles are used. These are good to use due to the stylet feature preventing the cortex from occluding the cannula during placement. In small birds such as cockatiels and conures, a 25-gauge needle can be placed in the distal ulna. To place a cannula in the distal ulna the patient will need to be anesthetized and sterile technique utilized (Procedure 3-1).

Blood Collection

Obtaining blood from a severely trimmed toenail is not acceptable. This is painful, stressful, and can yield abnormal cell distributions and cellular artifacts. A venous blood sample should be obtained. The medial metatarsal vein or leg vein is the vessel of choice for collecting blood in medium to large birds (Figure 3-29). The medial metatarsal vein is located on the medial side of the distal tibotarsus at the tibiotarsal-tarsometatarsal joint. This is an excellent venipuncture sight because it is a very stable vessel with little to no mobility, which helps reduce the risk of hematoma formations. Grasp the leg and syringe in one hand while collecting the sample; this will give you more control if the patient moves. Hemostasis can be achieved by bandaging. For best results a tuberculin syringe with a 26-25–gauge needle should be used.

The jugular vein is the method of choice for small birds such as budgies and lovebirds because the other vessels are usually too small. Birds do have two jugular veins; however, the right jugular is more prominent than the left. Usually a 1-ml tuberculin syringe with 26-25–gauge needle is used for the small birds and a 3-ml syringe equipped with a 25-gauge needle can be used in larger birds. The restrainer should hold the bird in left lateral recumbency. The phlebotomist should arch and extend the neck and lightly wet and part the feathers with alcohol and find the featherless

track and the jugular. Once the sample is collected, digital pressure must be applied by the restrainer to prevent large hematomas.

> **TECHNICIAN NOTE** The medial metatarsal vein or leg vein is the vessel of choice for collecting blood in medium to large birds.

The ulnar or basilic vein, also referred to as the wing vein, is an easily accessible vessel for venipuncture. Due to the severity of the complications that can occur, it is recommended to only attempt this on anesthetized patients. Patients that are not anesthetized have an increased chance of forming a large hematoma and/or fracturing the wing. This vein is located on the medial surface of the wing and runs across the radius and ulna. Place the patient in dorsal recumbency; lightly wet the feathers at the distal end of the humerus. Due to its location it is difficult to bandage this area for hemostasis, thus requiring that the bird be restrained until the bleeding has stopped. It can take 3 to 5 minutes or more to control the bleeding. This is, however, an excellent site to place IV catheters during anesthesia.

Once you have obtained your blood sample, the needle must be removed from the syringe prior to dispensing the blood into the appropriate tube for sampling. Cell lysis can occur if the blood is dispensed through the needle into the collection tube. Using blood collection tubes such as Microtainer® that are specially designed for small samples helps eliminate any anticoagulant dilution problems. The sample for CBC analysis should be collected in EDTA because heparin will cause clumping and staining artifacts. A blood film should be made if the blood is going to stay in the EDTA for any length of time. EDTA exposure may cause increased disruption of cells in the blood film. Biochemistries can be run on plasma in most laboratories. A larger plasma yield can be achieved by using a Microtainer containing lithium heparin.

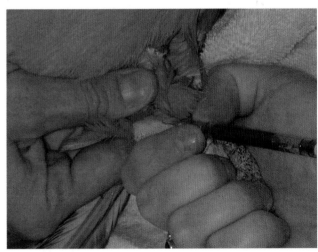

FIGURE 3-29. Venipuncture of the medial metatarsal vein. (From Sirois M: *Principles and practice of veterinary technology,* ed 3, St. Louis, Mosby, 2011.)

PROCEDURE 3-1   Intraosseous Catheter Placement

- Pluck a few feathers over the dorsal, distal ulna, and surgically prep the area (Figure 1).

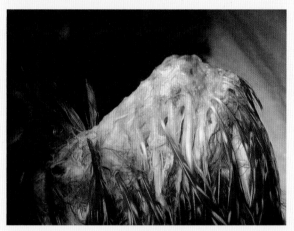

FIGURE 1

- Grasp the ulna with one hand and insert the cannula with the other.
- Palpate the dorsal condyle of the distal ulna, and insert the cannula just above this condyle (Figure 2).

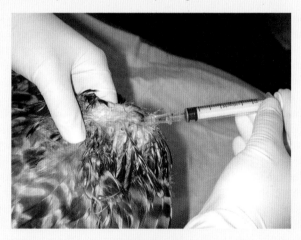

FIGURE 2

- Advance the cannula into the medullary cavity by applying steady firm pressure, with a slight rotating motion, on the cannula as it is positioned in a straight line with the ulna aiming toward the elbow.
- Once the cannula is in place, remove the stylette (Figure 3).

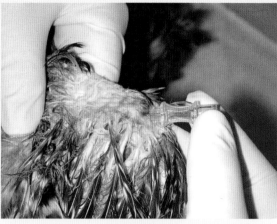

FIGURE 3

- Cap off the cannula with a sterile infusion plug.
- Flush with heparinized saline, and you will notice little to no resistance.
- As you flush the catheter, inspect the ulnar vein; it should be clear, demonstrating that you are in the correct location.
- The cannula should now be sutured into place (Figure 4).

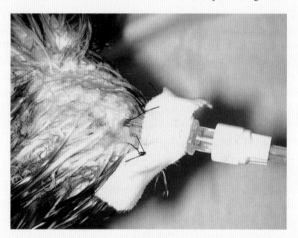

FIGURE 4

- The wing should be wrapped with a figure-eight bandage to secure the wing and keep the insertion site clean (Figure 5).

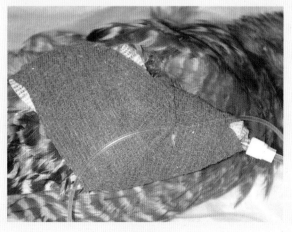

FIGURE 5

(From Sirois M: *Principles and practice of veterinary technology*, ed 3, St. Louis, Mosby, 2011.)

Blood Volume. Birds come in a wide range of sizes and therefore a wide range of blood volumes. Calculate how much blood can be safely taken from your patient. Blood volume in birds ranges from 6% to 12% of body weight, depending on the species of bird. It is safe to approximate a bird's blood volume to be 10% of the body weight measured in grams. Of the bird's total blood volume, you can safely take 10% for diagnostic sampling. Therefore, it is generally safe to take approximately 1% of the bird's body weight in grams in healthy birds and 0.5% in sick birds.

AIR SAC CANNULA PLACEMENT

Patients with tracheal or syringeal obstruction may require placement of an air sac cannula (Figure 3-30). The air sac cannula bypasses the obstructed upper airway and enters into the airway via the caudal thoracic or abdominal air sac. The patient should be anesthetized and placed in right lateral recumbency to utilize the left abdominal or caudal thoracic air sacs. The feathers are removed from the region of the last rib and caudal to the last rib. The insertion site is aseptically prepared, and a small incision made caudal to the last rib in the flank region. The muscle is bluntly dissected with a hemostat. The cannula is then inserted into the opening. Proper placement is verified by listening for air flow from the cannula or holding a feather over the opening. The cannula is secured to the body with tape that is sutured to the skin. An endotracheal adapter is placed over the end of the tube and covered with a piece material from a surgery mask. This will prevent debris from entering the air sac. A light bandage can be placed over the insertion site. The filter is changed daily and the insertion site cleaned. Any mucus that accumulates around the distal end of the tube must be removed.

ORAL MEDICATION

Medication and fluids may be administered to birds orally if the patient is alert and active. Primary regurgitation or vomiting, poor patient reflexes or recumbency, and oral and upper gastrointestinal trauma may exclude this method. This route of administering medication is practically stress free if the patient is tolerant. Some birds will love the attention of being hand fed and given medications. Medications mixed in mashed banana or fruit baby foods are often well accepted. Medication of the feed and water is unreliable for the majority of the patients in practice. However, this is the primary method of administering drugs to poultry and others in large flock situations.

Gavage Feeding

Fluid therapy, nutritional support, and medication administration can be provided by gavage or tube feeding. Limiting factors may include patients with crops stasis, ileus, gastrointestinal impactions, or other gastrointestinal abnormalities that reduce motility or absorption. A variety of flexible and rigid feeding needles and tubes are available (Figure 3-31).

> **TECHNICIAN NOTE** Fluid therapy, nutritional support, and medication administration can be provided by gavage or tube feeding.

Gavage feeding will require multiple people to complete in larger birds, but with the smaller birds a skilled person can usually do it alone (Figure 3-32). In larger birds one person holds the patient in an upright position, another opens the mouth, and another person advances the tube into place and administers the medications and food. In some instances this can be done with two people by scissoring the beak or putting the upper beak into the lower. These alternate methods are dangerous because the patient can bite the tube and potentially ingest it. To place the tube enter the oral cavity from the patient's right commissure of the mouth, and pass the tube/needle along the right side of the tongue, avoiding the glottis and advancing into the esophagus. Palpate the tube in the crop or visualize the glottis prior to administering any food or medications, ensuring that you did not place the tube in the trachea. While administering the medications or food, watch the back of the mouth. If food or liquid material appears in the oral cavity, the bird should be immediately

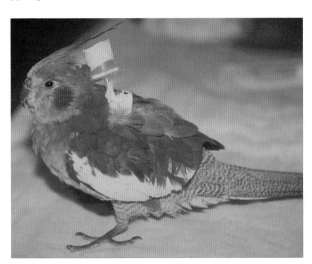

FIGURE 3-30. Cockatiel with air sac cannula. (From Sirois M: *Principles and practice of veterinary technology*, ed 3, St. Louis, Mosby, 2011.)

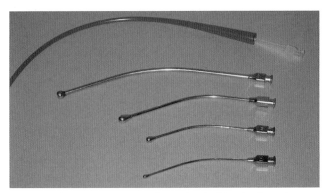

FIGURE 3-31. Gavage needles and red rubber feeding tubes can be used to provide fluid nutritional support and medications to hospitalized birds. (From Sirois M: *Principles and practice of veterinary technology*, ed 3, St. Louis, Mosby, 2011.)

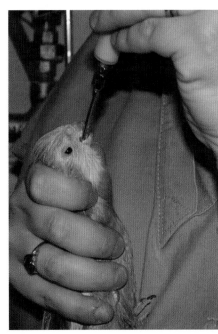

FIGURE 3-32. This experienced technician is able to gavage feed this cockatiel alone, which is the standard accepted method. (From Sirois M: *Principles and practice of veterinary technology*, ed 3, St. Louis, Mosby, 2011.)

placed back into its enclosure without further handling to prevent the risk of regurgitation and potential aspiration.

SURGERY AND ANESTHESIA
Anesthesia
Birds require anesthesia for some diagnostic procedures, such as radiographs, in addition to major surgical procedures. Avian patients must be closely monitored at all times. Most models of anesthesia machines are adequate for anesthetizing the avian patient. Requirements include an out-of-circuit vaporizer for administering Isoflurane or Sevoflurane in oxygen and a nonrebreathing circuit. Nonrebreathing circuits such as Magill, Ayre's T-piece, Mapleson systems, Jackson-Rees, Norman mask elbow, and Bain circuits are adequate for companion bird anesthesia. Sevoflurane produces a faster induction and recovery than Isoflurane and may be a safer choice for high-risk patients.

In preparation for anesthesia the crop should be empty. Birds have a high metabolic rate and poor hepatic glycogen storage and it has been recommended that birds be fasted no more than 2 to 3 hours, depending on the size and condition of the patient. Regurgitation can occur if the patient is not properly fasted. Fasting will help decrease the probability of aspiration of crop contents. In emergency situations, when there is no time for fasting, you can aspirate the crop contents and intubate to reduce the possibility of aspiration.

Preanesthetics, Analgesia, and Sedation
Routine administration of parasympatholytic agents such as atropine and glycopyrolate is usually contraindicated. These drugs tend to thicken the salivary, tracheal, and bronchial secretions creating a greater risk for airway obstructions during anesthesia. Benzodiazepines such as diazepam and midazolam will reduce anxiety but have no analgesic properties. Butorphenol is a useful analgesic in birds.

IV catheter placement and fluid therapy are essential for any lengthy procedure. A fluid rate of 10ml/kg is normally used, administered by continuous rate infusion with a syringe pump. During anesthesia two sites are optimal for placing an IV catheter: the wing (cutaneous ulnar vein) and the leg (medial metatarsal). These catheters can be secured with tissue glue, tape, or suture.

Induction. Most patients can be restrained and masked with gas anesthetics. In some cases the patient may need to be induced in a chamber (Figure 3-33). This type of induction prevents monitoring the heart rate of the patient, there is a risk the patient can be injured if the chamber is not padded adequately, and high concentrations of gas anesthetic are released into the clinic environment when the patient is removed from the chamber. When using a chamber for induction, cover the chamber to create a calming effect. Leave a small opening for monitoring the patient. The anesthetic vaporizer is usually set at 3% to 4% initially and oxygen flow rate of 4-5 liters/min. Once the patient begins to show evidence of anesthesia, such as droopy wings, eyes closing, loss of equilibrium, the vaporizer setting is reduced to 2% to 3%. When the patient is sedate, remove the patient from the chamber and continue the induction with a mask. If the patient shows any signs of respiratory distress during chamber induction, remove the patient from the chamber immediately and place an oxygen mask over the beak and nares. Place the mask over the beak and nares, or with smaller birds, place the entire head inside of the mask (Figure 3-34). A slow induction is the safest, starting with a low percentage of the anesthetic and working up until the desired depth of anesthesia is reached. Monitor the heart rate with a stethoscope and watch the respiration rate and depth during the entire induction; bradycardia and apnea are common if induction

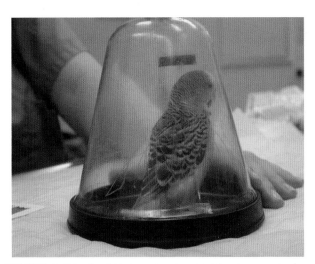

FIGURE 3-33. Small birds can be placed inside a large canine face mask for a chamber induction. The only disadvantage to this induction method is the lack of cardiac monitoring. (From Sirois M: *Principles and practice of veterinary technology*, ed 3, St. Louis, Mosby, 2011.)

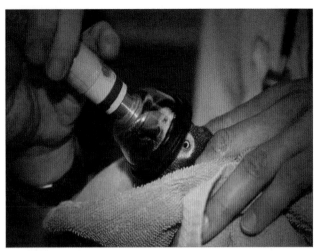

FIGURE 3-34. During a mask induction the patient should be held in an upright position, the masked placed over the nares and entire beak. (From Sirois M: *Principles and practice of veterinary technology*, ed 3, St. Louis, Mosby, 2011.)

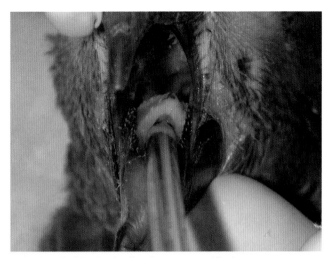

FIGURE 3-35. Tracheal intubation is not difficult in most companion birds, but tracheal trauma is easy to cause and cuffed endotracheal tubes should not be used. (From Sirois M: *Principles and practice of veterinary technology*, ed 3, St. Louis, Mosby, 2011.)

is too quick. The eyes will close, the wings will drop, and the legs will become more relaxed when the patient is feeling the effects of the anesthetic and is ready to be intubated. If bradycardia or apnea occurs, shut off the gas anesthetic immediately and administer straight oxygen until the patient's vital signs stabilize.

> **TECHNICIAN NOTE** Most patients can be restrained and anesthetized by mask induction or an anesthetic chamber can be used.

Intubation. Intubation should always be done with long procedures and high-risk patients to allow mechanical ventilation for birds that do not breathe adequately on their own when anesthetized. Birds have complete cartilaginous tracheal rings so tracheal necrosis can occur if the cuffs on cuffed endotracheal tubes are inflated; thus cuffed endotracheal tubes should not be used. Once the patient is relaxed from mask induction, with reduced jaw, wing, and leg tone, the patient can be intubated. Open the beak and either gently pull the tongue out with a pair of hemostats or place a laryngoscope blade on the tip of the tongue. This will expose the glottal opening. Gently place the noncuffed endotracheal tube lubed with sterile KY jelly into the opening (Figure 3-35). When the tube is in the trachea, secure it by taping once around the tube and then tape the tube to the lower beak. This allows easy access to the mouth for placement of monitoring equipment and removing any regurgitate. If the patient presents with a tracheal obstruction and an air sac cannula is placed, anesthesia can be administered via the cannula in the same manner as through the trachea.

> **TECHNICIAN NOTE** Always use uncuffed endotracheal tubes for avian patients.

Oxygen Flow Rate and Ventilation

Safe oxygen flow rates can range from 500 ml/min to 1 L/min; flow rates more than 1 L/min can damage the tracheal mucosa. Normal respirations should be slow, deep, and regular, approximately 10 to 40 breaths/min, depending on the size of the patient. Regardless of how the patient is ventilating or the length of the procedure, monitoring the patient's respiratory rate and effort is vital. When small endotracheal tubes are used, there is a chance that the mucoid secretions may thicken and consolidate inside the tube and block the airway.

Applying pressure to the bag in the anesthetic circuit and gently forcing air into the patient produces manual ventilation. Watch the patient's keel expansion to ensure that the pressure applied is not excessive. Air sacs can be ruptured if the respirations are too aggressive. The amount of pressure applied to the system should range between 5 to 8 cm H_2O. The rate can range between 8 to 20 breaths per minute. A positive pressure ventilator can also be used.

Manual ventilation, high oxygen flow rates, and high-pressure ventilation can cause tracheal mucosal damage if improperly used. Protect the trachea by keeping it moist. Humid Vents® can be placed between the endotracheal tube and the breathing circuit during the procedure. This device retains moisture in the hopes that the trachea will remain moist and prevents damage.

Body Temperature. Loss of body heat during anesthesia can delay recovery. Normal body temperature for birds ranges from 105 to 112° F. It is not unusual for the core temperature to drop dramatically during surgical procedures, especially when feathers have been plucked and alcohol used in preparation for surgery. An esophageal temperature probe placed as far as the proventriculus is usually needed for monitoring core body temperature; the crop and cloaca will not be representative of the patient's core body temperature but will provide evidence of trends. A forced-air heating blanket can be used to provide supplemental heat (Figure 3-36).

Recovery. During recovery, some birds will regain consciousness, vocalize and try to bite, then fall back into a stupor, and become apneic and bradycardic. Once the bird is extubated, supplemental oxygen can be provided by face mask for a few more minutes and monitoring of heart rate and respiratory must continue until the patient is able to ambulate in the cage. Continue to monitor the patient for at least ½ hour after any anesthetic procedure, from outside of the recovery cage.

Avian Surgical Techniques. Birds are challenging surgical patients. Anesthesia can be complex. The physical characteristics of birds make hypothermia, hypoglycemia, and blood loss significant factors. Surgeries are carefully planned to minimize time under anesthesia and complications. A thorough physical examination should be done on birds prior to anesthesia, including a fecal exam, a CBC, radiographs, and blood chemistries. Birds that are extremely ill or in poor physical condition may have elective surgery delayed until they can be treated medically.

Surgical Site Preparation and Drapes. The first step in preparation of the surgical site is the plucking of feathers to provide 2 to 4 cm of bare space surrounding the proposed incision. Once the bird is anesthetized, feathers are pulled individually in the direction of growth. If possible, removal of flight feathers is avoided. There is the possibility of damage to the feather follicle, resulting in growth of deformed or misdirected feathers. Once anesthetized, the patient will need to be positioned and prepared for surgery. The patient can be secured with masking tape on a plastic board or acrylic heating pad. Masking tape or painter's tape works very well for positioning birds because the adhesive is not too sticky but strong enough to hold the bird or feathers in position. Regular white porous or other tape can damage or remove more feathers than necessary or leave a residue.

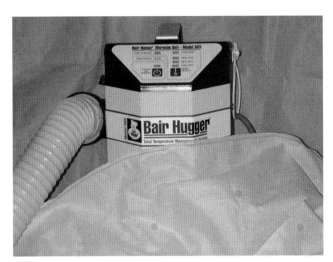

FIGURE 3-36. Forced air heating blankets are used to provide supplemental heat to the anesthetized patient. (From Sirois M: *Principles and practice of veterinary technology*, ed 3, St. Louis, Mosby, 2011.)

Any feathers adjoining the surgical site are held away from the incision site with masking tape or sterile, water-soluble lubricating gels. The surgical site is aseptically prepared. Alcohol is avoided because use may cause hypothermia to develop as it evaporates from the skin. Transparent adhesive disposable surgical drapes are often used in birds. They adhere directly to the prepped skin and the incision is made through the plastic drape material. The drape must be removed carefully to minimize trauma to the bird's skin.

Suture material in avian surgery needs to be minimally reactive and of a smaller size, 4-0, 5-0, and 6-0. Monofilament suture material is often preferred and has the advantage of minimizing trauma and cutting of tissue when compared to multifilament material. Taper-point needles are less traumatic than cutting needles since avian skin is thin and very friable. Cutting needles can be used for tougher skin such as the skin found on the feet of larger birds.

DIAGNOSTIC IMAGING
Radiographs
Most companion psittacine birds will require anesthesia or heavy sedation for diagnostic radiographs. Digital radiology is quickly becoming the standard in most clinics and will yield the best results. If digital radiology is not available, high-detail, rare earth cassettes with single-emulsion film provides the desired results. Mammography film will produce even better detail but does require a higher KVP and ma. A technique can be extrapolated from the tabletop technique used on small animal patients. For extremely small patients, a dental radiography unit can be used.

> **TECHNICIAN NOTE** Most companion psittacine birds will require anesthesia or heavy sedation for diagnostic radiographs.

The standard whole body views are a ventrodorsal (VD) and a right lateral. Plexiglas restraint boards can be used to aid in patient positioning. For the VD place the bird on its back, legs stretched down to expose the coelomic cavity, wings stretched out symmetrically to the sides, and place two pieces of masking tape or paper tape in the form of an X across each carpus. Palpate the keel to ensure it is in line with the backbone. If the patient is not positioned correctly, tissues and organs can be superimposed on the radiograph.

For the lateral view, the patient is placed in right lateral recumbency, legs stretched downward, and wings pulled back together. Paper or masking tape is placed across the carpus to keep the wings back and tape or gauze is used to keep the legs stretched downward. Once the plain films are reviewed, it may be necessary to isolate limbs for an individual view, perform a contrast study of the gastrointestinal system, or perform an ultrasound.

The VD and lateral views reveal the same lateral view of the wing. When two views of the wing are necessary, a caudocranial (CdCr) view needs to be obtained. The CdCr can be obtained by placing the bird in a downward position at a right angle to the table with its head on the plate and body up in the air. Extend the wing out as close to the plate as possible and collimate to the desired area (Figure 3-37).

The critically ill bird or one in respiratory distress may not be able to survive the stress of restraint required for a routine diagnostic radiograph. The bird can be placed in a cardboard box or induction chamber or allowed to stand on a low perch to obtain a standing radiograph. If the x-ray machine has horizontal beam capabilities, a lateral standing view can also be obtained.

Gastrointestinal Contrast Study

Contrast studies are often done when abnormalities are indicated on the standard x-ray images. These are done with the same positioning mentioned previously with the addition of barium. The preferred dose is 25-50 mL/kg of straight barium sulfate or Iohexol (240 mg/iodine/mL) diluted 50:50 with water. The barium is administered via a gavage tube into the crop. Due to the fast gastrointestinal transit time of the avian patient, an immediate radiograph may be taken with subsequent views taken at 15-, 30-, 60-, and 90-minute intervals. To reduce the risk of aspiration of barium from the crop, the patient can be elevated on the restraint board during positioning (Figure 3-38). The board can be placed level for the radiograph and then elevated again for patient repositioning.

Ultrasound

Ultrasound studies are limited in the avian species since ultrasound waves cannot penetrate the gas-filled air sacs throughout the bird's body. In some cases the patient is just too small to achieve a diagnostic image. Ultrasound can be used to demonstrate organomegaly and coelomic fluid and masses such as soft-shelled eggs and tumors.

Endoscopy

Endoscopes are fiberoptic probes that utilize magnification that can provide direct visualization of body structures. A 2.7-mm rigid fiberoptic endoscope can be successfully used in almost all size birds. Most endoscopic procedures are minimally invasive and patient recovery time is more rapid than with exploratory surgeries. Endoscopy can be used for the visual examination of any part of the body that has an

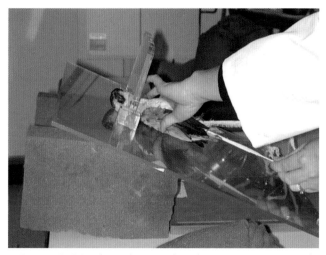

FIGURE 3-38. Elevated restraint board. (From Sirois M: *Principles and practice of veterinary technology*, ed 3, St. Louis, Mosby, 2011.)

orifice large enough to allow the insertion of the instrument. Laparoscopy, tracheoscopy, rhinoscopy, and cloacal endoscopy are common diagnostic procedures and the veterinarian can obtain tissue biopsies, apply interlesional and topical treatments and surgical interventions, and determine gender of monomorphic species.

> **TECHNICIAN NOTE** Endoscopy can be used for the visual examination of any part of the body that has an orifice large enough to allow the insertion of the instrument.

The bird will need to be anesthetized and the scope insertion site aseptically prepped and draped. The standard approach for diagnostic evaluation of the internal organs is right lateral recumbency. There are two approaches that can be used, one with the left leg pulled caudal and the other with the left leg pulled cranially. A small incision is made in the skin and the muscle layer is bluntly dissected with forceps. The scope and cannula are introduced into the incision through the cranial thoracic or abdominal air sac and organs can be viewed. Lung, reproductive organs, kidney, adrenal glands, ventriculus, and other organs will typically be visualized during this examination. Once the endoscopy is complete the area is sutured.

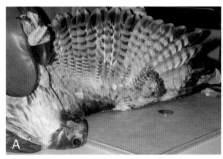
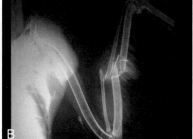
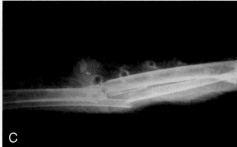

FIGURE 3-37. A, A red-tailed hawk in posterior/anterior wing position for radiographs. **B,** Lateral view of the wing with a fracture. **C,** Posterior/anterior view of the wing with the same fracture. (From Sirois M: *Principles and practice of veterinary technology*, ed 3, St. Louis, Mosby, 2011.)

Organs may be sampled using the endoscope's biopsy instrument. After collection, the tissues are often arranged on filter paper or closely woven cloth, which is then immersed in fixative solution. Alternatively, biopsy samples may be placed in fixative in a blood collection tube that does not contain anticoagulant.

The endoscope is very delicate and must be picked up by the eyepiece. Scope maintenance is essential. Proper cleaning and disinfecting will provide higher-quality diagnostics, and increase the longevity of the scope.

BANDAGING AND WOUND MANAGEMENT

The figure-of-eight bandage is used when a patient is presented with fractures or soft tissue injuries distal to the elbow, or when stabilization of a wing with an intraosseous catheter is needed (Figure 3-39). Soft roll gauze followed by a layer of self-adherent bandage material will provide the best results. With the wing in a flexed position, start the bandage at the carpus; wrap the gauze around the carpus thus creating the top of the 8 in the figure 8. Roll the gauze toward the elbow and wrap the gauze around the area proximal to the elbow. Make sure the gauze is high in the axillary region; this will help prevent slipping. This will create the lower end of the figure 8. Be careful not to make the wrap too tight or bulky or constrict the keel.

A body wrap is added in addition to the figure-of-eight bandage when the patient has a humeral or pectoral girdle fracture. When placing a body wrap, care must be taken not to place tension on the keel, which can cause inadequate breathing. Ensure that the body wrap is directly over the keel and not putting pressure on the crop or coelomic cavity or interfering with the movement of the legs. Use caution when placing a body wrap on anesthetized birds, due to the potential respiratory depression that can occur if the body wrap is placed too tight. Once the bandage is in place, the bird should be monitored for increased stress, dyspnea, and chewing or destroying the bandage.

Elizabethan Collar Placement

Elizabethan collars and other mechanical barriers are placed for many reasons including prevention of self-trauma such as feather picking and self-mutilation or to protect a bandage or wound. The collars can be fashioned from old x-ray film or insulation pipe found at the hardware store. The edges of the collar must be padded to prevent sores from forming and ensure that the bird cannot chew at the outside rim of the

collar. Crib-type collars have an attachable disk that prevents the bird from dropping its head far enough to pick at the upper and lower portions of the body. In some cases the bird can still reach the area just below the lower rim of the crib collar and the tips of the wings. The disk can be added to prevent any picking altogether; however, you should monitor the bird closely to ensure that it can still eat and drink. Commercially available bubble-style E-collars can be used but may not be as effective at keeping the bird from reaching the back half of its body (Figure 3-40).

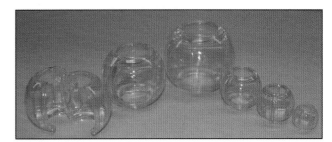

FIGURE 3-40. Commercially available bubble-style E-collars. (From Sirois M: *Principles and practice of veterinary technology*, ed 3, St. Louis, Mosby, 2011.)

When a collar is first placed on the bird, sedation and cage padding may be required until the collar is accepted. Some birds are highly stressed after the collar is placed and begin flipping in all different directions along with flapping uncontrollably and screaming. Once the bird has adjusted to the collar, you can return the bird to its owner, providing you counsel the owner on the possible complications regarding the collar. Complications can include trouble eating and drinking, trouble with balance and navigating around its normal environment, and pressure sores or abrasions from the collar.

DIAGNOSTIC TESTING
Fecal Examinations

Direct smear of the feces is used for detection of protozoa, especially *Giardia*. Fecal floatation is needed to detect helminthes, although these are extremely rare in pet birds. A Gram stain of the feces should be performed to detect yeast and bacteria. Grain- and fruit-eating psittaciformes should have a gram-positive bacterial flora with potentially some yeast. A few yeast or gram-negative bacteria per high-powered field could be considered normal, but budding yeast

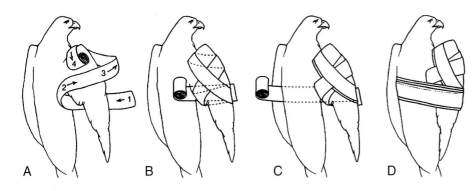

A B C D

FIGURE 3-39. The figure-of-eight bandage is one of the most common and useful bandages placed on avian patients. (From Mitchell M, Thomas T: *Manual of exotic pet practice*, St. Louis, WB Saunders Company, 2009.)

are not normal. Carnivorous or insectivorous passeriformes, raptors, galliformes, and anseriformes will have some gram-negative bacteria in their cloaca. A fecal occult blood test can be performed to look for blood.

> **TECHNICIAN NOTE** Fecal exam, choanal swab, cloacal swab, and nasal flush are commonly performed diagnostic procedures.

Respiratory System Diagnostics

A sample from the choana will demonstrate the presence of organisms in the sinuses of the bird. Excellent restraint and light are required to obtain the proper amount of exposure to obtain the sample. Open the oral cavity with tape or gauze strips and use a tongue depressor, or similar object, to keep the tongue out of the way. Insert a culturette or sterile cotton-tipped applicator into choanal slit (Figure 3-41). Gently advance the culturette into the rostral portion of the slit to collect the sample.

Nasal Flush

A nasal flush is performed to obtain a cytology sample representing the organisms of the sinuses. This procedure can also be therapeutic, flushing any debris or rhinoliths out of the sinuses or nares. The solution is injected directly into the sinus using a needle and syringe or flushed into the sinus through a nostril using a syringe without a needle (Procedure 3-2).

Tracheal Lavage

A tracheal wash is performed when tracheal or lower-respiratory system pathology is suspected. The glottis is not covered by an epiglottis as in mammals, making this procedure relatively simple (Procedure 3-3). Be sure to flush through the collection tube after collecting a tracheal wash sample. Sometimes debris can accumulate at the tip but never make it to the syringe. Flushing back out will push the debris into your sample container. This sample can be submitted for cytology as well as microbial culture.

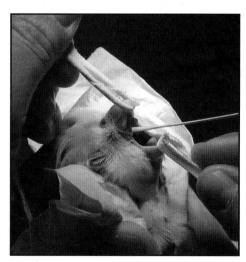

FIGURE 3-41. Obtaining a culture from the choanal slit of a cockatiel. (From Sirois M: *Principles and practice laboratory veterinary technology*, ed 3, St. Louis, Mosby, 2011.)

Hematology

The blood film is used to perform the differential WBC count; estimate platelet numbers; and evaluate the morphologic features of WBCs, RBCs, and platelets. Peripheral blood films can be prepared by using either a wedge smear technique or a coverslip technique. The coverslip technique is often used for preparing smears from blood samples obtained from avian species.

> **TECHNICIAN NOTE** RBCs of avian species are nucleated.

To prepare a blood film, a drop of blood is withdrawn from the EDTA-anticoagulated blood collection tube. Coverslip smears are made by putting one drop of blood in the center of a clean, square coverslip. Place a second coverslip diagonally on top of the first, causing the blood to spread evenly between the two surfaces. Then pull the coverslips apart in a single smooth motion before the blood has completely spread (Figure 3-42). Wave the smears gently in the air to promote drying. After they air dry, the blood smear can be stained with any of the Romanowsky-type stains. In avian species, the cell that is functionally equivalent to the neutrophil is referred to as a **heterophil**. Heterophils have distinct eosinophilic granules in their cytoplasm (Figure 3-43). Unlike the mammalian RBCs, RBCs of avian species are nucleated.

COMMON DISEASES AND DISORDERS

Infectious diseases that infect avian species include a number of serious bacterial and viral infections and some of these are zoonotic.

INFECTIOUS DISEASES
Avian Chlamydiosis

Chlamydiosis is caused by the obligate gram-negative intracellular bacterium, *Chlamydia psittaci*. This is a zoonotic disease that causes psittacosis in humans and avian

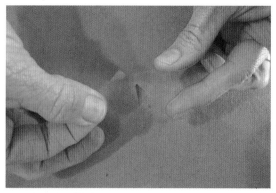

FIGURE 3-42. Pull the coverslips apart in a single smooth motion before the blood has completely spread. Wave the smears gently in the air to promote drying. After they air dry, the blood smear can be stained with any of the Romanowsky-type stains.

PROCEDURE 3-2 Nasal/Sinus Flush

Materials
- 3-ml, 6-ml, 12-ml, or 20-ml syringe, depending on the size of the bird and needle
- Preservative-free saline
- Sterile container to collect the sample
  It is best to wear protective eye gear and masks to prevent contaminated liquid from splashing into your face and eyes.

Procedure
- Depending on the size of the bird, fill the appropriate syringe with the saline and position the tip of the syringe so that it completely occludes one of the nares (Figure 1).

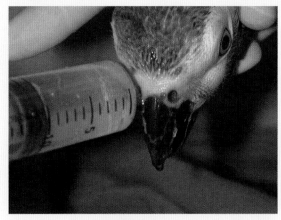

FIGURE 1

- Hold the patient in ventral or lateral recumbency and have the head pointing downward slightly.
- Flush with moderate force.

- The restrainer should monitor the eyes closely; sometimes you will have periorbital swelling during the flush. If this happens, decrease the amount of pressure you are using to flush the fluid through.
- As the sinus flush is performed, fluid should come out of the opposite naris and the choanal slit.
- Another person should be ready to collect the sample in a sterile container as it exits the bird (Figure 2).

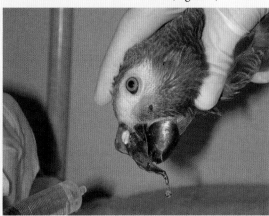

FIGURE 2

- In normal situations you will get fluid from the opposite naris and the choanal slit. Noninsectivorous passeriformes have no connection between the sinuses, so you will collect fluid only from the choanal slit.
- If you feel that the patient has severely packed sinuses, then nebulization before flushing might help loosen up the debris and increase your yield during the flushing.

(From Sirois M: *Principles and practice of veterinary technology*, ed 3, St. Louis, Mosby, 2011.)

PROCEDURE 3-3 Tracheal Lavage

Materials
- Gauze or tape strips for opening the mouth
- Focal light source
- Syringe
- Polypropylene catheter or red rubber feeding tube
- Sterile preservative-free saline (0.5-1.0 mL/kg)
- Sterile gloves

Procedure
- Restrain the patient in an upright position.
- Expose the oral cavity by gently retracting the beak with gauze or tape strips.
- Advance a sterile plastic or rubber tube down the trachea until resistance is met.
- Administer the calculated amount of fluid and immediately aspirate the contents.
- Place contents into a sterile container.

(From Sirois M: *Principles and practice of veterinary technology*, ed 3, St. Louis, Mosby, 2011.)

chlamydiosis in avian species. Bird owners, aviary and pet shop employees, poultry workers, and veterinary staff members are at greatest risk of infection. Outbreaks of psittacosis in poultry-processing plants have also been reported. The organism had been referred to as *Chlamydophila psittaci*, and active research into the antigens present on the surface of the organism indicate that there are at least nine species of *Chlamydia*. The disease is also referred to as ornithosis and parrot fever. The lungs, air sacs, liver, spleen, CNS, and heart may all be affected. Pneumonia, ocular and nasal discharge, greenish-yellow diarrhea, dehydration, and weight loss are typical signs. Some birds may be asymptomatic carriers of the disease and may shed the organism. Evidence indicates that the severity of the disease is likely related to the serotype as well as the species. Serotypes that are severe in one species of bird may be asymptomatic in another. Clinical signs and numerous clinical tests are used to diagnose chlamydiosis. Unfortunately, no one single test will determine whether a bird is acutely ill, a carrier, or uninfected. Available diagnostic tests include cell culture, immunofluorescence tests, and polymerase chain reaction tests. Human and avian

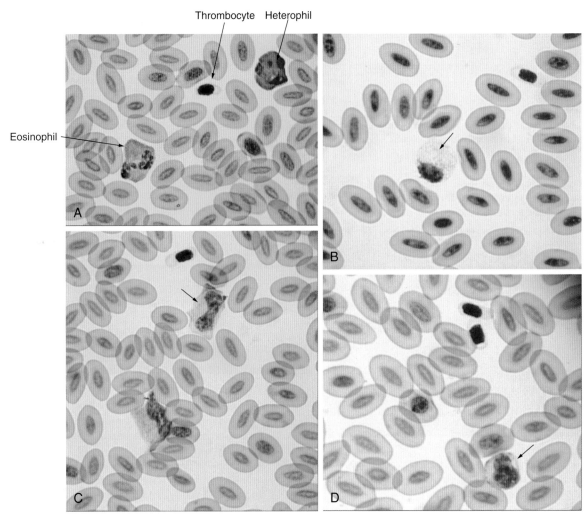

Thrombocyte   Heterophil

Eosinophil

FIGURE 3-43. In avian species, the cell that is functionally equivalent to the neutrophil is referred to as a heterophil. Heterophils have distinct eosinophilic granules in their cytoplasm. Unlike the mammalian RBCs, RBCs of avian species are nucleated.

chlamydiosis is a reportable disease and appropriate regulations must be followed (Box 3-2).

> TECHNICIAN NOTE | Veterinary staff members are at risk of infection with psittacosis.

Polyomavirus

The avian polyomavirus (APV) was first discovered in 1981 in fledgling budgerigars and is a nonenveloped virus that infects primarily young birds and causes acute death in psittacines. Older affected birds may show lack of blood clotting and gastrointestinal signs such as vomiting, diarrhea, and crop stasis. Surviving birds grow poorly, have abnormal feather development, and produce excessive and watery feces. Recovered asymptomatic birds shed the virus, keeping the facility contaminated. A test and vaccination are available for polyomavirus. Some veterinarians recommend vaccinating all susceptible birds in a breeding facility, or as soon as possible after purchasing the bird and before it is taken into a new home.

BOX 3-2	Infectious and Zoonotic Diseases of Birds

- Chlamydia psittaci (zoonotic)
- Psittacine beak and feather disease virus (PBFDV); circovirus
- Avian polyoma virus (APV)
- Psittacid herpes viruses (PsHVs) or Pacheco's disease
- Paramyxovirus 3 (PMV-3)
- Exotic Newcastle disease virus
- Psittacine proventricular dilatation disease (PDD)
- Papillomaviruses
- Adenoviruses
- Avian influenza
- West Nile virus (WNV)
- Eastern equine encephalitis (EEE)
- Poxviruses
- *Mycobacterium* sp. (zoonotic)
- Fungal infections such as *Aspergillus* sp.

(From Sirois M: *Principles and practice of veterinary technology,* ed 3, St. Louis, Mosby, 2011.)

Pacheco's Disease

Pacheco's disease is a highly contagious, acute disease of psittacines caused by a herpesvirus. It is associated with stress, which can cause clinically healthy carriers to shed virus and initiate infection in susceptible birds. It is spread by direct contact and by aerosol or fecal contamination of food or water. Macaws, Amazon parrots, monk parakeets, and conures are often involved in outbreaks. Terminal signs include acute death in well-fleshed birds and bright yellow urates with scant feces. Most affected birds will have an enlarged liver, splenomegaly, and renomegaly.

Cloacal Papillomatosis

Cloacal papillomatosis is associated with a herpesvirus of the strain that also causes the acute presentation of Pacheco's disease. Papillomatosis tends to occur as a flock problem. The disease is characterized by erythematous prolapsed cloacal tissue. Surgical removal or chemical cautery is indicated, but relapses may occur.

Proventricular Dilatation Disease

Proventricular dilatation disease (PDD) occurs most frequently in African grey parrots, cockatoos, and conures and is a disease first seen as early as 10 weeks of age. Clinical signs of disease vary significantly. Inflammation of the central and peripheral nervous systems are responsible for the characteristic signs of crop stasis, anorexia, cachexia, and incoordination. A virus is suspected to cause this disease, and the avian bornavirus (ABV) has recently been proposed as the infectious agent. PCR testing is being developed. Treatment trials with NSAID drugs have shown promise in halting the disease.

Psittacine Beak and Feather Disease

Psittacine beak and feather disease (PBFD) is caused by a circovirus that may first be seen in neonates in an infected nursery. The large majority of birds with the chronic form first develop lesions between 6 months and 3 years of age. Abnormal feather growth and lack of powder on the beak are the main signs, and it is easily spread by feather dust, dander, and feces to other birds. The germinal tissues of the beak are also affected, resulting in a misshapen and crumbly beak. Birds are most susceptible up to age 2 or 3. Diagnosis is based on gross appearance, PCR, and biopsies of affected feather follicles. Young birds that test positive must be removed from the flock. The contagious nature of PBFD and its generally terminal outcome in clinically affected birds warrant isolation and likely euthanasia in most clinical cases. Strict hygiene with attention to dust control, screening protocols (including PCR testing of both the birds and the environment), and lengthy quarantines are highly recommended in breeding facilities with susceptible species. All young birds must be tested before they are transferred to new owners or into a breeding situation. New birds are often tested when they receive their postpurchase veterinary examination.

Poxvirus

There are many poxviruses, and each one has its own host range. Poxviruses need an injury or vectors such as mosquitoes to allow the virus to enter the body. Poxvirus is most often associated with imported Amazon parrots and macaws, but other species such as canaries may be infected if housed outside in temperate or subtropical climates. Clinical presentation of this disease can be lesions around the face, eyelids, and commissures of the mouth, on the feet, and under the wings. Treatment is supportive therapy.

West Nile Virus

The West Nile virus is a mosquito-borne disease that primarily infects horses, humans, and birds. It has spread rapidly throughout the United States in the past few years. Psittacines appear to be somewhat resistant, as only a few cases have been reported from endemic areas. However, keeping pet birds inside or in screened areas is suggested to prevent exposure. An avian vaccine is not commercially available in North America.

NONINFECTIOUS DISEASES

Many of the noninfectious diseases that afflict birds are caused by improper husbandry, including poor nutrition, trauma, and exposure to toxic agents. Toxicities can be aerosolized toxins, plants, or other ingested substances. Trauma can result from flying into windows or ceiling fans, attacks by animals, or becoming entangled in cage toys.

Burns

Burns on birds commonly occur on the feet and legs. Birds that are left to free fly through the house can run the risk of landing in a pot of boiling hot liquid or on the burners of the stove causing severe burns to the legs and feet. Burns to the oral cavity and tongue may occur by biting electrical cords. Treatment for burns involves flushing the areas with copious amounts of cool water or saline and removal of surrounding feathers.

Crop Burn and Crop Trauma

A crop burn is normally caused by poorly mixed microwave foods that are fed to neonates. Once the burn has occurred, normally in the right ventral portion of the crop, crop and skin necrosis occurs, forming a fistula (Figure 3-44). Food will leak from this fistula, creating a very alarming situation for the client that may be an emergency. If the bird is not able to retain enough food or water, then there is a risk of dehydration and starvation. This will require anesthesia and a surgical closure, but the recovery is usually rapid. Client education on how to properly heat the food is essential to prevent future crop burns.

Timing of surgery on damaged crops will depend on the severity of injury. Birds with extreme trauma from ceiling fans or animal bites must be operated on immediately in order to stabilize the patient. Surgery on baby birds whose crops were burned with excessively hot formula often is deferred for 7 to 10 days until a fistula develops and the extent of the injury is obvious. After surgery the birds are fed small volumes of formula more frequently until healing occurs.

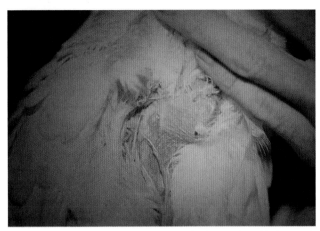

FIGURE 3-44. Crop fistula leaking food in a hand-fed juvenile cockatoo. (From Sirois M: *Principles and practice of veterinary technology*, ed 3, St. Louis, Mosby, 2011.)

> **TECHNICIAN NOTE** Many of the noninfectious diseases that afflict birds are caused by improper husbandry.

Toxicity

Birds are naturally curious and like to investigate unfamiliar objects with their mouths. When this behavior is combined with the bird given free run of the house, the potential of ingesting foreign objects is greatly increased. In addition, some materials used to create cages or toys may contain zinc or lead. Because there is no quality control for toys manufactured for birds, the toys themselves can be made from toxic materials and the client is unaware. Typically, ingestion of curtain weights, lead clappers from bells, old-style solder, lead-based paints, plaster, foil from wine bottles, and calcium-rich dolomite or bone meal can result in signs of lead poisoning. Galvanized cage wire is the usual source of ingested zinc. Diagnosis may be based on signs and radiographic findings of heavy metal densities within the body. Whole blood samples can be sent to an outside lab to analyze for heavy metals. Testing may take a number of days, so treatment is started before the blood levels are received if radiographs and signs suggest poisoning. Treatment for lead and zinc toxicosis is supportive with chelation therapy using calcium EDTA. If large amounts of metal are present, they need to be removed endoscopically or surgically. Response is usually rapid, and improvement may be seen in a few hours or days.

Other ingested poisons can include cleaning products, prescription medications, toiletries, tobacco, matches, and plants. Plant poisoning is not common. Birds often will tear leaves without eating them, decreasing the amount ingested. The avian gastrointestinal tract empties quickly, further reducing chances of poisoning. Owners may unintentionally expose their birds to poisonous plant materials in the feed, materials used as perches that may be toxic or use of plants for house decoration. Some common plants that are toxic to birds are listed in Box 3-3. Symptoms of toxicity can

---

| **BOX 3-3** | Toxic Plants |

- Avocado
- Black locust (should not be used for perches)
- Oak (should not be used for perches)
- Oleander (should not be used for perches)
- Rhododendron (should not be used for perches)
- Clematis
- Dieffenbachia
- Foxglove
- Lily of the valley
- Lupine
- Philodendron
- Poinsettia
- Yew
- Crown vetch

---

range from gastrointestinal upset to seizures, depending on the agent consumed and amount ingested. Treatment is usually supportive.

Egg Stasis

Egg retention is defined as the failure of an egg to pass through the oviduct at a normal rate. This is a commonly seen emergency in budgies, canaries, cockatiels, finches, and lovebirds. These birds typically have been laying eggs for some time, thus depleting their calcium stores. This causes decreased muscle activity in the oviduct, and the egg becomes trapped. Malformed eggs, vitamin deficiencies, and obesity are among other causes of egg stasis. Signs can include abdominal distention and straining, lack of droppings, depression, sitting on the cage bottom, tail wagging, and walking with widespread legs. In some cases the bird may be limping due to the pressure placed upon the pelvic plexus. The treatments for egg retention may include supportive care or surgery. Egg stasis is one possible cause of a space-occupying mass. Other causes include tumors, organ enlargement, or fluid buildup in the coelom (Figure 3-45). If a space-occupying mass is putting pressure on the air sacs, then the bird will present in respiratory distress.

Bleeding Emergencies

A variety of conditions may cause bleeding emergencies. Broken blood feathers will often be the result of a traumatic fall or injury to the bird. The bird may be covered in blood, from flapping or with an area covered with matted, bloody feathers. Immediately locate the broken blood feather. You may need to clean the site with saline or water while trying to locate the feather in question. If the bird is stable, apply direct pressure or styptic powder to stop the bleeding and try to save the feather from removal. If the bleeding will not cease, then remove the feather using hemostats or needle-nosed pliers. With one hand hold the wing stable and pull in the same direction that the feather is growing. Apply direct pressure to the feather follicle if bleeding continues.

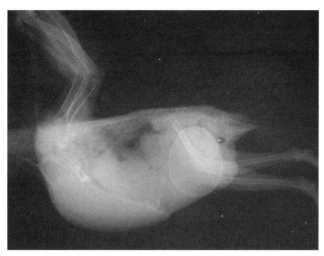

FIGURE 3-45. Space-occupying masses, such as the egg in the bird, can displace air sacs that are needed for air exchange. (From Sirois M: *Principles and practice of veterinary technology*, ed 3, St. Louis, Mosby, 2011.)

Prolapsed Cloaca

In case of prolapsed cloaca, the most important immediate therapy is to keep the prolapsed tissue moist and clean. If the patient is too stressed to restrain, place the patient in a cage lined with clean towels or gauze moistened with sterile saline. There are many aliments that can lead to a prolapsed cloaca, including egg stasis, papillomas, chronic masturbation, and coelomic masses. It is very important to determine the cause of the prolapse to insure that it will not be a recurring problem.

Animal Bites

This accident normally occurs when a larger animal attacks a smaller bird, and in some cases, when a bird attacks another bird. Mammal bites are usually from a pet dog or cat and are true emergencies. Oral bacteria from dogs and cats can be detrimental to the avian patient. The oral cavity of the cat is especially dangerous because it carries *Pasteurella multocida* on the gingival tissue and teeth. Immediate antibiotic therapy is commonly indicated. Evaluating a patient that has been attacked by a cat or dog can be challenging. The puncture wounds may be very small and concealed by the multiple layers of feathers. Blow on the feathers to part them, enabling you to view the skin beneath, or wet the feathers with saline and part them. To avoid hypothermia take care not to get the patient too wet. Once the wound is located, remove any surrounding feathers by plucking. Be careful when attempting to flush while cleaning the wound, due to the possibility that the puncture may communicate with an air sac.

Fractures

Birds are commonly presented with fractures that can result from a variety of situations, including being attacked by a larger animal, being caught in its cage or cage toys, leg band entrapped in toys or other objects, flying into a window or ceiling fan, and being stepped or sat on. Place the patient in a quiet, dark, well-padded environment until stable enough to restrain. Provide analgesics and determine the best method to stabilize the fracture. The condition, age, and personality of the bird have to be considered before proceeding with fracture treatment. The patient should be evaluated for any preexisting or concurrent medical conditions that prevent immediate repair.

Bandages and splints are used when some support of the fracture is all that is necessary. This method will make the bird more comfortable but may not allow proper healing and return to full function. Fractures commonly stabilized with this treatment are some wing and foot breaks. Alternatively there are many different surgical methods and approaches to fracture repair. In extreme cases, a traumatized leg or wing cannot be salvaged. In this instance, amputation may be the only choice. Most psittacines do well after losing a leg because they can use their beaks to move around. Most birds will perch comfortably but do run the risk of developing pododermatitis on the remaining foot. In pet birds, removal of a wing may cause some loss of balance, but most seem to manage rather well. The majority of birds are not troubled by toe amputations.

Wing Fractures. Fractures of the wing usually are immobilized with a figure-of-eight bandage. This holds the flexed wing snug against the body. If the humerus is fractured, a body wrap is also applied. An open fracture should also be cleaned and flushed using caution due to the pneumatic bones of birds (flushing could introduce fluid into the airway). Appropriate supportive, antimicrobial, and analgesic therapies should be implemented as soon as possible. Most broken wings will need to be bandaged for 3 to 5 weeks with routine changes. The bandage should be removed as soon as healing is complete. Complications include stiffness, muscle atrophy from disuse, and loss of flight feathers. Physical therapy will help the bird become limber and recover muscle mass.

Some severe fractures are best treated by surgery. The wing will need to be stabilized until surgery can be performed.

Leg Fractures. Some lower leg fractures are stabilized with a splint until healing occurs, usually 4 to 6 weeks. Because of the bird's anatomy, splints will often worsen fractures of the femur and upper tibiotarsus. These often require prompt surgical repair. Toe fractures can be treated in large birds by taping the broken toe to the neighboring intact toe.

An open fracture should also be cleaned and flushed with caution. Due to the pneumatic bones of birds, flushing could introduce fluid into the airway. Appropriate supportive, antimicrobial, and analgesic therapies should be implemented as soon as possible. Surgical correction will generally be required. Splints will be used to support the repaired break. The Schroeder-Thomas splint can be used to treat fractures of the lower third of the tibiotarsus and the entire tarsometatarsus. The bandage is changed every 1 to 2 weeks and is accompanied by passive physical therapy. A Robert Jones bandage can be used for simple lower leg fractures. Although these are heavily padded, additional splinting materials such as tongue depressors may be needed. The bandage needs to be changed at least every 2 weeks. A ball bandage is used for broken toes or pododermatitis. A ball formed of gauze sponges is placed so the toes curl around it. The foot is covered with cotton padding and wrapped with stretchy self-adherent bandaging. Very small birds can be difficult to splint. Materials such as pipe cleaners, toothpicks, paperclips, and wooden applicator sticks are used to stabilize their fractures. With all splints it is necessary to assess circulation in the foot. Look for swelling of the toes, blue coloration, and coldness. The bandage will need to be changed if any of these occur. Bandages need to be checked often for signs of chewing or moisture. Clients should be advised to bring the bird in to the clinic for a bandage change. Removal of leg bands is advised because they may cause fractures when they become caught on the cage or other objects.

Head Trauma

Head trauma cases where the bird flies into a window or a ceiling fan require immediate supportive therapy and evaluation. Evaluate for signs of shock and neurologic signs. Closely examine the eyes, ears, nose, and nares for hemorrhage or bruising. Place the patient in a dark, quiet, and (contrary to other situations) cool environment to prevent vasodilation of the intracranial vessels. Provide supportive care as needed. Monitor the patient closely for neurologic symptoms such as circling, head pressing or tremors, and seizures.

EUTHANASIA

Euthanasia is sometimes necessary to alleviate patient suffering and should be done in a humane manner. Acceptable methods should include anesthesia to create an environment where the patient is unaware of the injection. In some cases the patient may be incoherent enough that only heavy sedation is necessary and in others gas anesthesia is required. When the patient is unconsciousness, a commercially available euthanasia solution (barbiturate) can be administered. In a research setting, euthanasia methods other than barbiturate overdose require review and approval by the IACUC. Routes of administration for euthanasia solution are intravenous, intracardiac, or intraperitoneal. The patient must anesthetized if intracardiac or intraperitoneal routes are to be used, and in all cases the patient must be monitored until the heart stops. If the client is present, you must make them aware that some patients may experience agonal breaths, muscle twitching, or vocalizations and that the eyes may not close and gastrointestinal contents may release through the cloaca. In most cases the patient will have a peaceful release of tension, as if going to sleep.

KEY POINTS

- Most species encountered in exotic companion animal practice are passerines or psittacines.
- Psittacines are known as hookbills and their feet are zygodactyl.
- Passerines have a pointed or slightly curved beak and their feet are anisodactyl.
- The uropygial gland has one duct opening found dorsally at the base of the tail and secretes a lipoid sebaceous material that is spread over feathers during preening to help with waterproofing.
- Birds have several types of feathers: contour, semiplume, down, filoplume, and bristle.
- The avian skeleton is lightweight due to the presence of many pneumatized bones.
- The choana is a V-shaped notch in the roof of the mouth that directs air from the mouth and nasal cavities to the glottis.
- The crop serves to soften food and allows continuous passage of small amounts of food to the proventriculus.
- The cloaca is the common terminal chamber of the gastrointestinal, urinary, and reproductive systems.
- Urates are the major excretion product in birds and comprise the white portion of the droppings.
- Many avian behaviors that owners wish to modify are the result of instinctive avian reactions or related to the stresses of captivity.
- Common avian behavior problems include chewing, biting, excessive vocalization, dominance, and self-mutilation.
- The primary bird enclosure must be large enough for the bird to spread its wings, should be wider than it is tall, and maintained in a draft-free area.
- Ideal environmental temperature for birds is between 61° and 81° F with humidity levels in the range of 30% to 70%.
- For most companion birds, pellets should comprise approximately 70% of the diet and a variety of fresh fruits and vegetables approximately 30%.
- Individual birds may be identified with leg bands or with microchips.
- A terry cloth towel is used when capturing and restraining birds.
- The physical examination includes observation from a distance and may also include a systematic hands-on examination.
- Beak, nail, and wing trimming are common procedures performed on pet birds.
- The inguinal region is the preferred site to administer subcutaneous fluids and medications.
- For intramuscular injections the pectoral muscles are most commonly used.
- The medial metatarsal vein or leg vein is the vessel of choice for collecting blood in medium to large birds.
- Fluid therapy, nutritional support, and medication administration can be provided by gavage or tube feeding.
- Most patients can be restrained and anesthetized by mask induction or an anesthetic chamber can be used.
- Always use uncuffed endotracheal tubes for avian patients.
- Most companion psittacine birds will require anesthesia or heavy sedation for diagnostic radiographs.
- The standard whole-body x-ray views are a ventrodorsal (VD) and a right lateral.

- Endoscopy can be used for the visual examination of any part of the body that has an orifice large enough to allow the insertion of the instrument.
- The figure-of-eight bandage is used when a patient is presented with fractures or soft tissue injuries distal to the elbow or when stabilization of a wing with an intraosseous catheter is needed.
- Direct smear of the feces is used for detection of protozoa.
- A sample from the choana will demonstrate the presence of organisms in the sinuses.
- In avian species the cell that is functionally equivalent to the neutrophil is referred to as a heterophil. RBCs of avian species are nucleated.
- Infectious diseases that infect avian species include a number of serious bacterial and viral infections and many of these are zoonotic.
- Noninfectious diseases that afflict birds include those caused by improper husbandry, including poor nutrition, trauma, and exposure to toxic agents.

REVIEW QUESTIONS

1. The _____ _____ gland secretes a lipoid sebaceous material that is spread over the bird's feathers during preening.

2. A parakeet is an example of a _____.

3. The anatomy of this organ varies from species to species, ranging from a dilation of the esophagus to a single or double pouch.

4. List the common behavior problems associated with companion birds.

5. A _____ room and a _____ are helpful to reduce stress during capture and restraint of a bird.

6. Obtaining a detailed _____ of husbandry and diet is an essential part of the avian physical examination.

7. Observing _____ and _____ is important to evaluate prior to physical restraint of a bird.

8. The safest way to determine the sex of a bird is _____ _____.

9. When performing a beak trim, the bird should be monitored closely for _____ and _____.

10. Care must be taken to avoid cutting a _____ _____ during a wing trim.

11. Blood volume in birds ranges from _____% to _____% of body weight, depending on the species of bird.

12. The _____ jugular vein is the more prominent vessel in birds.

13. Which type of endotracheal tube should be used when intubating an avian patient?

14. The most common radiologic views used in avian patients are _____ and _____.

15. List the infectious diseases that affect the avian species and indicate if they are bacterial or viral and if they have zoonotic potential.

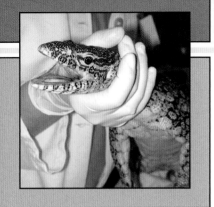

4 Reptiles

LEARNING OBJECTIVES

After studying this chapter, you will be able to:

- Describe the unique features of the anatomy of reptiles.
- Discuss the basic behavior of reptiles.
- Discuss the basics of client education, husbandry, and nutrition for reptiles.
- Describe how to obtain a complete and thorough history of the reptile patient.
- Explain the different capture and restraint techniques used for reptiles.
- Identify methods of sample collection for laboratory analysis.
- Describe how to obtain high-quality diagnostic images of reptile patients.
- Discuss nursing care and supportive therapy techniques for the reptile patient.
- Identify and discuss some of the common diseases and presentations of the reptile patient to the veterinary clinic.
- List the common infectious diseases, noninfectious diseases, and zoonoses found in the reptile patient.
- Describe the routine clinical procedures performed on reptile species.
- Explain the unique aspects of reptile anesthesia and surgery.

Reptiles are a diverse group of animals that include more than 7000 species. Those most likely to be seen in veterinary practice and in research include snakes, lizards, and chelonians. Chelonians seen in practice are in the taxonomic superorder Chelonia, order Testudines. These include box turtles, red-eared sliders and other water turtles, and various tortoises. The order Squamata contains the snakes and lizards. Commonly encountered animals include boas, pythons, king snakes, rat snakes, corn snakes, and gopher snakes. Other reptile orders include the crocodilians and rhynchocephalians. These are not commonly encountered in veterinary practice or research.

USES IN RESEARCH

Snakes and their venoms are used in biomedical research as a source of proteins for the study of biologic activity at the surface of cell membranes. Snakes are the most commonly used reptiles in biomedical research. Similarities between human skin and snake skin have been evaluated, and some researchers are working on techniques to use the skin shed by snakes for transdermal research. Snakes are also used in ecologic research, embryology, and natural history research.

UNIQUE ANATOMIC FEATURES

Most reptiles are ectothermic, meaning they derive the vast majority of their body heat from outside heat sources. Reptiles have one visceral cavity called the **coelom** with no diaphragm to separate the thoracic and abdominal cavities. Significant differences in anatomy and physiology exist among different families and species of reptiles. A complete review of all potential variations is beyond the scope of this discussion.

INTEGUMENTARY SYSTEM

Reptiles have a protective layer of keratinous scales or scutes covering the skin. Scales are formed from epidermal folds that overlap. Scutes are found in turtles and form a hard external plate with nonoverlapping sections. The outermost layer of the skin is shed on a regular basis. This process is referred to as **ecydysis**. Species such as snakes shed their skin all at once. Prior to ecdysis, the skin becomes very sensitive and turns an opaque color (Figure 4-1). Unlike snakes, lizards and chelonians shed in pieces. Some reptiles have **chromatophores**, which are specialized pigment-containing cells in the integument that allow for changing of skin color and pattern.

> **TECHNICIAN NOTE** Snakes shed their skin in one piece while lizards and chelonians shed in pieces.

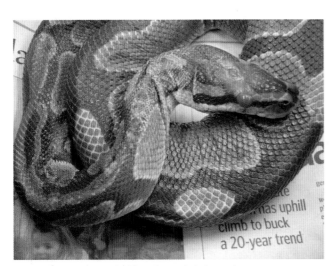

FIGURE 4-1. Prior to shedding, the snake's skin and eyes turn an opaque, blue color. The snake should not be handled just before and during the shed because this can damage the delicate, new skin. (From Sirois M: *Principles and practice of veterinary technology*, ed 3, St. Louis, Mosby, 2011.)

MUSCULOSKELETAL SYSTEM

The skulls of the different reptile orders exhibit significant diversity. Chelonian skulls do not have temporal openings (**anapsid** skulls) while other reptiles do have temporal openings (**diapsid** skulls). In snakes, the mandibular symphysis is connected by ligaments rather than fused. The jaws can move independently, and this allows for the ingestion of large prey. The spines of reptiles are extremely flexible, and a single occipital condyle forms the articulation between the skull and spine. This allows for increased mobility of the head on the spine.

The bony shell of chelonians is made up of the dorsal **carapace** and the ventral **plastron** covered by scutes. Some chelonians, like box turtles, have hinged plastrons that allow them to withdraw into their shells and close up completely for protection. The shell of chelonians is composed of the dorsal carapace and ventral plastron. Hinged plastrons are present in some chelonians that allow them to close up completely into the shell for protection from predators or prevention of desiccation.

Most reptiles have five digits on both front and rear feet and the hind limbs are longer than the forelimbs. Some species of snakes have vestigial limbs, referred to as spurs, used in courtship behaviors. Snakes have well-developed epaxial muscles, as well as segmental muscles that attach the ventral scutes to the ends of the ribs.

RESPIRATORY SYSTEM

The anatomy and physiology of the reptilian respiratory system differ significantly from those of mammals. Reptiles are capable of surviving for long periods of time without breathing. The glottis of the turtle and tortoise is located behind the tongue. The position of the lizard glottis is variable. The snake glottis is located on the floor of the oral cavity just caudal to the tongue and is mobile (Figure 4-2). This mobility allows for snake respiration while ingesting prey. Reptiles do not have vocal cords and can only hiss or grunt. The trachea of chelonians contains complete cartilaginous tracheal rings. Tracheal rings are incomplete in other reptile species. Snakes and some lizards have a simple, sac-like lung with one lobe. Chelonians and some lizards have bilobed lungs.

DIGESTIVE SYSTEM

Great diversity in feeding strategies exists among reptiles. Lizards and chelonians can be carnivorous, omnivorous, or herbivorous. Snakes are strict carnivores. Some reptiles are very specific in their feeding strategies and consume only specific foods. For example; the king cobra preys exclusively on other snakes. Nutritional deficiencies occur when incorrect food is offered to captive reptiles.

The forked tongue of snakes and lizards functions to deliver scent particles to the vomeronasal organ, also referred to as Jacobson's organ. In snakes and lizards, it is connected to the oral cavity by a duct. The tongue of some reptiles is projectile and can be extended to capture prey. Salivary glands in the oral cavity release enzymatic secretions that lubricate

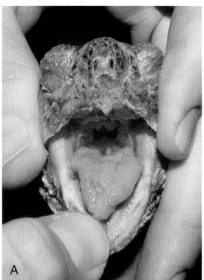
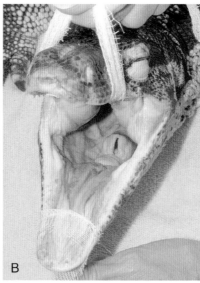
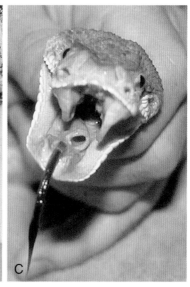

FIGURE 4-2. **A,** The turtle and tortoise glottis is situated behind the fleshy tongue. **B,** The position of the lizard glottis varies depending on species and can range from a rostral position that is readily visualized, as seen in this monitor, to a more caudal location behind the fleshy tongue, as is seen in the turtles. **C,** The snake glottis is located cranially on the floor of the oral cavity just caudal to the tongue. (From Mader DR: *Reptile medicine and surgery,* ed 2, St. Louis, Saunders, 2006.)

prey to ease ingestion in addition to aiding in digestion. Venom glands of some snakes are a type of salivary gland. Dentition of reptiles is widely variable. Chelonians have no teeth and use their **tomia** or keratinized beaks to acquire and tear their food. The fang teeth of venomous species contain modifications for delivery of venom. A duct at the base of the fang delivers venom to the teeth. Snake teeth are curved backwards to allow anchoring of prey.

> **TECHNICIAN NOTE** Lizards and chelonians can be carnivorous, omnivorous, or herbivorous, while snakes are strict carnivores.

In most carnivorous reptiles, the esophagus and stomach are thin and distensible to allow for passage of prey. The specific structure of the intestinal tract of reptiles varies with the type of diet consumed. Those that are herbivorous generally have a very large colon.

UROGENITAL SYSTEM

The kidneys of reptiles are variable in structure. In turtles and most lizards, the kidneys are oblong and smooth while in snakes, they are lobulated. A urinary bladder may be present, or urine may be stored in the cloaca or rectum. The nephron cannot concentrate the urine by removing water. Water can be absorbed from the urine through the wall of the urinary bladder, rectum, or cloaca. Uric acid is the principle end product of protein metabolism and is excreted in the urine combined with calcium salts (urates).

> **TECHNICIAN NOTE** Reptile excrement includes three components; urine, urates, and feces.

Most species of reptiles have a renal portal system. This is a network of vessels associated with the kidneys. The renal portal system is clinically significant because medications injected caudal to the kidneys can be carried directly back to the kidneys before being distributed to the rest of the body. This can result in damage to the kidneys if the drug is nephrotoxic or excretion of the drug before it has been distributed throughout the body. The cloaca is the common opening through which the urinary, digestive, and reproductive systems empty.

Male reptiles have internal testes and possess copulatory organs that have no function in urination. Chelonians have a phallus composed of erectile tissue that originates in the floor of the cloaca. Male snakes and lizards possess paired structures, called **hemipenes**, that can be everted from the tail base through the vent. Although all turtles and most lizards and snakes lay eggs (**oviparous**), some species of lizards and snakes give birth to live young (**viviparous**). Most species of reptiles do not care for eggs or offspring.

> **TECHNICIAN NOTE** All turtles and most lizards and snakes lay eggs. Some species of lizards and snakes give birth to live young.

CIRCULATORY SYSTEM

Snakes, lizards, and chelonians have a three-chambered heart with two atria and one ventricle (Figure 4-3). The right atrium receives deoxygenated blood through the sinus venosus, which receives blood directly from the right and left precaval veins the postcaval vein and the left hepatic vein. The left atrium receives oxygenated blood from the lungs via the left and right pulmonary veins. The ventricle is divided

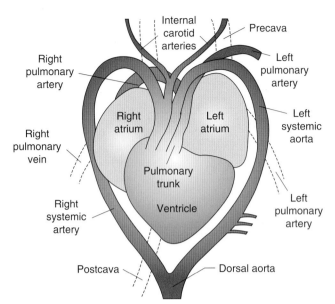

FIGURE 4-3. Ventral view of a lizard heart. (From Colville TP, Bassert JM: *Clinical anatomy and physiology for veterinary technicians*, ed 2, St. Louis, Mosby, 2008.)

into three subchambers separated by muscular ridges. The cavum venosum directs oxygenated blood into the paired aortic arches. The cavum pulmonale receives blood from the right atria and directs it into the pulmonary circulation. The cavum arteriosum receives blood from the pulmonary veins and directs it into the cavum venosum.

> **TECHNICIAN NOTE**   Reptiles have a three-chambered heart with two atria and one ventricle.

SPECIAL SENSES

Like birds, reptiles have voluntary control over the muscles that change the opening of the iris. The lower eyelids of some lizard species are very thin, allowing limited vision even when the eyes are closed. In most species, the lower lid is more mobile than the upper. The third eyelid is well developed and mobile in many reptiles. Snakes and lizards do not possess true eyelids.

The ears are found on both sides of the head and caudal to the eyes in most amphibians and reptiles. The tympanum is easily observed in most species but lies in a depression and may be covered by folds of skin in some lizards. Like birds, reptiles have a single bone in the middle ear called the columella.

Reptiles possess semicircular canals comparable to those found in mammals and birds; these fluid-filled canals control balance and equilibrium. Snakes do not have external ears. Their unique anatomy allows snakes to be sensitive to ground vibrations.

BEHAVIOR

The unique behaviors seen in reptiles are specific adaptations that evolved to allow them to obtain food, escape predation,

or reproduce. Defensive behaviors include death-feigning, tail displays, squirting blood, **tail autonomy**, color changes, skin sloughing, and coiling (balling up).

In response to a threat, some groups of snakes and lizards will writhe with the tongue hanging out. They may regurgitate and defecate and the mouth us usually hung open. The snake will then turn over onto its ventrum in an effort to appear dead (Figure 4-4). Most species of lizards have a unique feature to their tails called tail autonomy. The lizard can drop its tail as a defensive mechanism when pursued. The muscles of the tail contract to minimize bleeding. The discarded piece of tail usually continues to wiggle and draws the attention of the pursuer away from the lizard as it makes its escape. The tail will regenerate, although it will be smaller and more rigid than the original (Figure 4-5).

Some snakes and horned lizards may squirt blood from their eyes or cloaca to deter predators. Tail displays are seen

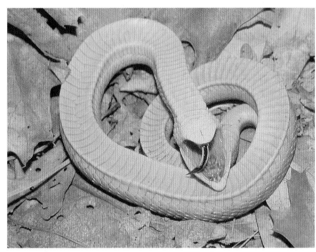

FIGURE 4-4. This eastern hog-nosed snake, *Heterodon platirhinos,* is death feigning. Note the characteristic position of dorsal recumbency, with gaping mouth, protruding tongue, and gaped cloaca. If placed upright, the snake immediately rolls onto its back, as if to prove it is still dead. (Photograph courtesy S. Barten.) (From Mader DR: *Reptile medicine and surgery*, ed 2, St. Louis, Saunders, 2006.)

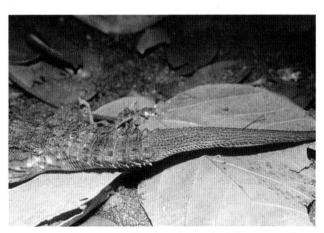

FIGURE 4-5. Regrown tail in a lizard. Note the difference in scalation and markings between the original and regrown portions. (Photograph courtesy R.D. Bartlett.) (From Mader DR: *Reptile medicine and surgery*, ed 2, St. Louis, Saunders, 2006.)

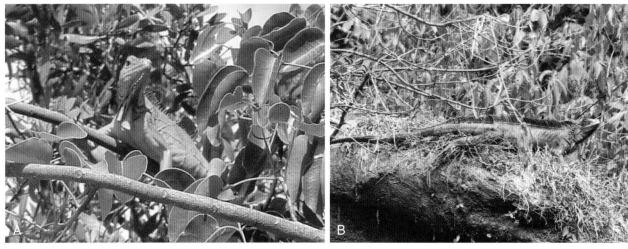

FIGURE 4-6. A, The Green Iguana *(Iguana iguana)* is generally bright green in early morning hours, before it thermoregulates and warms the core body temperature. **B,** Within minutes of positioning the body to incident rays of the sun, the skin darkens to help absorb radiant energy. (**A,** Photograph courtesy C. Givens; **B** Photograph courtesy D. Mader.) (From Mader DR: *Reptile medicine and surgery*, ed 2, St. Louis, Saunders, 2006.)

in many species of snakes and some lizards. These usually involve the animal hiding its head beneath its body and then waving the tail so that it mimics a head about to strike, sometimes accompanied by writhing. Tail vibrating is seen in rattlesnakes and some nonvenomous snakes. Bluff and threat displays are also seen in many reptiles. The animal will puff up its body to increase its size. Skin sloughing occurs in some lizards. When grasped, most of the skin tears away, allowing the animal to escape.

Behaviors that result from the unique physiology of reptiles include salt spraying and behaviors associated with thermoregulation and reproduction. Accessory salt glands are present in many species of reptiles and serve to aid in conserving water. When excess salts accumulate, the reptile will sneeze a fine spray, resulting in white deposits around the nares or on the walls of the enclosure. Thermoregulatory behaviors involve movement between warmer and cooler areas as needed but may also involve lifting parts of the body to expose the skin or huddling beneath objects to warm the body. Some species undergo color changes associated with thermoregulation (Figure 4-6). Courtship behaviors include head-bobbing, dewlap extension, and biting. Iguanas may become highly aggressive during breeding season.

HUSBANDRY

HOUSING

Many pet reptiles can be housed in a simple terrarium. Appropriate cage furniture should be placed in the terrarium as well. Cage furniture will vary based on the species and includes items such as logs, plants, hide boxes, and rocks (Figure 4-7). Commercially available reptile enclosures are suitable for most species. Reptiles that are normally terrestrial can be housed in a shallow cage with a tight-fitting lid. Arboreal reptiles (those that live in trees) require a cage that has greater vertical space.

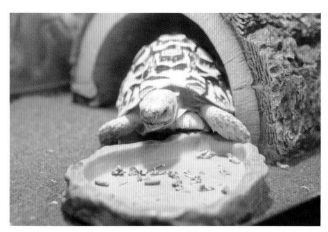

FIGURE 4-7. Appropriate cage furniture must be provided.

Each species has a specific temperature range at which they thrive (Table 4-1). This is referred to as the **preferred optimum temperature zone** (POTZ) or preferred optimum temperature range (POTR). Most aspects of reptile physiology are tied to body temperatures and, therefore, also tied to their behavior and overall health. A thermal gradient must be provided that allows for both warmer and cooler areas within the enclosure. A heat source is generally provided using heat lamps or heating pads (Figure 4-8).

In addition to temperature, the duration (**photoperiod**) and quality of light to which a reptile is exposed has an effect on overall health. If the reptile is housed without exposure to natural light, an artificial light source must be present. The light should be placed on a timer set to provide the duration of light that the reptile would be exposed to at the latitude where it would exist in the wild and modified throughout the year to mimic seasonal changes. Most reptiles also require ultraviolet light in order to produce vitamin D₃. Humidity requirements vary among different species of reptiles. Some tropical species such as the green iguana require extremely high levels of humidity to stay healthy. An area of high

TABLE 4-1	Preferred Optimum Temperature Ranges for Commonly Housed Captive Reptiles	
COMMON NAME	**DAY (° F)**	**NIGHT (° F)**
Boa constrictor	Mid-80s	70-80
Ball python	Mid-80s	70-80
Cornsnake	77-84	67-75
Green iguana	84-90	67-77
Leopard gecko	77-85	65-75
Bearded dragons	84-88	68-74
Blue-tongued skink	80-85	67-75
Monitor lizard	84-88	74-78
Tegus	80-86	70-78
Tropical turtles	82-86	74-80
Box turtles	78-89	60-70

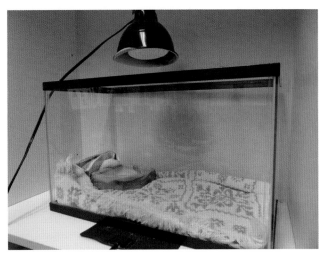

FIGURE 4-8. A simple terrarium with a heat lamp can be used for maintaining many species of reptiles.

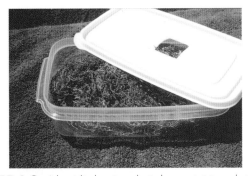

FIGURE 4-9. A humidity box is a plastic box containing substrate that holds some moisture. The most commonly used substrate for this purpose at this time is sphagnum moss. (From Mader DR: *Reptile medicine and surgery*, ed 2, St. Louis, Saunders, 2006.)

humidity can be created within the reptile enclosure by placing soaked sphagnum moss in a sealable plastic box with a hole cut into it for access (Figure 4-9). Appropriate substrates also vary depending on the species. Ideal substrates are readily available, nonabsorbent, nontoxic, and large enough to not be ingested by the reptile. Absorbent substrates such as

wood chips should only be used when cage ventilation is sufficient to prevent the absorption of moisture that can encourage bacterial growth. Examples of appropriate substrates include newspaper, butcher's paper, large stones, artificial turf, and shredded coconut shells.

> **TECHNICIAN NOTE** The reptile enclosure must have a thermal gradient that allows for both warmer and cooler areas within the enclosure.

Proper sanitation of the reptile enclosure is very important. The cage should be cleaned thoroughly and disinfected on a routine basis. Excrement should be picked up daily. Owners should be aware that all reptiles have the ability to shed *Salmonella* species if they are positive carriers of the bacteria. Salmonellosis is a significant zoonotic disease. Owners should take precautions by wearing examination gloves during cleaning and handling of the pet. Handling the animal and cleaning of the enclosure should never take place near food or where food for human consumption is prepared or stored.

> **TECHNICIAN NOTE** All reptiles have the ability to shed *Salmonella*.

NUTRITION

A complete review of nutritional requirements of all reptile species is beyond the scope of this text. Snakes, some species of lizards, and some aquatic chelonians are carnivorous and should be offered euthanized prey of the type they would consume in the wild. Live prey should not be fed due to the likelihood that the prey would attack and injure the reptile. Feeding duration is generally every 7 to 21 days depending on the species and age of the reptile. Herbivorous lizards and tortoises eat a variety of grasses, fruits, and leaves. Most herbivorous lizards benefit from a varied diet. Commercially available diets may not contain all the nutrients required. Insectivorous reptiles thrive on a diet composed primarily of insects such as crickets and mealworms. Some lizards and many chelonians are omnivores and should be fed a varied diet that includes prey, insects, and vegetables. Commercially available diets can be used to supplement natural food sources in captive chelonians.

Clean, fresh water should be available at all times. Water should be provided in a manner consistent with how the reptile would obtain water in the wild. For example, reptiles that live primarily in tress (arboreal) should have tree branches misted periodically or a water bowl mounted in a tree limb. Reptiles that would reside in desert environments are likely to obtain water by licking it from rocks and may not be able to use a water bowl. The water bowl must not be taller than the animal and the water should not be deeper than the length of the reptile's legs.

IDENTIFICATION

In research and in exotic pet practice, reptiles are usually housed individually so identification can be maintained with cage cards. Microchips can also be used as well as description of distinctive markings of an individual reptile.

RESTRAINT AND HANDLING

SNAKES

Most snakes can be easily captured directly out of their carrier or cage. Nonaggressive snakes can simply be picked up and pulled out of the cage. If the snake is aggressive, it may be necessary to use a towel along with leather gloves to safely capture it. In these cases it is easiest to gently toss the towel over the snake and find the head. Once the head has been isolated and restrained, the snake can be safely taken out of the enclosure. If the snake is extremely aggressive or if it is a venomous snake, a snake hook should be used to pin down the head of the snake long enough to safely grasp its head and body. Improper use of the snake hook can cause trauma to the patient; therefore, extreme caution should be taken.

Snakes are commonly brought into the clinic in pillowcases (Figure 4-10). It is important that the veterinarian or technician does not just open the pillowcase and quickly pull the snake out, especially if unfamiliar with the patient. It is important to first know what type of snake is in the pillowcase. To safely remove the snake from the pillowcase, first find the snake's head and gently grasp it from the outside of the pillowcase. Once the snake is restrained, the restrainer should put his or her free hand into the pillowcase and transfer the head to the free hand. After this is accomplished, it should now be safe to take the entire snake out of the pillowcase. Hold the snake directly behind the head with one hand and support the body with the other hand (Figure 4-11). If the snake is large, more than one person may be needed to restrain it. The general guideline is to have one restrainer per 3 feet of snake.

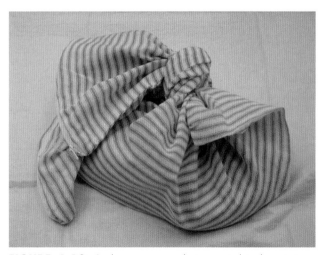

FIGURE 4-10. Snakes are commonly transported to the veterinary hospital in a pillowcase. (From Sirois M: *Principles and practice of veterinary technology,* ed 3, St. Louis, Mosby, 2011.)

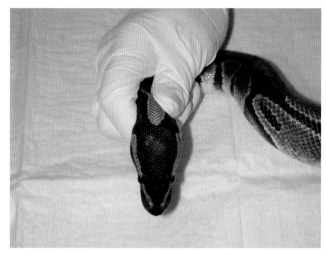

FIGURE 4-11. The snake's head is restrained by placing your hand behind the base of the skull. This will keep the snake from turning around and biting you. (From Sirois M: *Principles and practice of veterinary technology,* ed 3, St. Louis, Mosby, 2011.)

CHELONIANS

Although chelonians are usually the easiest to capture, they are the hardest to restrain. With the exception of extremely large tortoises, most chelonians can just be picked up with both hands and placed on the examination table. When examining large tortoises, it is easiest to set up an examination area within the animal's enclosure or on the floor in the clinic's examination area. Because there is such a great deal of variation in size and strength, restraint techniques may vary between small and large chelonians. Once the animal's body is under control, it is imperative that the head is properly restrained. Although this is relatively easy when the animal is sick, it can be difficult on strong, healthy chelonians, especially large tortoises and box turtles.

There are several ways the restrainer can gain control of the animal's head. Many turtles and tortoises are very curious. If they are set down on the table or the ground, they may just start walking around to check things out. If this is the case, the technician can just walk up to them and grasp the head with one hand while restraining the body with the other hand. To keep control of the head, it is best to position your thumb on one side of the cranial portion of the neck and position the rest of your fingers (or just the index finger for smaller species) on the other side of the neck just behind the base of the skull (Figure 4-12). Healthy chelonians are strong so it may take a lot of constant but gentle force to keep the turtle or tortoise's head out of the shell. If the animal is extremely active, an additional person may be necessary to help restrain the limbs and body.

Another way to gain control of the head is by trying to coax the animal out of its shell. Many chelonians will extend their head out of the shell if food is offered to them or if they are placed in a container of shallow warm water. Once the head is extended, the same techniques mentioned above can be used to gain and keep control of the

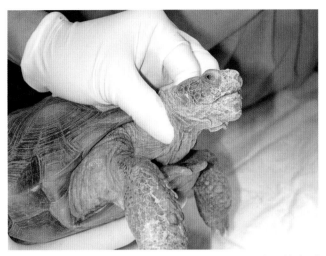

FIGURE 4-12. The tortoise is restrained by placing one hand behind the base of the skull to help keep the head and neck extended. The other hand should be used to support the body. (From Sirois M: *Principles and practice of veterinary technology*, ed 3, St. Louis, Mosby, 2011.)

animal's head. If these techniques fail, it may be possible to slip a small, blunt ear curette or spay hook under the horny portion of the upper beak, known as the rhinotheca. Once the probe has been placed, it can be gently pulled back to extend the neck to a position for the restrainer to grasp. It is important to note that this technique can be dangerous. The beak can be chipped or broken if the animal struggles or is in poor health. If a spay hook is the tool of choice, apply padding to the hooked portion of the instrument. Padding can simply consist of tape or an elastic wrap cut to the appropriate size. Caution should be taken when dealing with any aquatic turtle, especially snapping turtles. These species of turtles have a tendency to bite, and many of the larger turtles can cause serious bodily harm to the people working with them.

Box turtles can be the most challenging chelonians to properly restrain. Because box turtles have a hinge on their plastron, many species are able to completely tuck themselves into their shells. The easiest way to extend their head is to gently prop open the cranial portion of the carapace (upper shell) and the plastron (lower shell). Extreme care must be taken when trying to prop the shell open. It is suggested that a well-padded object be used when attempting this. This will help avoid traumatizing or fracturing the shell. Another way to extend a box turtle's head is to grasp one of the forelimbs, keeping the leg extended out of the shell until the head can be successfully pulled out and properly restrained. This method works well because once the leg is extended, the turtle will usually not close its shell down on its own leg. It is important to remember that any of these capture and restraint techniques can potentially cause a fair amount of stress to the turtle or tortoise. If initial attempts at capture and restraint are not successful, chemical restraint may be necessary for any reptile, especially large tortoises and box turtles.

LIZARDS

Lizards can be challenging animals to both capture and restrain. Smaller lizards are generally easy to capture but can be difficult to restrain because they tend to wiggle and squirm while they are being held. Most small lizards can simply be picked up with both hands and taken out of the enclosure. This is also true of the larger lizard species as well. However, some of the larger lizards can be both difficult to capture and restrain, especially if they are aggressive. If the lizard is aggressive, a towel or blanket along with leather restraint gloves should be used. It is important to remember that lizards can scratch and bite when they are scared or nervous. Therefore, it is a good idea to wear long sleeves. Long-necked lizards like monitors can easily turn around and bite if their head is not properly restrained during capture. Keeping one hand on the neck, just behind the base of skull, will help prevent getting bitten (Figure 4-13). Never pick up any species of lizard by its tail. Some lizards voluntarily "drop" or autotomize their tail in an attempt to escape predation.

Generally, lizards can be restrained by placing one hand around the neck and pectoral girdle region while the other hand can be used to support the body near the pelvis (Figure 4-14). Although it is sometimes difficult, try to avoid pressing down and damaging the dorsal spines of lizards such as iguanas when they are being restrained. It is also important to remember that not all lizards have durable and tough skin. Some lizards such as geckos have extremely delicate skin that can easily be damaged by capture and restraint. Make sure only soft towels are used on geckos.

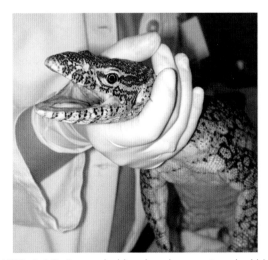

FIGURE 4-13. Long-necked lizards such as monitors should be restrained by placing one hand behind the base of the skull and the other hand supporting the body. Placing your hand behind the skull base will help keep the animal from biting you. (From Sirois M: *Principles and practice of veterinary technology*, ed 3, St. Louis, Mosby, 2011.)

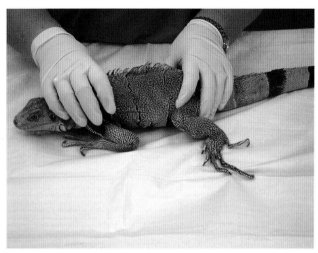

FIGURE 4-14. Restraint of a large lizard, with one hand around the pectoral girdle and the other hand around the pelvic girdle. (From Sirois M: *Principles and practice of veterinary technology*, ed 3, St. Louis, Mosby, 2011.)

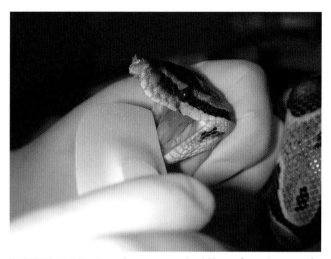

FIGURE 4-15. An oral examination should be performed as part of a complete physical examination. A soft plastic spatula is commonly used to gently open the mouths of snakes. (From Sirois M: *Principles and practice of veterinary technology*, ed 3, St. Louis, Mosby, 2011.)

CLINICAL PROCEDURES

PHYSICAL EXAMINATION

Performing a physical examination on reptiles is comparable to performing a physical examination on most mammalian species. All items needed for the physical examination should be ready and within reach. This will help decrease the time that the patient must be restrained and provide a less stressful experience for both the animal and the veterinary staff. Always begin by performing a visual precapture examination. This can provide an overview of the animal's attitude and mentation before it has been potentially stressed by handling.

> TECHNICIAN NOTE   The physical examination always begins with visual observation of the reptile.

To perform a thorough physical examination, start at the head and work toward the tail. This method will help ensure that nothing is overlooked. The eyes, ears, and oral cavity should be thoroughly examined. The eyes should be bright, clean, and free of any discharge. A pen light and ophthalmoscope should be used to visually observe and examine the eyes. The sclera should be observed for any signs of redness or irritation. Any opacity should also be noted during the ophthalmologic examination. The ears or tympanic membranes should be observed with a pen light during the physical examination. They should be clean, clear, and free of any debris.

The oral cavity can be safely opened with either porous tape stirrups or a soft plastic instrument such as a spatula (Figure 4-15). Metal specula can be used, but caution should be taken to avoid causing trauma to the mouth. The oral cavity should be moist, pink, and free of any lesions. Sometimes mucous membranes in snakes are paler then one would expect. Pale mucous membranes could be a sign of a medical problem, but many times this coloration is considered "normal." The mouth should be observed for signs of erythema, stomatitis, fractured teeth, and evidence of plaques on the mucous membranes.

Palpation of the coelomic cavity, extremities, and tail should then follow (Figure 4-16). The same techniques used to palpate dogs and cats can be used to palpate most reptiles. It is important to note any abnormalities such as soft tissue swellings, space-occupying masses such as urinary calculi, developing eggs, neoplasia, and any current or old injuries such as fractures. Obtain an accurate heart rate and respiratory rate (Table 4-2). A heart rate is most easily obtained by using a Doppler. Most reptile patients cannot be auscultated with a stethoscope. The Doppler probe can be placed directly on the heart (Figure 4-17) or either over the carotid artery or into the thoracic inlet in some species (Figure 4-18).

> TECHNICIAN NOTE   A heart rate is most easily obtained by using a Doppler.

In most snakes you can commonly palpate the heart, gall bladder, and a prey item or feces if present. If the animal has a systemic infection or is septic, petechiae and ecchymosis can often be observed on the ventral aspect of the snake along the scutes.

Turtles and tortoises usually present the biggest challenge when trying to perform a complete physical examination. The shell makes it difficult to palpate most of the organs. Depending on the size of the animal, one or two fingers may be placed in the inguinal area between the hind limbs and the shell. This enables palpation of the coelomic cavity for any abnormalities such as cystic calculi, foreign bodies, neoplasia, or eggs. Note the shell quality and color. If the animal has a systemic infection or is septic, petechiae and ecchymosis can often be found on the shell, especially the plastron.

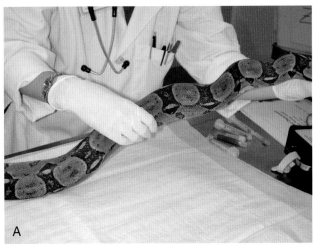

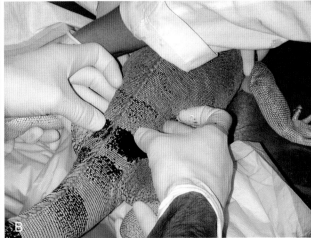

FIGURE 4-16. A, The entire length of the snake should be palpated while performing a complete physical examination. **B,** The coelom of lizards can be easily palpated and is done in a manner comparable to that used with dogs and cats. (From Sirois M: *Principles and practice of veterinary technology,* ed 3, St. Louis, Mosby, 2011.)

TABLE 4-2	Obtaining a Heart Rate with a Doppler
SPECIES	**PLACEMENT OF THE DOPPLER**
Lizards	Lateral cervical region over the carotid artery
	Cranial thorax over the heart
	Medial aspect of thigh over femoral artery
	Ventromedial aspect of the carpus over the artery
Snakes	Ventral aspect of the body directly on the heart
	Carotid artery
	Tail artery
Chelonians	Directly over the carotid artery
	Directly into the thoracic inlet
Amphibians	Ventral aspect of the body directly over the heart

(From Sirois M: *Principles and practice of veterinary technology,* ed 3, St. Louis, Mosby, 2011.)

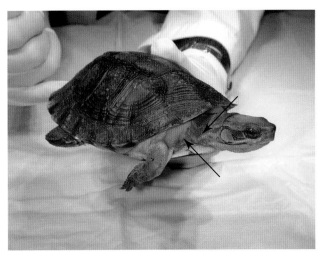

FIGURE 4-18. The Doppler probe is placed either over the carotid artery or into the thoracic inlet as indicated by the two black arrows. (From Sirois M: *Principles and practice of veterinary technology,* ed 3, St. Louis, Mosby, 2011.)

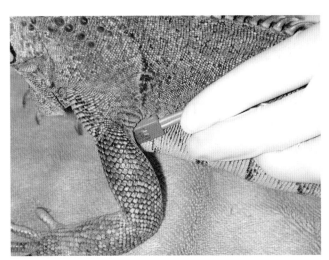

FIGURE 4-17. The Doppler probe is placed in the axillary region to obtain a heart rate on most lizard species. (From Sirois M: *Principles and practice of veterinary technology,* ed 3, St. Louis, Mosby, 2011.)

In lizards it is sometimes difficult to palpate many of the organs. In some of the larger lizards, the kidneys can be palpated via a rectal examination. The kidneys sit in the pelvic girdle and are almost impossible to palpate unless they are enlarged or mineralized. If the animal has a systemic infection or is septic, petechiae and ecchymosis can often be observed. In some lizards such as iguanas, petechiae and ecchymosis are commonly seen on the dorsal spines along the animal's back.

DETERMINING GENDER

It is relatively easy to determine gender in many species of reptiles. For example, male iguanas and bearded dragons have very large femoral pores compared with females (Figure 4-19). Many species of male tortoises have a concave plastron making it easier to mount the female. Several male water turtles have elongated nails that are dangled in front of the female to impress her. Some species of male box turtles have brilliant red eyes.

The gender of snakes can be determined using a well-lubricated metal or plastic probe inserted into the cloaca and then directed caudolaterally (Figure 4-20). In male snakes the probe will enter the cavity where the inverted hemipenis is located. In female snakes the probe will enter a blind diverticula. Once the probe has been inserted, it is slowly and gently advanced until it will not advance any further. Place your thumb on the scale where the end of the probe is located. Remove the probe and count the number of scales from the cloacal opening to the thumb. If the number is greater than 7, it is a male and if it is less than 5, it is a female. If the number is in between, it is very hard to say whether the animal is a male or female.

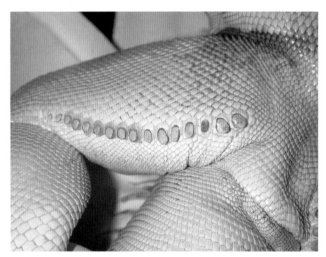

FIGURE 4-19. The femoral pores are commonly used to sex lizards such as iguanas and bearded dragons. The males (pictured) have large femoral pores, while females have tiny femoral pores. (From Sirois M: *Principles and practice of veterinary technology*, ed 3, St. Louis, Mosby, 2011.)

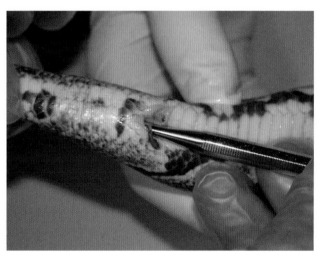

FIGURE 4-20. Snakes can be sexed using a well-lubricated metal or plastic probe inserted into the cloaca. (From Sirois M: *Principles and practice of veterinary technology*, ed 3, St. Louis, Mosby, 2011.)

INJECTIONS

Injections are most often administered intramuscularly or subcutaneously. To avoid the renal portal system, injections are usually given in the front limbs. Subcutaneous injections can be given in the lateral coelomic body wall between the scales or in the inguinal or ventral skin folds in chelonians. Fluids can be administered intravenously into the caudal tail vein in most reptiles or the jugular vein in chelonians (Table 4-3). Needle and catheter size generally ranges from 27 to 20 gauge, depending on the size of the patient. An indwelling catheter can be placed in the jugular vein in chelonians. For lizards, intraosseous fluids can be given a 25- to 20-gauge spinal needle that is placed into the distal portion of the femur or humerus or into the proximal portion of the tibia (Figure 4-21). The catheter is placed using aseptic technique and is sutured to the skin for stability. It is then bandaged to protect the catheter site. This procedure is painful and requires either sedation with analgesia, general anesthesia, or the use of a local anesthetic.

The intracoelomic (ICe) route can also be used for administration of fluids and is often preferred. The patient should be placed in lateral recumbency, with the hind leg extended away from the body. The needle is then placed under the skin and into the coelomic cavity. Aspirate before administering any fluids to verify that the needle has not penetrated the bladder or lungs.

> **TECHNICIAN NOTE** Fluids are commonly administered by the intracoelomic (ICe) route.

TABLE 4-3	Common Intravenous Catheter Sites in Reptiles
SPECIES	**CATHETER SITES**
Chelonians	Jugular vein
Lizards	Ventral and lateral aspects of the caudal tail vein
Snakes	Ventral aspect of the caudal tail vein

(From Sirois M: *Principles and practice of veterinary technology*, ed 3, St. Louis, Mosby, 2011.)

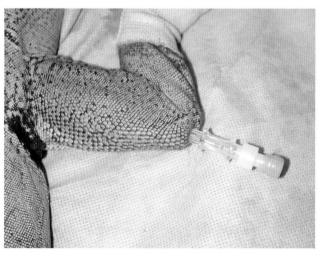

FIGURE 4-21. Intraosseous fluids in a lizard. (From Sirois M: *Principles and practice of veterinary technology*, ed 3, St. Louis, Mosby, 2011.)

ORAL MEDICATION

Oral medications can be given using a feeding tube or just titrated in with a syringe. Nutritional supplementation of hospitalized patients is generally given using syringe feeding. Tube feeding is comparable to that in birds. The mouth is opened with a speculum such as a plastic spatula. The tube is premeasured to estimate where the stomach is located before inserting it into the patient. As opposed to the metal tubes that are usually used in birds, a red rubber feeding tube is usually used with most reptile species (Figure 4-22). An esophagostomy tube can be placed in chelonians that will need long-term assisted feeding. Tube placement is done in a similar manner as it is in mammalian species.

> **TECHNICIAN NOTE** Oral medications can be given using a feeding tube or a syringe.

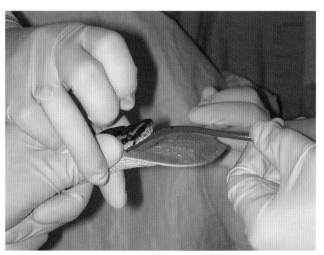

FIGURE 4-22. Tube feeding is best accomplished by opening the mouth with a soft plastic spatula, plastic card, or tape stirrups. (From Sirois M: *Principles and practice of veterinary technology*, ed 3, St. Louis, Mosby, 2011.)

Specific syringe-feeding diets are available, such as Oxbow Carnivore Care for carnivores or Oxbow Critical Care for herbivores. Omnivorous animals can have a mixture of the two. Other diets can be used as well, as long as they are complete and balanced. Insectivores can be fed an appropriate meat-based baby food.

ANESTHESIA

Preanesthetics should always be given to reptile patients before any anesthetic induction. Preanesthetics are given intramuscularly cranial to the kidneys to avoid the renal portal system and should be given at least 30 to 60 minutes before anesthetic induction. It is important to keep the patient warm to enable it to properly metabolize the drugs.

Common equipment used to monitor reptiles during anesthesia includes an electrocardiogram (ECG), Doppler, end tidal carbon dioxide monitor, and a temperature probe. The ECG is placed in the same manner as in mammals. The end tidal carbon dioxide monitor is attached to the endotracheal tube, and the temperature probe is placed either rectally or into the esophagus. Pulse oximetry is not reliable in reptiles and is therefore not commonly used. An intravenous catheter should be placed when possible. Lactated Ringer's solution or Normosol-R is commonly given intravenously at a rate of 5 ml/kg/hour.

Propofol is the most common injectable induction agent used in reptiles. Propofol is given intravenously slowly over a few minutes. Once the patient has been induced, it should be intubated and placed on isoflurane in oxygen at an appropriate percentage. Snakes do not have an epiglottis, making it very easy to intubate them after anesthetic induction. Once the endotracheal tube is placed, it is taped around either the mandible, maxilla, or around the back of the head to properly secure it (Figure 4-23).

The patient should be placed on a ventilator or bagged by hand to provide intermittent positive pressure ventilation (IPPV) throughout the procedure because reptiles do not breathe well on their own while under anesthesia. It is very important to keep the patient at an appropriate temperature during the surgical procedure. For most species of reptiles, core body temperature should be kept between about 80° and 90° F. If the patient is kept too cold, the drugs will take longer to metabolize and the patient will have a prolonged recovery time.

> **TECHNICIAN NOTE** For most species of reptiles, core body temperature should be kept between about 80° and 90° F during anesthesia.

Once the procedure is over, the inhalant anesthetic is turned off and the patient taken off of pure oxygen. The reptile's respiratory drive to take a breath is more oxygen driven than carbon

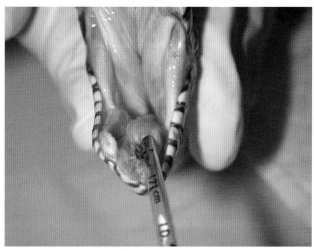

FIGURE 4-23. Endotracheal intubation in a snake. (From Sirois M: *Principles and practice of veterinary technology*, ed 3, St. Louis, Mosby, 2011.)

dioxide driven as in mammals. If kept on pure oxygen, the reptile patient has little drive to take a breath on its own and recovery will be very prolonged. An Ambu bag should be attached to the endotracheal tube, and the patient should be given a breath about four to six times per minute until the patient is awake and can be extubated. Postoperative analgesic medications should be given at the conclusion of the surgical procedure.

DIAGNOSTIC IMAGING

Diagnostic imaging is an important component of the evaluation of skeletal and soft tissues of reptiles. Radiographs of reptiles often have poor image contrast due to the superimposed scales, lack of separation of thorax and abdomen, and small amount of internal fat present. Digital radiology is quickly becoming the standard in most hospitals and will yield the best results. However, if digital radiology is not yet available in your hospital, high-detail, rare earth cassettes with single-emulsion film provide appropriate results. Mammography film will produce even better detail, but does require a higher KVP and MA. For extremely small patients, a dental radiology unit can be used. The recommended views for reptile patients are summarized in Table 4-4.

Snakes

Unless the snake is very sick, heavy sedation or general anesthesia is needed to obtain diagnostic-quality radiographs. A plastic tube can be used to immobilize the snake, or the snake can be taped to a padded board. Two views are normally taken, which include a dorsoventral (DV) or ventrodorsal (VD) and a lateral. If the entire body is to be imaged, the radiographs are taken in sections from head to tail and labeled with numbered lead markers to delineate each section.

Chelonians

Three views are normally taken, which include a dorsoventral (DV), horizontal lateral, and horizontal craniocaudal views. The craniocaudal view is taken to evaluate the left and right lung fields. A horizontal beam is essential to obtain good radiographs. Because chelonians do not have a diaphragm, placing them in lateral recumbency causes shifting of the organs into the lung cavity, which leads to poor radiographs. Most chelonians do not need to be sedated for radiographs, but chemical restraint can be used if necessary. In most cases the patient will just sit there, or it can be placed on a plastic dish with its feet hanging in the air.

Lizards

Two views are normally taken and a horizontal beam is necessary. As with chelonians, placing lizards in lateral recumbency causes shifting of the organs into the lung cavity. Anesthesia is recommended when obtaining radiographs from lizards due to their high activity level. Avian restraint boards can be used to restrain nonanesthetized lizards. Vagal stimulation or the "**vagal response**" to calm the patient if needed. The vagal response in iguanas and other medium to large lizard species can be induced by gently applying digital pressure to both eyes for a few seconds to a few minutes. The patient will usually respond with a decrease in heart rate and blood pressure. The vagal response can also be induced by placing cotton balls over the eyes (Figure 4-24). The vagal response induces a short-term, trancelike state, allowing time to take radiographs and in some cases even draw blood.

TABLE 4-4	Recommended Radiographic Exposures for Reptiles		
	DORSOVENTRAL*	CRANIOCAUDAL†	LATERAL†
Chelonians			
Respiratory tract		♦	♦
Digestive tract	♦		
Genitourinary system	♦		
Carapace and plastron	♦	♦	♦
Skeleton	♦		
Snakes			
Respiratory tract			♦
Digestive tract	♦		♦
Genitourinary system	♦		♦
Skeleton	♦		♦
Lizards			
Respiratory tract			♦
Digestive tract	♦		♦
Genitourinary system	♦		♦
Spine	♦		♦
Extremities	♦		

*Vertical radiograph beam.
†Horizontal radiograph beam.
(From Mader DR: *Reptile medicine and surgery*, ed 2, St. Louis, Saunders, 2006.)

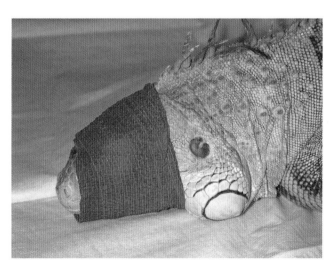

FIGURE 4-24. To induce the vagal response, place cotton balls over the eyes and lightly wrap an elastic wrap around the head. This wrap takes the place of digital pressure. (From Sirois M: *Principles and practice of veterinary technology*, ed 3, St. Louis, Mosby, 2011.)

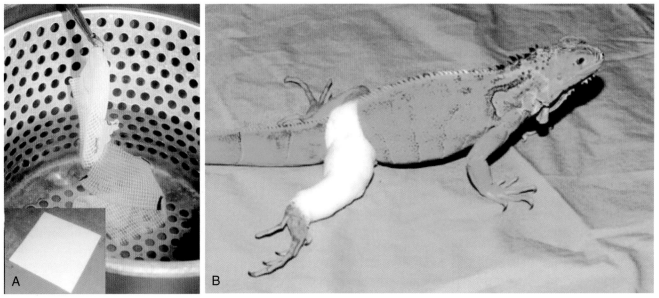

FIGURE 4-25. A, Several commercially available plastics are available that are designed for making lightweight, rigid casts and splints. Vet Thermoplastic comes as a rigid plastic square. When placed in hot water, it turns clear, softens, and can be manipulated like a standard cloth tape. The plastic hardens when it cools. **B,** These plastics can be cut off, reheated, and reused. (Photograph courtesy D. Mader.) (From Mader DR: *Reptile medicine and surgery*, ed 2, St. Louis, Saunders, 2006.)

BANDAGING AND WOUND MANAGEMENT

Some wounds are left open to heal in a clean environment. Bandages must not be bulky and interfere with normal behavior. When necessary, lightweight bandages and splints can be used. Tape cannot be used on reptiles with fragile skin. Plastic materials are commercially available that can be fashioned into light splints (Figure 4-25).

DIAGNOSTIC TESTING

Blood Collection

Venipuncture sites and maximum blood draw volume vary with different species (Table 4-5). The blood volume of most reptiles ranges between 5% and 8% of their total body weight, and 10% of the circulating blood volume can be withdrawn safely. Because only a small amount of blood is generally obtained, blood collection tubes such as Microtainers should be used. These tubes are made specifically for small amounts of blood and the anticoagulant is powdered rather than liquid. This helps to not dilute out the blood sample. The most common anticoagulants are EDTA (ethylenediaminetetraacetic acid) and lithium heparin. Heparin is preferred for collection of samples for biochemistry because plasma yield is higher than serum obtained from a plain tube. Clipping toenails to obtain a blood sample is painful for the animal and may introduce infection.

> TECHNICIAN NOTE Plasma collected in heparin is more commonly used than serum for biochemistry testing in reptiles.

TABLE 4-5	Common Venipuncture Sites in Reptiles
SPECIES	**VENIPUNCTURE SITES**
Chelonians	Radialhumoral plexus sinus (brachial sinus)
	Dorsal venous sinus (coccygeal vein)
	Jugular vein
	Subcarapacial venous sinus
	Femoral vein
Lizards	Ventral and lateral aspects of the caudal tail vein
Snakes	Heart
	Ventral aspect of the caudal tail vein

(From Sirois M: *Principles and practice of veterinary technology*, ed 3, St. Louis, Mosby, 2011.)

Lizards. The most common vessel used for lizard venipuncture is the caudal tail vein, also called the ventral coccygeal vein. The cephalic, jugular, and ventral abdominal vessels are not commonly used to obtain a blood sample. However, the cephalic vein is usually very small, and a surgical cut-down may be necessary. The jugular vein is not readily palpable or visible and may also require a surgical cut-down to access. The ventral abdominal vein is not generally used (especially in awake animals) because of the inability to both properly restrain the animal and control hemorrhage. Lizards usually struggle when they are placed on their backs, making it difficult to draw blood from them. Therefore, it is important to keep the animal in sternal recumbency while obtaining the blood sample. During the blood draw, it is also important that the phlebotomist gently restrain the caudal portion of the tail with one hand and obtain the blood sample with the other.

There are two different techniques commonly used to obtain blood from the caudal tail vein. These techniques include a lateral and ventral approach. For either method, a 1- or 1½-inch 27- to 20-gauge needle attached to a 1-ml or 3-ml syringe should generally be used. Insulin syringes can be used on very small lizards.

For a lateral approach, the needle should be inserted into the tail (between two scales) at approximately a 90-degree angle. Slowly insert the needle into the tail, keeping slight negative pressure on the syringe until either blood enters the syringe or the needle touches the vertebrae. If the needle is touching the vertebrae, slowly back the needle off the bone (still keeping slight negative pressure on the syringe) and redirect the needle into the vessel. It is important to put only slight negative pressure on the syringe while obtaining the blood sample. Too much negative pressure may collapse the vessel.

The technique for the ventral midline approach is very similar to that for the lateral approach. The needle is slowly inserted into the tail between two scales at approximately a 90-degree angle, keeping slight negative pressure on the syringe until either blood enters the syringe or the needle touches the vertebrae. The blood vessel is located just ventral to the vertebrae. If the needle is touching the vertebrae, slowly back off of the bone until the needle is seated within the vessel.

Snakes.
The caudal tail vein is a commonly used blood collection site in snakes. Drawing blood from the tail vein can be difficult in small snakes because of the size of the vessel. The same method used to draw blood from the ventral midline approach in lizards is used in snakes as well. Cardiocentesis can also be used for collection of blood samples and yields a greater volume of blood. The snake should first be placed in dorsal recumbency. The heart can then be located in the cranial one third of the body. The heart can move both cranially and caudally. Place your thumb and index finger on either side of the heart to minimize this movement. The needle insertion site is two scutes (scales) below the caudal portion of the heart. Insert the needle between two scutes at a 45-degree angle (Figure 4-26).

Chelonians.
The radial-humoral plexus (brachial plexus sinus), subcarapacial venous sinus, dorsal venous sinus (coccygeal vein), and jugular vein are the major sites where blood can be obtained from a turtle or tortoise. The venipuncture site will depend on the size and species of the patient and the preference of the phlebotomist. If blood is to be drawn from the jugular vein, the turtle/tortoise should be placed in lateral recumbency. The head and neck should be pulled away from the shell. The jugular vein can be found in the same plane as the eye and the tympanum. To obtain the sample, the phlebotomist will hold the head while the restrainer will keep the patient in lateral recumbency. A 27- to 20-gauge needle attached to a 1- to 3-ml syringe is used and will vary depending on the size of the patient.

The subcarapacial venous sinus is generally used when jugular venipuncture is not an option (Figure 4-27). Depending on the size of the patient, a 1- to 1½-inch, 27- to 20-gauge needle or a 2-inch spinal needle attached to a 1- to 3-ml syringe is used to obtain the blood sample. The needle is inserted upward at about a 60-degree angle just dorsal to the neck. Slight negative pressure should be applied on the syringe until either blood enters the syringe or bone is encountered. If bone is encountered, back away from the bone and redirect the needle.

The radial-humoral plexus sinus is generally used in larger chelonians. Pull the front limb away from the body and palpate the tendon near the radiohumeral joint. A 22- to 20-gauge needle attached to a 1- to 3-ml syringe is inserted at a 90-degree angle to skin and angled toward the radiohumeral joint.

When drawing blood from the dorsal venous sinus, the phlebotomist should place the patient in sternal recumbency. The tail should be held as straight as possible, and the needle should be inserted on midline. A 1- to 1½-inch 27- to 20-gauge needle attached to a 1- to 3-ml syringe should be used. The size of the syringe and needle will depend on the size of the patient. The needle should be inserted at a 45-degree angle into the tail. Slight negative pressure should be placed on the syringe, and the needle

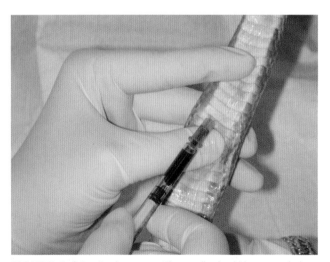

FIGURE 4-26. Cardiocentesis. The needle should be inserted about two scutes caudal to the last beating scale. (From Sirois M: *Principles and practice of veterinary technology*, ed 3, St. Louis, Mosby, 2011.)

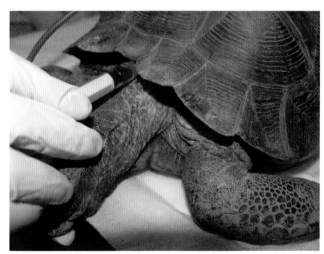

FIGURE 4-27. Blood collection from the subcarapacial venous sinus. (From Sirois M: *Principles and practice of veterinary technology*, ed 3, St. Louis, Mosby, 2011.)

should be inserted until it is either in the vein or touches bone. If bone is hit, slowly back the needle off the bone until blood enters the syringe.

Cloacal Wash

Cloacal washes are used to collect feces for laboratory analysis. A red rubber feeding tube of appropriate size is attached to a 1-ml syringe. The tube is well lubricated with a water-based jelly and placed into the cloaca. Saline is infused into the cloaca and aspirated back out. This lavage will often yield enough fecal material for microscopic analysis. A similar technique can be used to collect samples from the esophagus and stomach (Figure 4-28).

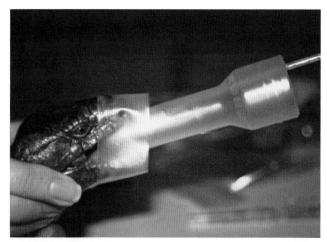

FIGURE 4-28. Gastric lavage of a conscious Solomon Island skink (*Corucia zebrata*). The cut-off syringe casing acts as a mouth gag and protects the lavage catheter. (From Mader DR: *Reptile medicine and surgery*, ed 2, St. Louis, Saunders, 2006.)

Skin Scrape and Touch Imprints

Performing skin scrapes and touch imprints is an easy way to obtain information on potential bacterial and fungal infections of the skin. A coverslip edge is gently scraped across the skin and then placed on a slide with saline, making a wet mount. This sample should be analyzed immediately to obtain accurate results. A touch or impression smear is primarily used on specific lesions such as ulcers or other damaged tissue. A microscope slide is touched to skin in an attempt to collect histologic data. The smear is then stained for analysis.

Tracheal Wash

To perform a tracheal wash, the mouth is gently opened using an appropriate mouth speculum. Using aseptic technique, the tracheal wash is performed by inserting a sterile red rubber feeding tube or polypropylene urinary catheter into the trachea. The patient must be anesthetized for the procedure because it can be very stressful and the tissues are very delicate. Generally, a small amount of saline is infused and then aspirated from the trachea. The volume will depend on the size of the patient. The sample should be smeared onto a slide and stained for analysis.

COMMON DISEASES

There are a large number of common conditions for which reptiles may be presented to the veterinary practice. Many of these are related to poor husbandry practices. A complete review of all reptile diseases is beyond the scope of this text. The most commonly encountered disorders are discussed below.

INFECTIOUS DISEASES

Reptiles are susceptible to infection with a number of bacterial, viral, and fungal agents as well as parasites of the blood and gastrointestinal system and ectoparasites. In some cases, the reptile is an asymptomatic carrier, and disease develops when the animal is under stress or kept in inappropriate husbandry conditions. Some of these organisms have significant zoonotic potential. Bacterial infections are probably the most common infectious disease observed in reptiles. Most gram-positive bacteria are considered nonpathogenic in reptiles. Gram-negative bacteria that may infect reptiles include *Escherichia coli, Pseudomonas* spp., *Aeromonas* spp., *Citrobacter, Proteus* spp., *Serratia* spp., *Klebsiella* spp., *Enterobacter* spp., *Yersinia* spp., *Mycobacterium* spp., *Pasturella* spp., and *Salmonella* spp.

TECHNICIAN NOTE Reptiles are susceptible to infection with a number of bacterial, viral, and fungal agents as well as parasites of the blood and gastrointestinal system and ectoparasites.

Parasites

Ectoparasites of reptiles include ticks and mites. Leeches may parasitize aquatic reptiles.

Protozoal endoparasites of reptiles include those in the genera *Entamoeba, Isospora, Eimeria, Sarcocystis,* and *Cryptosporidium.* The most commonly found hemoparasites are in the genera *Plasmodium, Haemoproteus, Haemogregarina, Hepatozoon,* and *Trypanosoma.* Although reptiles can be infected with trematode parasites, most do not result in clinical signs. A large number of cestodes and nematodes are able to parasitize reptiles. Diagnosis of endoparasitism is usually made by direct fecal examination, fecal flotation, or cloacal wash.

Pneumonia

A number of bacterial, viral, and fungal agents are capable of infecting the lower respiratory tract of reptiles. In general, reptiles are most susceptible when their enclosures are not properly sanitized or when environmental conditions are not appropriate. Poor nutrition may also be a predisposing factor. Clinical manifestations include open-mouth breathing or breathing with the head and neck extended. Diagnosis involves a complete physical examination, thorough patient history, radiographs, and endoscopy. A transtracheal wash is often indicated.

NONINFECTIOUS DISEASES

Dysecdysis

Some reptiles will have problems shedding the skin. This is called dysecdysis. If the patient is having problems shedding the skin, the humidity and/or temperature in the cage should be increased or the animal can be soaked in a warm water bath. Always examine the toes of lizards such as leopard geckos if they are having problems shedding their skin as the skin can become wrapped around the digits, cutting off circulation and causing necrosis. The shed skin should be examined to verify that all of the skin has been shed. Snakes and some geckos have eye caps or spectacles that represent fused eyelids. Incomplete shedding can result in retained spectacles and give a dull and dry appearance to the eye caps. This can occur on one or both eyes.

> **TECHNICIAN NOTE** Examine the skin after it has been shed to verify a complete shed.

Thermal Injury

Captive reptiles are prone to thermal burns from heat lamps and hot rocks. This may be due to malfunction of or inappropriate use of these items, poor cage ventilation, or may simply result from an animal falling asleep under the heat lamp. The temperature of the heat source and duration of exposure affect the severity of the burns as well as the prescribed treatment (Table 4-6). First-degree burns are superficial and involve only the epidermis. The epidermis is completely destroyed in second-degree burns and damage to the underlying dermis may be present. Third-degree burns are characterized by complete destruction of the skin. If the underlying muscle is also involved, the burn is classified as

TABLE 4-6	Treatment of Burns

First-Degree Burns
Brief cool-water rinses, cold compresses.
Do not open blisters; if open, keep clean.
Antibiotics/analgesics usually not necessary if burn is minor.

Second-Degree Burns
Analgesics (butorphenol, nonsteroidal antiinflammatory drugs [NSAIDS]).
Antibiotics (systemic ceftazidime, amikacin, topical silver sulfadiazine; can switch to oral antibiotics for chronic treatment as needed).
Daily debriding and wound care (with or without anesthesia, wet-to-dry, sugar or honey bandages).
Fluid therapy (intravenous [IV], intracoelomic [ICe], oral).
Ensure adequate nutrition (assist-feed as needed).

Third-Degree (and Fourth-Degree) Burns
As in second-degree burns, just more extensive.
Pay close attention to analgesia as the wounds start to heal because pain usually intensifies.

(From Mader DR: *Reptile medicine and surgery*, ed 2, St. Louis, Saunders, 2006.)

fourth-degree. Aseptic technique and proper pain management is an important aspect of burn treatment.

> **TECHNICIAN NOTE** The temperature of the heat source and duration of exposure affect the severity of the burns as well as the prescribed treatment for thermal burns.

Shell Trauma

Shell damage in chelonians can occur as a result of poor water quality, inappropriate substrates, inadequate nutrition, stress, and insufficient ultraviolet light exposure. Damage due to trauma from being dropped or being bitten by domestic or wild animals also occurs. Treatment varies but generally includes evaluation of husbandry conditions and correction of inappropriate environmental parameters. Fractures can be stabilized with orthopedic wire.

Bite Wounds

Bite wounds can occur as a result of exposure to domestic or wild animals or from live prey in the enclosure (Figure 4-29). Reptiles housed in groups may also be subject to bites from cagemates. Bacterial infections are common, and wounds must be carefully treated using aseptic technique. Antibiotics and pain management are also important components of treatment.

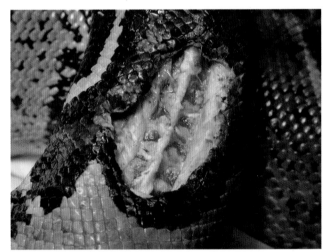

FIGURE 4-29. This wound was caused by offering live prey. The snake did not eat the rat and was left alone with it for a few days. When the owner returned, the rat had caused severe damage to the flesh and vertebrae. (From Sirois M: *Principles and practice of veterinary technology*, ed 3, St. Louis, Mosby, 2011.)

Organ Prolapse

Cloacal prolapses and prolapse of the copulatory organs can occur in reptiles. In addition to the cloaca itself, the bladder may also prolapse from the cloaca. Any condition that causes straining (e.g., gastroenteritis, impactions) can lead to prolapse. Treatment varies depending on the specific tissues involved. Exposed tissues must be kept clean and moist. It is possible to replace the tissues through the cloaca. Trauma to the penis or hemipenis during copulation may be severe enough to cause swelling sufficient to prevent retraction of the organ. Should the trauma be severe and the tissues become dessicated or necrotic, the organ may require amputation.

Nutritional Diseases

Metabolic Bone Disease. **Metabolic bone disease (MBD)** is usually the result of long-term dietary deficiency of calcium or vitamin D, a lack of exposure to UV light, and/or a negative dietary calcium-to-phosphorus ratio. Common dietary causes include a lack of bone in the diet of carnivorous animals and a lack of calcium with excess phosphorus in herbivorous diets. Common clinical signs include a pliable mandible or maxillae, kyphosis, scoliosis, fractures, tremors, lameness, abnormal shell development and pyramiding of the shell in chelonians, or the overall inability to move.

Hypovitaminosis A. This disorder is most commonly seen in chelonians that are fed a diet of vitamin A–poor foods such as iceberg lettuce and cucumbers. The disease can affect numerous epithelial tissues. The most common clinical sign is edema of the eyelids (**blepharedema**) (Figure 4-30). Conjunctivitis, anorexia, nasal and ocular discharge, and rhinitis can also occur.

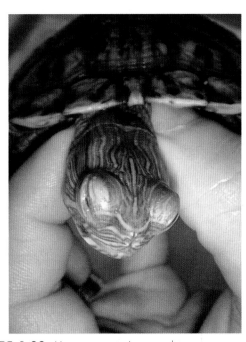

FIGURE 4-30. Hypovitaminosis A can result in squamous metaplasia of various tissues in a chelonian. In this box turtle, the animal presented with blepharedema. (Photograph courtesy Dr. David Sanchez-Migallon Guzman.) (From Mitchell M, Thomas T: *Manual of exotic pet practice,* St. Louis, WB Saunders Company, 2009.)

Gout. **Gout** results from an increase in uric acid in the bloodstream that results in the deposition of the excess uric acid crystals around the joints, in the subcutaneous space, and in the viscera. Risk factors that contribute to the development of gout include dehydration and kidney damage that lead to decreased excretion of uric acid. Excessive protein intake, such as occurs when herbivorous animals are fed an animal protein source diet (e.g., iguanas fed a cat food diet) can also result in gout.

EUTHANASIA

Euthanasia can be difficult because it can sometimes be hard to access a vessel. A euthanasia barbiturate solution can be given into any vessel, the heart, or into the coelomic cavity. If the injection is into the heart, the patient must be anesthetized. An electrocardiograph or Doppler can be used to check for a heartbeat. However, the heart may continue to beat for several minutes to several hours after administration of the euthanasia solution, even though the patient may be clinically dead. The patient should be kept in the clinic overnight to ensure it has been properly euthanized before sending it home with the owner if that is the owner's preference.

KEY POINTS

- Reptiles include those in the order Squamata (snakes and lizards) and those in the superorder Chelonia (turtles and tortoises).
- Lizards and chelonians can be carnivorous, omnivorous, or herbivorous. Snakes are strict carnivores.
- Reptile excrement includes three components: urine, urates, and feces.
- Reptiles have a three-chambered heart with two atria and one ventricle.
- The unique behaviors seen in reptiles are specific adaptations that evolved to allow them to obtain food, escape predation, or reproduce.
- The reptile enclosure must have a thermal gradient that allows for both warmer and cooler areas within the enclosure, as well as an area of high humidity in the enclosure.
- Food and water should be provided in a manner that mimics what the reptile would encounter in the wild.
- A thorough physical examination begins with visual observation then proceeds to an evaluation of all systems starting at the head and working toward the tail.
- Injections are most often administered intramuscularly or subcutaneously. To avoid the renal portal system, injections are usually given in the front limbs.
- Oral medications can be given using a feeding tube or a syringe.
- Common equipment used to monitor reptiles during anesthesia includes an electrocardiogram (ECG), Doppler, end tidal carbon dioxide monitor, and a temperature probe.
- Venipuncture sites and maximum blood draw volume vary with different species.
- Plasma collected in heparin is more commonly used than serum for biochemistry testing in reptiles.
- Ectoparasites of reptiles include ticks and mites.

- Protozoal endoparasites of reptiles include those in the genera *Entamoeba, Isospora, Eimeria, Sarcocystis,* and *Cryptosporidium.*
- The most commonly found hemoparasites in reptiles are in the genera *Plasmodium, Haemoproteus, Haemogregarina, Hepatozoon,* and *Trypanosoma.*
- Diagnosis of endoparasitism is usually made by direct fecal examination, fecal flotation, or cloacal wash.
- Noninfectious diseases of reptiles include dysecdysis, thermal injury, shell trauma, bite wounds, organ prolapse, and nutritional diseases.
- Nutritional diseases of reptiles include metabolic bone disease, hypovitaminosis A, and gout.

REVIEW QUESTIONS

1. Give an example of a type of animal commonly seen in veterinary practice that belongs to the order of Squatmata.

2. Shed snake skins are used in _____ _____ research.

3. Reptiles have one visceral cavity called a _____ and lack a _____ to separate the thoracic and abdominal cavities.

4. The process of shedding the outermost layer of skin is referred to as _____.

5. The shell of chelonians is comprised of the dorsal _____ and ventral _____.

6. Reptiles have a network of vessels associated with the kidneys referred to as the _____ _____ _____.

7. Most reptiles require ultraviolet light in order to produce _____.

8. List examples of appropriate substrates that can be used in reptile cages.

9. _____ is a significant zoonotic disease carried by reptiles.

10. Why should live prey not be fed to captive carnivore reptiles?

11. Why should injectionable medications be given in the front limbs of reptiles?

12. List the common equipment used to monitor reptiles under anesthesia.

13. List the radiographic views that should be taken on chelonians.

14. It is safe to collect _____ percent of the circulating blood volume in reptiles.

15. List and explain the noninfectious diseases of reptiles.

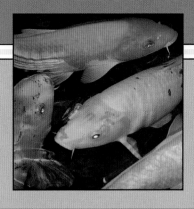

5 Amphibians and Fish

LEARNING OBJECTIVES

After studying this chapter, you will be able to:

- Describe the unique features of the anatomy of common amphibian and fish species.
- Explain the different capture and restraint techniques used for amphibians and fish.
- Identify methods of sample collection for laboratory analysis.
- Describe how to obtain high-quality diagnostic images of amphibian and fish patients.
- Discuss nursing care and supportive therapy techniques for the amphibian and fish patient.
- Describe the routine clinical procedures performed on fish and amphibian species.
- Identify and discuss some of the common presentations, emergencies, and critical care.

There are more than 20,000 species of fish that vary significantly in their appearance, physiology, genetics, behavior, and ecology. Both freshwater and saltwater species may be seen in the veterinary practice and in the research setting. **Amphibians** are a large class of vertebrates that live at least part of their life cycle in water. They are a diverse group of animals that have become popular pets over the last several years. While there are over 4000 species alive today, only a few are commonly seen in most clinical practices.

TAXONOMY

There are three taxonomic orders of amphibians, with some variation in terminology used to describe the groups. The Anurans, also known as Salentia, are the largest group of amphibians and include the frogs and toads. The Urodela, also known as Caudata, consist of the newts and salamanders. One common member of this group is the Axolotls. This species is unique in that it retains a tadpolelike appearance throughout its adult life. The third group is the Apoda, or Gymnophiona. These are commonly referred to as the "legless" amphibians and are not generally used in biomedical research. The amphibian species most commonly used for biomedical research are *Xenopus laevis* (African clawed frog), *Necturus* (mudpuppies), *Rana pipiens* (leopard, meadow, or grass frogs), and *Ambystoma* (salamander). *Xenopus* species are also commonly seen in veterinary practice. Other popular amphibians that may be seen in practice include dwarf clawed frogs (*Hymenochirus* species), ornate horned frogs (*Ceratophrys* spp.)

(Figure 5-1), toads (*Bufo* spp.), poison dart frogs (*Dendrobates* spp., *Phyllobates* spp., *Epipidobates* spp.), frogs (*Rana* spp.), and tree frogs (*Hyla* spp.).

Taxonomic groups of fish represent the largest number of vertebrate species with more than 25,000 different species. Several hundred different species are commonly kept in captivity. Both freshwater and marine species are available in the pet trade and kept in homes as well as used in biomedical research. Goldfish *(Carassius auratus auratus)* and koi *(Cyprinus carpio)* (Figure 5-2) are some of the more commonly kept species in homes. Biomedical research facilities commonly keep zebrafish (Danio rerio), as well as trout, salmon, and catfish.

Fish and amphibians may be wild caught or farm or laboratory reared. In some cases, the use of wild-caught animals requires special permits from fish and wildlife divisions of the federal or state government. Aquatic animals, especially those that are wild caught, can harbor a number of potential

human pathogens. This is a particular problem when the animals are maintained in a closed system in a laboratory environment because any microorganisms that may be present are concentrated in a small space. Newly acquired amphibians are usually quarantined for 30 days before introduction into a colony. Regular visual inspections occur during the quarantine period. Organisms that have been associated with human disease include *Aeromonas hydrophila*, atypical *Mycobacteria, Campylobacter* species, *Pseudomonas* species, *Salmonella* species, and *Vibrio* species. To minimize the potential for these infections, caretakers must practice good hygiene. Hands should always be washed with an antimicrobial soap after handling animals or working in their environment. Open wounds must be covered to prevent inoculation.

> **TECHNICIAN NOTE** Aquatic animals, especially those that are wild caught, can harbor a number of potential human pathogens.

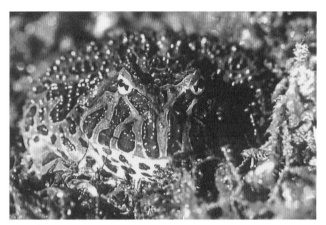

FIGURE 5-1. An Argentine horned frog *(Ceratophrys ornata)*. (From Rabinowitz PM, Conti LA: *Human-animal medicine: clinical approaches to zoonoses, toxicants and other shared health risks*, St. Louis, Saunders, 2010.)

ANIMAL MODELS

Amphibians or their tissues have been used in studies of embryology, pharmacology, skin permeability, and limb regeneration. The unique susceptibility of amphibians to dissolved toxins has made them useful in research of agricultural waste and its effect on surface and ground water.

The use of fish in biomedical research has been steadily increasing, in part because of an increasing focus on finding replacement animal models for higher vertebrate species. Research into aquaculture methods has expanded, and interest in keeping pet fish has increased. Studies of fish health and husbandry have focused on increasing the availability of fish as a high-quality food source as well as addressing concerns regarding environmental pollution, conservation, and protection of the freshwater estuarine and marine environment.

The diversity among species is one reason why fish have been useful animal models. One of the earliest studies on renal tubular secretion used the aglomerular toadfish. Arctic species of fish contain antifreeze-like molecules of interest to researchers. Other research involving fish include studies of electrical activity in muscles of the electrical eel and copper accumulation in white perch. Fish are also used as models for research on aging, vision, locomotion in cells, and leukemia. Species are also evaluated for pharmacologically active compounds, such as Indian catfish venom and antineoplastic agents in shark tissue. Other uses of fish as animal models include research into type 1 diabetes in carp and monkfish, hepatocellular carcinoma in rainbow trout, muscular dystrophy in the Japanese puffer fish, and malignant melanoma in swordtail and platyfish hybrids.

Zebrafish are one of the most common fish used in biomedical research. Studies of neuroscience, carcinogenicity, mutagenesis, toxicology, and genetics have been performed with zebrafish. Part of what makes the zebrafish a valuable animal model includes its nearly transparent embryo, which

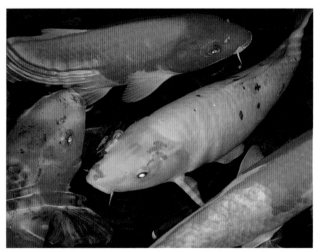

FIGURE 5-2. Koi *(Cyprinus carpio)* represent one of the most coveted groups of fish. These animals are prized for their color, size, and longevity. Their desirability is reflected in their value, with prized individuals selling for tens to hundreds of thousands of dollars. (From Mitchell M, Thomas T: *Manual of exotic pet practice*, St. Louis, Saunders, 2009.)

allows for easy observation of development. An artificial hemophilia has been induced in zebrafish, and research into new treatments for hemophilia are being evaluated.

UNIQUE ANATOMIC AND PHYSIOLOGIC FEATURES

The three orders of amphibians show considerable variation in anatomy. Common characteristics of amphibians include highly glandular, permeable skin. Characteristics of common amphibians are located in Table 5-1. Two types of skin glands are present: mucous and granular. Mucous glands keep the skin surface moist to allow respiration through the skin, but they also put the animals at risk of desiccation. The granular glands secrete toxins and function primarily for defense.

Amphibians have a three-chambered heart, and gas exchange occurs both at the alveoli and through the skin. Amphibians are ectotherms and therefore require external heat sources. Hypothermia can result in lethargy and immunosuppression. Hyperthermia is often fatal. Sexual dimorphism is common. In most species, eggs are fertilized externally and hatch to the larval form, such as the tadpole. Amphibian larvae possess gills.

Fish are a highly diverse group of animals and few generalizations can be made regarding their anatomy. Fish have cells in their integument that secrete a mucus coating that serves as a barrier to pathogens. Overlapping scales protect the underlying musculature. Fish also have gills that serve as the primary organs of respiration. They are nearly all **ectothermic** and use fins for locomotion (Figure 5-3). A **swim bladder**

is used for buoyancy, allowing the fish to rise or fall within the water by altering the volume of air in this structure. The digestive system varies depending on diet, with herbivorous fish having a longer digestive tract than carnivorous fish. The reproductive system is also highly variable, with both oviparous ad viviparous species. The circulatory system is characterized by a simple two-chambered heart. Blood leaves the ventricle and is pumped through the arteries to the gills. Gas exchange takes place in the small blood vessels of the gills. The blood then continues through the rest of the body, delivering oxygen and picking up nutrients that are also transported to other organs. Carbon dioxide is also transferred into the blood, which eventually travels back to the atrium of the heart.

> **TECHNICIAN NOTE** Fish and amphibians have an outer coating of mucoid material.

HUSBANDRY, HOUSING, NUTRITION

The primary species of amphibians used in biomedical research are aquatic or partly aquatic. Pet amphibians can also include those that are partly **arboreal**. All can be maintained in either a plastic cage or aquarium. The enclosure must have smooth sides because the delicate skin of amphibians is easily damaged by rough surfaces. Bottled spring water or conditioned tap water may be used for housing. Conditioned water can be obtained by allowing an open container of water to sit for 24 hours before use. Chlorine and other additives contained in tap water are toxic to many amphibians.

Regardless of the type of enclosure or species, the native habitat should be mimicked whenever possible. The best way to provide a proper habitat is to do ample research about the species involved. For example, a terrestrial cage may consist of mosses, various plants, rocks, logs, and a small amount

TABLE 5-1	Characteristics of Selected Amphibian Species		
FAMILY	**NUMBER OF SPECIES**	**EXAMPLE**	**COMMENTS**
Order Anura			
Bufonidae	350	American toad	Terrestrial species
Pipidae	26	Xenopus	Aquatic frogs; tongueless
Ranidae	700	Leopard frog	Worldwide distribution
Order Urodela (Caudata)			
Ambystomatidae	35	Mole salamanders	Axolotl (*Ambystoma mexacanum*) is unmetamorphosed (neotenous)
Sirenidae	3	Sirens	Lack hindlimbs; external gills
Order Gymnophiona			
Ichthyophiidae	37	Koh Tao island caecilian	Limbless; nocturnal

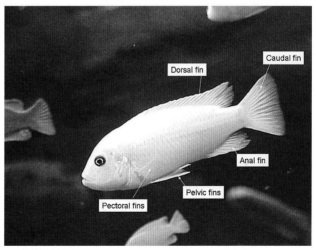

FIGURE 5-3. Fish generally have two sets of paired fins, the pectoral and pelvic, and three unpaired fins, the dorsal, anal, and caudal. (From Mitchell M, Thomas T: *Manual of exotic pet practice*, St. Louis, Saunders, 2009.)

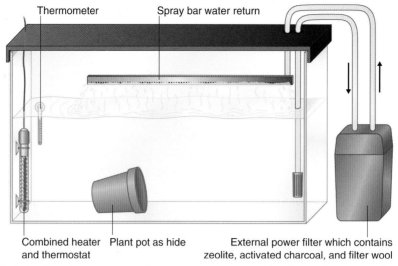

Thermometer   Spray bar water return

Combined heater   Plant pot as hide
and thermostat

External power filter which contains
zeolite, activated charcoal, and filter wool

FIGURE 5-4. Clinical aquarium setup. (From Jepson L: *Exotic animal medicine*, St. Louis, Saunders, 2009.)

of water in the cage. An aquatic cage will have a completely different set of criteria. If the amphibian is arboreal, you must provide height in the cage so it can climb into a planted canopy. Many species also need a temperature and humidity gradient in the cage. Optimal temperatures for housing vary tremendously because amphibians originate in a wide variety of climates.

> | **TECHNICIAN NOTE** Chlorine and other additives contained in tap water are toxic to many amphibians.

Most require a fairly high relative humidity of approximately 80%. Whether the cage is set up for an aquatic species or a terrestrial species, you must maintain proper lighting, heating, humidity, water quality parameters, and cleanliness. Most diseases in exotic animals are caused from poor husbandry and improper diet.

NEWTS AND GRASS FROGS

Newts and grass frogs require both a wet and a dry area in the same cage. This can be provided by adding an inclined shelf to the cage bottom. Newts can be housed in groups of 10 to 15 animals. Clear plastic or glass aquariums are suitable for housing. Water is usually changed every few days, and cages are completely cleaned weekly.

XENOPUS FROGS

Several species of *Xenopus* are used in biomedical research. These include *X. laevis* (South African clawed toad), *X. borealis* (Kenyan clawed toad), *X. tropicalis,* and *X. epitropicalis* (Nigerian clawed toad). All these species are entirely aquatic. They are usually housed singly or in breeding groups with a maximum of one adult animal per gallon of water. The water should be changed several times each week and the inside of the cage cleaned with a soft brush at least weekly. Care must be taken to avoid the use of harsh detergents because even a slight residue of this in the cage can be toxic to the frogs.

When changing cages, it is important to protect the skin of the frog from desiccation. The new tank should be set up in advance and the animals moved into it with a fish net. An alternative mechanism for housing can be accomplished by using a continuous water flow system. Conditioned water is provided through a tap or faucet above the cage. Water passes from the faucet into the cage, and excess is removed by a drainpipe in the cage. The flow rate is set to provide a twice daily water change in the tank. Conditioned water is continuously provided for these tanks through a faucet above each tank. Carbon filters can be used in this system to improve the water quality. Debris and waste materials can be removed from the tank with a small net. Tanks do not have to be emptied or disinfected unless new groups of animals are being placed in the tank. This system is somewhat more complicated to maintain, and the water must still be tested regularly. An advantage of this system is that the animals do not need to be handled as often, so injuries are less likely to occur.

Many fish species in the pet trade and in biomedical research originate in tropical or subtropical areas. Ambient water temperatures in the range of 76° to 78° F are suitable for most species. Goldfish and koi are coldwater species with a preferred ambient temperature of 65° to 68° F. Fish are kept in acrylic or glass aquariums. A variety of sizes and shapes are available. Figure 5-4 shows an aquarium setup that may be used in the veterinary practice for convalescing aquatic species.

WATER QUALITY

All aquatic animal enclosures must have regular water quality assessment to ensure the health of the animals. The use of municipal tap water should be avoided due to the likely presence of chorine, which is toxic to aquatic species. Ideal water quality parameters for amphibians are presented in Table 5-2. Recommended water quality parameters for koi and goldfish are presented in Table 5-3.

Animals excrete waste products, such as ammonia, that alter the chemical composition of the water. In addition, food particles can remain in the water and affect water quality. A filtration system must be used that helps to remove some of

TABLE 5-2 | Water Chemistry Parameters for Amphibians

PARAMETER	NORMAL	SUBLETHAL	LETHAL
Dissolved oxygen	≥5 mg/L	2-4 mg/L	<2 mg/L
Ammonia (unionized)	<0.01 mg/L	0.5 mg/L	>1 mg/L
Nitrite	<0.1 mg/L	0.015-0.1 mg/L	>0.1 mg/L
Nitrate	0-5 mg/L	20-50 mg/L	Species dependent
pH	Species specific (~6.5-8.5)	5.5-6.5; 8.6-9.5	5.5-6.5; 8.6-9.5
Gas pressure	28 mmHg	28-78 mmHg	>78 mmHg
Hardness	75-150 mg/L	>150-250 mg/L skin lesions can occur	Unknown
Alkalinity	20-100 mg/L	>100 mg/L	Unknown
Chlorine (tadpoles)	0-2 ppm	2-4 ppm	>5 ppm

(From Mitchell M, Thomas T: *Manual of exotic pet practice*, St. Louis, Saunders, 2009.)

TABLE 5-3 | Recommended Water Quality Parameters for Koi and Goldfish

PARAMETER	VALUE
Temperature (°C)	10-30 (preferred range = 22-28 for koi)
pH	6.0-8.4 (preferred 7.0-8.0)
Hardness (CaCO$_3$) (mg/L)	100-250
Conductivity (mS/cm)	180-480
Ammonia (total) (mg/L)	<0.02
Nitrite (mg/L)	<0.2
Nitrate (above ambient tapwater levels) (mg/L)	<40
Oxygen (mg/L)	5.0-8.0
Chlorine (mg/L)	0.002

(From Jepson L: *Exotic animal medicine*, St. Louis, Saunders, 2009.)

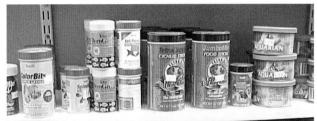
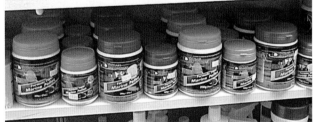

FIGURE 5-5. A wide variety of fish food is commercially available. (From Mitchell M, Thomas T: *Manual of exotic pet practice*, St. Louis, Saunders, 2009.)

these components from the water. A variety of filtration systems are commercially available and more than one type of system can be used at the same time. Aquarium water should be regularly assessed for pH, temperature, ammonia, nitrites, hardness, and alkalinity.

NUTRITION

Adult amphibians are carnivorous or insectivorous; tadpoles are usually herbivorous. Fish species can be herbivorous or carnivorous. The goal should be to replicate the animal's natural diet as much as possible. The key to providing a healthy diet is offering a variety of different types of food. For example, just crickets or just neonatal mice should not be offered every single day. Providing an improper diet will lead to severe life-threatening nutritional disorders. Some species eat daily while others do not. Some species will eat only in the water, other species may eat only flying insects, and still others will eat only prey that is alive and moving around.

Detailed information on the nutritional requirements of many ornamental fish is not readily available. Pelleted feeds are available for some species (Figure 5-5). They may also be fed meat diets or live invertebrates.

> **TECHNICIAN NOTE** A nutritional goal for fish and amphibians is to replicate the natural diet as much as possible.

HANDLING AND RESTRAINT

Fish should be transported in a plastic, sealed container. The container must be clean and thoroughly rinsed. Water from the home aquarium should be used to fill the container. The client should be advised to bring an additional water sample in case water quality must be tested.

Whenever possible, an amphibian patient should be transported to the veterinary clinic in its primary enclosure. This will allow the veterinary staff to evaluate the overall environment of the animal. Transport cages are also available for small amphibians (Figure 5-6).

A small net can be used to handle amphibians. Amphibian skin is covered with a layer of slimy mucus. This serves to protect the animal from infections and the environment. It also makes the animals particularly slippery and

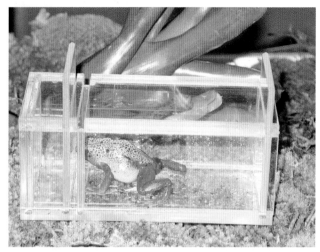

FIGURE 5-6. A blue poison dart frog *(Dendrobates azureus)* shifting into a transport crate. (From Mader DR, Divers SJ: *Current therapy in reptile medicine and surgery,* St. Louis, Elsevier, 2013.)

TABLE 5-4	Routes of Medication Administration in Amphibians
ROUTE	**COMMENTS**
Intracoelomic route	Injections can be given into the coelom in larger amphibians.
Intramuscular route	Medications can be given IM, but some medications can cause damage to the muscle or internal organs.
Oral route	If the GI tract works, use it. Oral medications can be given using a feeding tube or just titrated in with a syringe.
Subcutaneous route	Subcutaneous injections can be given if needed. This is usually performed in large toads and salamanders.
Topical route	Many medications can be given topically owing to systemic absorption.

(From Sirois M: *Principles and practice of veterinary technology,* ed 3, St. Louis, Mosby, 2011.)

difficult to handle. Amphibians should always be held with wet hands or gloves to prevent abrading the skin. Gloves should be nonpowdered to avoid damaging the skin and mucus coating. Aquatic salamanders should be handled gently to prevent damage to the exposed gill fronds.

Fish can be captured with a net and examined on a wet towel. The fish must be sedated when performing a complete examination.

CLINICAL PROCEDURES

ADMINISTRATION OF MEDICATIONS

Common routes for administration of medications to amphibians are located in Table 5-4.

Sedation or anesthesia can be achieved by immersing the animal in a tank of water containing an anesthetic or be placing an anesthetic-soaked gauze pad on the skin. Many medications can simply be added to the water and are absorbed through the skin. After anesthesia, the animals must be placed in a large tank with copious amounts of fresh water to allow the anesthetic to disperse. *Xenopus* species may also be given injections into the dorsal lymph sacs. Intramuscular injections can be given in the epaxial muscles of fish (Figure 5-7). Intraperitoneal (intracoelomic) injections are commonly used to administer medications to fish (Figure 5-8).

> **TECHNICIAN NOTE** Intraperitoneal (intracoelomic) and intramuscular injections can be administered to fish and amphibians.

BLOOD COLLECTION

Blood collection can be very challenging in amphibians and fish. Alcohol should not be used to clean the venipuncture site.

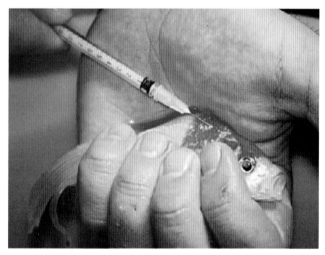

FIGURE 5-7. Intramuscular injections are routinely given in the epaxial muscles. (From Mitchell M, Thomas T: *Manual of exotic pet practice,* St. Louis, Saunders, 2009.)

This can irritate and/or desiccate the patient's skin. A 1:40 diluted 2% chlorhexidine solution should be used to cleanse the site instead.

Venipuncture in salamanders is generally performed using the caudal tail vein. This is the same technique described previously for both lizards and snakes. It is important to remember that the vessel is very small and can collapse easily; therefore, do not place a large amount of negative pressure on the syringe during collection. A 25- to 27-gauge needle attached to a 1-ml syringe should be used. An insulin syringe

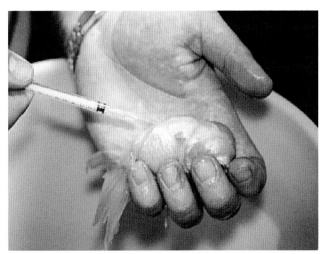

FIGURE 5-8. Intraperitoneal (intracoelomic) injection in a fish. (From Mitchell M, Thomas T: *Manual of exotic pet practice*, St. Louis, Saunders, 2009.)

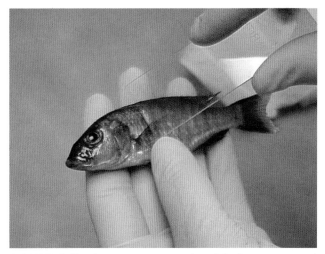

FIGURE 5-9. Skin scraping using a glass slide drawn in a cranial to caudal direction. (From Mitchell M, Thomas T: *Manual of exotic pet practice*, St. Louis, Saunders, 2009.)

can also be used for very small patients. The blood sample should be placed in a heparinized Microtainer tube for analysis.

Venipuncture sites in frogs and toads include the femoral vein, ventral abdominal vein, and the lingual vein. The femoral and lingual veins are rarely used. The ventral abdominal vein is by far the easiest vessel to obtain a blood sample from. The frog or toad is gently positioned on its back with the restrainer holding the pectoral girdle. The person drawing blood can hold the pelvic girdle with one hand and draw blood with the other hand. Some amphibians will need to be anesthetized for venipuncture. A 1-ml syringe with a 25- to 27-gauge needle is generally used to obtain the sample although an insulin syringe can be used as well. The blood sample should be placed into a heparinized Microtainer tube for analysis.

The caudal tail vein, which runs midline just below the caudal vertebrae, is the primary site for venipuncture in fish. In small fish this can be accessed via the ventral midline while in larger fish a lateral approach is usually used.

Blood volume needs to be considered in these small patients. No more than 1% of the body weight should be taken in blood volume from healthy fish and amphibians, and no more than 0.5% should be taken from sick patients.

Cloacal Wash

Cloacal washes are used to collect feces for laboratory analysis. This is very common because fresh stool is often not available. A red rubber feeding tube of appropriate size is attached to a 1.0-mL syringe. The tube is well lubricated with a water-based jelly and placed into the cloaca. Isotonic saline (0.6%) is infused into the cloaca and aspirated back out. In most species, approximately 0.5 to 1.0 mL of fluid is used. This lavage will often yield enough fecal material for microscopic analysis.

Culture Collection

Culture collection is accomplished by simply swabbing the area in question with a sterile culture swab. Both bacterial and fungal cultures can be performed. Blood cultures can be performed in amphibian species provided they have enough blood to take for the sample.

Endoscopy

Rigid endoscopy can be performed in many amphibians by passing the endoscope through the oral cavity and into the stomach. This is generally only done in larger amphibians that are under anesthesia. Endoscopy is primarily used to obtain gastric biopsies or to retrieve foreign bodies from the stomach.

Fecal Examination

Performing a fecal examination in amphibians is done in the same manner as in dogs and cats. The two most common fecal examinations include the fecal flotation and direct smear. For a fecal flotation, the feces are examined using standard commercial fecal flotation solutions. To perform a direct fecal smear, the feces are smeared onto a slide and 0.9% saline is applied to examine the feces under a microscope. Common ova include nematodes, trematodes, coccidian, protozoans, and lung worm larvae.

Skin Scrape and Touch Smears

Performing skin scrapes or touch (impression) smears is an easy way to obtain information on potential bacterial, fungal, or protozoal infections of the skin. A coverslip edge or glass slide is gently scraped across the skin and then placed on a slide with saline making a wet mount (Figure 5-9). This sample should be analyzed immediately to obtain accurate results. Skin scrapes should not be performed on specific lesions because this can cause more damage to the skin. A touch or impression smear is primarily used on specific lesions such as ulcers or other damaged tissue. A microscope

BOX 5-1	Common Diseases and Presentations in Amphibians

- Cutaneous bacterial infection (red leg)
- Egg binding
- Foreign body obstruction
- Metabolic bone disease
- Mycobacteriosis
- Parasitic infestations
- Poor husbandry and diet
- Toxin exposure
- Trauma
- Ulcerative dermatitis
- Various bacterial and fungal infections

(From Sirois M: *Principles and practice of veterinary technology*, ed 3, St. Louis, Mosby, 2011.)

slide is touched to skin in an attempt to collect histologic data. The smear is then stained for analysis.

DIAGNOSTIC IMAGING

Standard x-ray machines can be used to obtain images from fish and amphibians. Dental radiography units can also be used. Mammography films are also useful if available. Small fish and aquatic amphibians can be radiographed while being held in a small volume of water in either a glass or acrylic container placed on top of the film cassette. Larger species can be anesthetized and placed directly on a cassette for a brief period of time. A minimum of two whole body views should be taken.

COMMON DISEASES

A complete review of all disease of fish and amphibians is beyond the scope of this text. The most common diseases and conditions in amphibians presented to the veterinary clinic are summarized in Box 5-1.

Bacterial disease is very common in captive amphibians and fish, and the majority of pathogens are gram-negative organisms. A summary of common bacterial pathogens of fish is located in Box 5-2. Red-leg bacterial syndrome is a common infectious disease of amphibians and is characterized by hyperemia of the ventral skin (thighs, abdomen, digits), subcutaneous edema, petechia, and ecchymotic hemorrhage. A variety of disease agents have been implicated in development of this disease including *Aeromonas hydrophila*, *A. aerogenes*, *A. aerophila*, *A. salmonicida*, *Citrobacter freundii*, *Flavobacterium* sp., *Klebsiella* sp., *Proteus* sp., and *Pseudomonas* sp.

Parasites of fish and amphibians include a variety of nematodes, trematodes, and protozoa. One common ectoparasite of freshwater fish is *Ichthyopthirius multfiliis*. Affected fish contract what is referred to as white spot disease and appear to be covered with white nodules due to the presence of this parasite. This ciliated protozoal organism feeds on the skin and gills of the fish, then leaves the fish when fully mature and develops into large numbers of free-swimming young that then infect another fish. Affected fish will rub against hard surfaces, lose

BOX 5-2	Principle Bacterial Pathogens Isolated from Captive Fish

PATHOGEN	DISEASE
Enterobacteriaceae (Gram-negative)	
Edwardsiella tarda	Red pest disease
E. ictaluri	Enteric septicemia in catfish
Yersinia ruckeri	Enteric red mouth
Vibrionaceae (Gram-negative)	
Vibrio anguillarum	Vibriosis
V. salmonocida	Hitra
V. viscossus	Winter ulcer disease
Vibrio spp.	Larval infections
Aeromonas salmonocida	Furunculosis
A. hydrophila	Septicemia
Pasteurellaceae (Gram-negative)	
Pasteurella piscida	Pseudotuberculosis
Pseudomonadaceae (Gram-negative)	
Pseudomonas anguilliseptica	Red spot disease
Flavobacteriaceae (Gram-negative)	
Flexibacter columnaris	Columnaris
Flavobacterium psychrophilium	Coldwater disease
Mycobacteriaceae (Gram-positive, acid-fast)	
Mycobacterium spp.	Tuberculosis
Nocardiaceae (Gram-positive)	
Nocardia kampachi	Nocardiosis
Nocardia spp.	Nocardiosis
Coryneforms (Gram-positive)	
Renibacterium salmoninarum	Bacterial kidney disease
Cocci (Gram-positive)	
Streptococcus spp.	Septicemia
Aerococcus viridans	Gaffkemia
Rickettsia-like organisms	
Piscirickettsia salmonis	Piscirickettsiosis

(From Mitchell M, Thomas T: *Manual of exotic pet practice*, St. Louis, Saunders, 2009.)

scales, and hemorrhage in the area of parasite attachment. The organism can be treated with appropriate chemicals placed in the water but only the free-swimming life stage is susceptible.

EUTHANASIA

An overdose of the anesthetic agent MS222 is normally used for euthanasia of fish and amphibians. Intracoelomic administration of barbiturates can also be used.

KEY POINTS

- Hundreds of different species of fish and amphibians are kept in cavity.
- Goldfish (*Carassius auratus auratus*) and koi (*Cyprinus carpio*) are some of the more commonly kept species in homes.

- Biomedical research facilities commonly keep zebrafish *(Danio rerio)*, as well as trout, salmon, and catfish.
- Common characteristics of amphibians include highly glandular, permeable skin and a three-chambered heart.
- Common characteristics of fish include an outer mucus coating, overlapping scales, the presence of fins and a swim bladder, and a simple two-chambered heart.
- Chlorine and other additives contained in tap water are toxic to many amphibians and fish.
- All aquatic animal enclosures must have regular water quality assessment to ensure the health of the animals.
- Adult amphibians are carnivorous or insectivorous; tadpoles are usually herbivorous.
- Fish species can be herbivorous or carnivorous.
- Amphibians and fish should be handled only when absolutely necessary and never with bare hands.
- No more than 1% of the body weight should be taken in blood volume from healthy fish and amphibians.
- Bacterial disease is very common in captive amphibians and fish.

REVIEW QUESTIONS

1. While only a few species of amphibians are seen in veterinary practices, there are over _____ species known.

2. _____ is the unique amphibian species that remains in a tadpolelike appearance for its adult life.

3. The scientific name for the African clawed frog is
_____ _____.

4. Biomedical research facilities often keep _____ in addition to salmon, trout, and catfish.

5. Aquatic animals that are _____ _____ can harbor many potential zoonotic pathogens.

6. Carp and monkfish are used as animal models in
_____ _____ _____ research.

7. List two unique features of the circulatory and respiratory system of amphibians.

8. Goldfish and Koi prefer ambient water temperatures of _____ to _____ °F.

9. Intramuscular injections can be given in the _____ muscle in fish.

10. One common ectoparasite of freshwater fish is _____ _____, which causes a condition referred to as *white spot disease*.

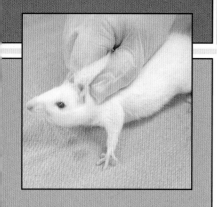

6 Rats and Mice

LEARNING OBJECTIVES

After studying this chapter, you will be able to:

- Identify unique anatomic and physiologic characteristics of rats and mice.
- Describe breeding systems used for rats and mice.
- Identify unique aspects of rat and mouse behavior.
- Explain routine procedures for husbandry, housing, and nutrition of rats and mice.
- Describe various restraint and handling procedures used on rats and mice.
- Describe methods of medication administration and blood sample collection.
- List and describe common diseases of rats and mice.
- Describe appropriate methods of euthanasia that may be used on rats and mice.

Rats and mice belongs to the order Rodentia, suborder Myomorpha. There are more than 2000 species of rodents in approximately 30 families. In fact, nearly 40% of all mammalian species are rodents. Both mice and rats are in the superfamily Muroidea. The term murine refers specifically to mice and rats. Their small size, short gestation, and ease of housing and care have made mice and rats popular as pet and research animals. The word rodent is derived from the Latin word rodere, meaning "to gnaw." All animals classified as rodents have a single pair of incisors in each jaw.

The taxonomic name for the laboratory mouse is *Mus musculus*, also known as the Swiss albino mouse or the house mouse. The Swiss albino is the most popular pet mouse, but various colors, coat varieties (including satin, spotted, and longhaired), and exotic species are becoming more common. Spiny mice as well as African pygmy mice are also available as pets. Mice and rats are also raised as feeder animals for carnivorous species such as snakes.

The African pygmy mouse is one of the smallest of all rodents. The deer mouse and cotton mouse belong to the genus *Peromyscus*. Grasshopper mice make up the genus *Onychomys*. Members of these two genera may occasionally be encountered in biomedical research. The common wood mouse of Europe is classified as *Apodemus sylvaticus*. American harvest mice make up the genus *Reithrodontomys*. The harvest mouse of Europe is classified as *Micromys minutus*.

There are two common species of rats: *Rattus norvegicus* and *Rattus rattus*. Other species of rats include the wood rats (*Neotoma* species), the rice rats (*Oryzomys* species), and the cotton rats (*Sigmodon* species). A large number of rat breeds have been developed and are available in pet stores and through private rat breeders. Box 6-1 contains information on coloration and markings that may be seen in pet rats.

Rattus rattus is commonly known as the black, house, roof, or ship rat. This species originally inhabited Southeast Asia and the spread to Europe and then the Americas in the sixteenth century. The infamous "black death" of the fourteenth century was spread by flea-infested rats of this species. Descendants of the black rat are not often used in laboratory animal studies. *Rattus norvegicus* is commonly known as the brown or Norway rat. The majority of laboratory rats are domesticated varieties of this species. The Norway rat is thought to have originated in China and spread to Western Europe by the Norwegian peninsula. The two species of rats differ in a number of characteristics. The diploid chromosome number of the brown rat is 42 and that of black rats is 38. Black rats thrive primarily in tropical climates, whereas brown rats live in nearly all climates. This chapter focuses on information specifically related to *Rattus rattus* and *Mus musculus*.

ANIMAL MODELS

Rats and mice are used extensively as animal models. Many decades of breeding for specific characteristics have provided a vast array of genetic variants that are well characterized anatomically and physiologically. As a result, the mouse is the most widely used research animal. Their high **fecundity** (reproductive potential), short gestation, and short life span make them useful animal models for studies of teratology, genetics, and gerontology. The availability of mice that are susceptible to specific viruses and the development of specific tumors makes them useful oncology and virology subjects. Studies of tissue histocompatibility are possible because of the availability of well-characterized **inbred** strains of mice. This has greatly enhanced research related to organ transplantation.

BOX 6-1	Markings and Colorations of Rats

Coat Colors

Agouti: Normal, "wild" color; black eyes
Amber: Light gold color; red eyes
Beige: Grayish-tan color; dark ruby eyes
Black: Black with black eyes
Black-eyed white: White rat with black eyes
Blue: Slate-blue color; black or dark ruby eyes
Blue agouti: Like normal agouti, but with blue base; black eyes
Blue beige: Grayish tan with hints of blue; dark ruby eyes
Blue point Siamese: Ivory body with slate-blue points; red or ruby eyes
Champagne: Similar to beige but more orange; red eyes
Chinchilla: Like agouti but with gray base; black eyes
Chocolate: Dark chocolate color; black eyes
Coffee: Light brown; black or dark ruby eyes
Cinnamon: Like agouti, but missing black bands; black eyes
Cinnamon pearl: Like cinnamon, but with a golden hue; black eyes
Fawn: Golden-orange color; dark ruby eyes
Himalayan: White body with sepia points; red eyes
Lilac: Dove gray, blue cast; ruby or black eyes
Lynx: Gray/tan with slate base; dark ruby eyes
Merle: Light background with dark splotches
Mink: Gray/brown color; black eyes
Pearl: Pale silver; black eyes
Pink-eyed white: White body; red eyes
Platinum: Dove gray; ruby or dark ruby eyes
Russian blue: Dark slate color; black eyes
Seal point Siamese: Medium beige with sepia points; red or light ruby eyes

Coat and Body Types

Standard: A rat with normal ears and normal coat
Rex: A rat with curly hair and curly whiskers
Hairless: A bald rat
Satin: Shiny, satinlike coat
Dumbo: The ears are set lower on the head
Manx: Tailless rat

Markings

Bareback: Similar to hooded rat, but without spine stripe; eyes match body color
Berkshire: Any color body, white belly, white spot between ears; eyes match top color
Blaze: White blaze, any color body; eyes match body color
Capped: White body, colored head; eyes match head color
Dalmatian: White body, colored splashes over body; eyes match marking color
English Irish: White triangle on chest, any body color; eyes match body color
Irish: White marking on belly, any body color; eyes match body color
Hooded: White body, colored stripe on back, head, shoulders, chest; markings any color; eyes match color of hood
Masked: White body, mask on face, any color; eyes match mask color
Variegated: Uneven markings on body, any color; eyes match color of markings
Odd-eyed rats: Any color or marking; one red eye, the other black or dark ruby

Because of their small size and relatively low cost, mice are also used in toxicity testing and carcinogenicity studies when data from a large number of animals are required (e.g., when meeting legal requirements of drug testing). Mice are also used in studies of diabetes, renal disease, behavior, giardiasis, obesity, and a variety of autoimmune diseases.

> **TECHNICIAN NOTE** The mouse is the most widely used research animal.

The molars of rats closely resemble those of humans, and the rat is often used as a model for dental research. Rats have been purpose-bred to be susceptible to specific human diseases, including hypertension, diabetes insipidus, cataracts, and obesity. Because of their unique ability to adapt to new environments, rats are also used for behavioral studies. Other research involving rats includes studies of audiology, oncology, teratology, embryology, gerontology, endocrinology, and immunology.

UNIQUE ANATOMIC AND PHYSIOLOGIC FEATURES

GENERAL CHARACTERISTICS

Rats and mice have a number of unique features that distinguish them from other mammals. Table 6-1 contains a summary of unique physiologic data. Rats and mice have tails that are longer than their body length. In mice, the tail is covered with a sparse hair coat while the tail of rats is usually hairless and covered with overlapping scales. The tail functions as both an organ of balance and mechanism for heat

TABLE 6-1	Normal Physiologic Reference Values	
	RATS	**MICE**
Average life span (mo)	26-40	12-36
Average adult body weight (g)	Male: 267-500 Female: 225-325	Male: 20-40 Female: 22-63
Heart rate (beats/min)	313-493	427-697
Respiratory rate (breaths/min)	71-146	91-216
Rectal temperature (°C)	37.7	37.1
Daily feed consumption (g)	15-20	3-5
Daily water consumption (ml)	22-33	5-8
Recommended environmental temperature (°C)	21-24	24-25
Recommended environmental relative humidity (%)	45-55	45-55
Average age at puberty (weeks)	6-8	5-8
Estrus cycle length (days)	4-5	4-5
Length of gestation (days)	21-23	19-21
Average litter size	6-13	7-11
Weaning age (days)	21	18-21

loss. Rats and mice do not pant and lack sweat glands. They dissipate heat through their tail and ears. Forelimbs each contain four digits, and hindlimbs each contain five digits. Because the epiphyses of the bones do not close in most rats, the rat grows continuously throughout life. In older rats, much of the marrow is replaced with fat. Estrogens may cause closure of epiphyses of females late in life. Unlike rats and most other mammals, the marrow of the long bones of mice remains active throughout life.

THE HEAD AND NECK

Eyes of rats and mice are somewhat bulging. Rats and mice possess a type of lacrimal gland called a **harderian gland** that occupies much of the orbit. Secretions from this gland contain porphyrin, a red-pigmented substance commonly referred to as "red tears" (Figure 6-1). The discharge is sometimes confused with blood but is a normal secretion of this gland. Secretions of the gland may increase when the animal is ill or under stress. This is termed **chromodacryorrhea**. A retroorbital venous plexus is present in rats while mice have an orbital sinus. Rats and mice are **hypsodontic**, meaning the teeth grow continuously throughout life. The nares of rats can close when underwater, which is why wild rats living in a sewer can swim for long distances.

> **TECHNICIAN NOTE** Secretions from the harderian gland contain porphyrin, a red-pigmented substance commonly referred to as "red tears."

THORAX AND ABDOMEN

The lungs are divided unevenly, with the left lobe being smaller and single. The right lobe is significantly larger and divided into four sections: cranial, middle, accessory, and caudal. Rats and mice possess a large store of brown fat, sometimes referred to as hibernation tissue. The brown fat is located diffusely around

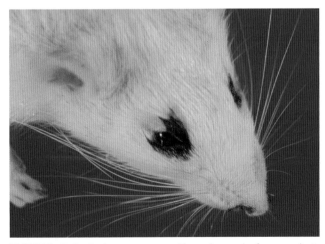

FIGURE 6-1. Red tears in a rat. The color results from porphyrin pigments in the harderian gland secretions, which are visible around the eyes and occasionally the nares. (From Quesenberry K, Carpenter JW: *Ferrets, rabbits, and rodents: clinical medicine and surgery*, ed 3, St. Louis, Saunders, 2012.)

the neck and between the scapulae and provides approximately 10 times the energy storage than other types of fat.

Rats and mice are semicontinuous feeders. A large portion of the esophagus extends caudal to the diaphragm. A monogastric stomach is divided into a glandular portion and a thin-walled nonglandular forestomach. A ridge, referred to as the limiting ridge, separates the two portions and covers the opening from the esophagus and makes the animal unable to vomit. The pancreas is highly diffuse and located throughout the mesentery and has many ducts that supply digestive enzymes directly to the small intestine. Rats do not have a gallbladder; bile continuously enters the duodenum. The small intestine contains a large, well-developed cecum that is functionally similar to the rumen of herbivores. The liver of mice and rats contains four lobes.

> **TECHNICIAN NOTE** The limiting ridge in the rodent stomach is responsible for the animal's inability to vomit.

UROGENITAL SYSTEM

The kidneys of rats contain only one papilla and one calyx. The right kidney is more anterior than the left. Female rats possess four to six pairs of mammary glands located in the thoracic and inguinal regions. The mammary glands of mice extend to the sides and back. Five pairs of glands are present. Male mice also have mammary glands but nipples are insignificant. The uterus is bicornuate, and each horn has a separate cervical canal. A membrane covers the vaginal opening until the female reaches sexual maturity. Male rats and mice have a number of accessory sex glands. These include the coagulating glands, vesicular glands, preputial, ampullary, bulbourethral (Cowper's), and prostate glands. Most of the glands are paired and located in the lower abdominal cavity. The male has an os penis that may be bony or cartilaginous. The inguinal canal remains open throughout life. Testicles can be retracted into the abdomen in colder temperatures.

REPRODUCTION

Millions of rats and mice are bred for use in research each year. Pet shop suppliers are also involved in breeding and raising rats and mice for the pet market. Female rats and mice are spontaneous ovulators and continuously polyestrous, with a 4- to 5-day estrous period. The female also undergoes a postpartum estrus approximately 20 to 24 hours after parturition. Determination of gender can be accomplished at birth. Males have a larger genital papilla than females and a greater distance between the papilla and anus (Figure 6-2). Female mice develop five pairs of conspicuous nipples by approximately 9 days of age. The age at puberty varies somewhat among different strains but is generally 35 days for mice, with sexual maturity complete by 50 days in males and 50 to 60 days in females. Puberty occurs in female rats between 37 and 67 days and between 40 and 75 days in male rats. Gestation is 19 to 21 days for mice, with an average litter size of 10 to 12 pups. In rats, the gestation period

is approximately 22 days, and litter sizes range from 6 to 12 pups. Rat and mice pups are hairless, blind, and deaf at birth. Ears open between 3 and 5 days, and eyes open between 7 and 14 days. The pups are fully haired by 7 to 10 days and begin eating solid food by the end of the second week. Weaning occurs at approximately 3 to 4 weeks in rats and approximately 11 to 14 days in mice.

Breeding normally occurs at night. The dried semen mixes with secretions from the vagina, forming a copulatory (vaginal) plug. The vaginal plug persists for 12 to 24 hours after mating and is used to confirm mating. There are a number of different mating and breeding systems that can be used with rats and mice. Monogamous mating involves one female bred to a single male. Polygamous systems usually involve two or more females bred to a single male. Breeding systems may be described as intensive systems or nonintensive systems.

Intensive breeding systems involve continuous housing of male and female animals. This may be either a monogamous mating or a polygamous mating with several males and many females. The polygamous system requires the least space and effectively takes advantage of the postpartum estrus. Disadvantages include a higher incidence of fighting between adults and a greater likelihood of injury to offspring. This system also results in somewhat higher stress to females because they are nearly always pregnant or nursing. A modification of the intensive system involves pairs or groups of animals that have been housed together since weaning. This reduces the probability of fighting.

Nonintensive breeding systems involve separate housing for the male and female while the female is pregnant. The female is not bred again until the litter is weaned. This results in fewer total offspring in a colony but minimizes the possibility of injury to offspring and fighting among adults.

Pheromones seem to play a significant role in breeding behavior. When large groups of female mice are housed together without the presence of male mice, the females will all enter a period of anestrus. When subsequently exposed to a male or the odor of a male, the females will all begin

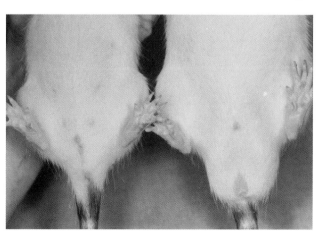

FIGURE 6-2. A male juvenile rat (right) and a female juvenile rat (left). Note the greater anogenital distance, the prominent presence of the scrotum, and the absence of nipples in the male. (From Quesenberry KE, Carpenter JW: *Ferrets, rabbits, and rodents: clinical medicine and surgery,* ed 2, St Louis, 2004, Saunders.)

estrus within 3 days. This phenomenon is referred to as the **Whitten effect** and allows for timed mating of large groups of females. Another unusual pheromone-related aspect of reproductive physiology in mice is referred to as the **Bruce effect**. If a pregnant female mouse is exposed to a new male or its odor within four days of breeding, the existing pregnancy will usually be aborted and the female will return to estrus. This effect has been documented in some species of rats and a few other mammals.

Genetics and Nomenclature of Laboratory Rats and Mice

Rats and mice have been used in medical research for many years. Because their genetic makeup has been well characterized, a large number of strains and stocks are available. These have been bred specifically for their susceptibility to specific diseases. Unique nomenclature has been developed to describe the characteristics of various stocks and strains of laboratory rats. Table 6-2 lists some common stocks and strains of laboratory rats and mice.

The term **stock** refers to a type of rat or mouse that has been randomly bred or, more specifically, not inbred. These animals are also referred to as outbred. Animals from outbred stocks have similar characteristics but are not genetically identical, in much the same way that the

members of a certain breed of dog are similar. Commonly used outbred stocks of rats include the Sprague-Dawley (SD), Long-Evans (LE), and Wistar (WI). Commonly used outbred stocks of mice include the Swiss, Swiss-Webster, CD-1, CFI, SKH1 (hairless). When describing stocks, a colon is used to separate the description of the stock and its source. For example, an animal designated as Crl:SD is a Sprague-Dawley rat maintained at Charles River Labs, whose symbol is Crl.

The term **strain** refers to a type of rat or mouse that has been inbred. A strain is considered inbred when at least 20 generations of brother-sister or parent-offspring mating have occurred. The goal of an inbred breeding program is to develop a strain of animals that is genetically homozygous. Inbred animals should all respond the same way to medical treatment or other experimental manipulation. Some inbred efforts fail because of the phenomenon referred to as inbreeding depression, which is a decrease in the reproductive capability of successive generations. In addition, as with all inbred programs, inbreeding concentrates undesirable traits as well as desirable ones. Occasionally, these undesirable genes are lethal. Common inbred rats include the Albany (ALB), used for research into mammary tumors, the spontaneous hypertensive rat (SHR), used for studies of high blood pressure, the brown (BN), used for study of myeloid leukemia, the Buffalo (BUF), used for the study of autoimmune disease, and the Fisher 344, used for the study of esophageal and bladder carcinoma. Substrains of inbred rats are also available. At least 500 distinct strains of inbred mice are available with a variety of specific genetic characteristics, such as immunodeficiency and diabetes.

TABLE 6-2	Common Strains of Laboratory Rats and Mice
Rats	
Strain	Description
Wistar	Albino, outbred
Sprague-Dawley	Albino, outbred
Long-Evans	Hooded, black and white, inbred
Gunn	Hooded, inbred
Fischer 344	Albino, inbred
Lewis	Albino, inbred
Buffalo	Albino, inbred
ACI	Brown, inbred
Mice	
ICR	White, outbred
Swiss-Webster	Albino, outbred
C57-BL	Black, inbred
C57-BR	Brown, inbred
C57-L	Lead colored, inbred
C3H	Brown, inbred
DBA/2	Gray, inbred
Balb/C	Albino, inbred
A	Albino, inbred
FVB	Albino, inbred
New Zealand black	Black, inbred
New Zealand white	White, inbred
SCID	Severe combined immunodeficient; most strains are albino
nu/nu	Athymic nude mice (BALB/C, C57-BL), lack body hair

> **TECHNICIAN NOTE**   A strain is considered inbred when at least 20 generations of brother-sister or parent-offspring mating have occurred.

Strains and substrains are also described by a specific system of nomenclature. A strain is designated with upper case letters. A substrain will have a slanted line after the strain designation. In some cases, methods of production of the animal (e.g., hand-reared, foster-reared) will be included in the name of the substrain. For example, a substrain of the ALB rat strain that is maintained at the NIH is designated ALB/N. The designation ALB f BUF indicates an Albany rat foster-reared on a Buffalo strain. Other types of inbred strains include coisogenic, congenic, and F1 **hybrid**. Coisogenic strains develop as a result of genetic mutation in existing strains. The mutation is then perpetuated in future generations. Congenic strains are those in which a mutation that arises in one strain is transferred to another through a series of backcross mating. Athymic animals (nude) were developed in this manner.

Hybrid animals are the direct result of mating between two different inbred strains. Hybrid animals are named with the female parent first, followed by the male parent, and then the designation F1 (denoting the F1 generation). For example, a cross between an Albany female rat and a Buffalo male would have the designation ALBBUFF1.

Transgenic animals are derived by removing specific DNA sequences from one strain or species and inserting them into an ovum just after fertilization. The ovum is then transplanted into a pseudopregnant female that serves as a surrogate. Animal models for a large number of gene-related disorders, including retinitis pigmentosa, Huntington's disease, and Alzheimer's disease, have been developed in this fashion.

Genetic Monitoring

A method for verification that a strain remains genetically pure is a critical component of rat and mice breeding programs. Common strategies used to confirm genetic purity include protein electrophoresis, serologic testing, mandible measurement, and backcross mating. Another method often used for genetic monitoring in inbred mice is transplantation of tissues. Genetically identical animals of the same strain or substrain should never develop signs of transplant rejection.

BEHAVIOR

Rats and mice are primarily nocturnal animals but can acclimate readily to changes in their environment and are sometimes active throughout the day and night. They are highly social animals and do well when caged in pairs or groups. A small percentage of rats and mice, especially intact males, will develop aggressive tendencies. Adult males will often fight, especially when kept in overcrowded enclosures. Female rats housed together are much more likely to fight than males housed together. Females with litters tend to be particularly aggressive toward other females. Most rats and mice are docile and respond well to regular, gentle handling. They usually enjoy interacting with their human caretakers.

A group of rats or mice is called a mischief. They may also be sometimes referred to as a horde, a family, or pack. Neonatal rats and mice that receive regular, gentle handling remain quite tame throughout life. Rats and mice prefer environments in which they can burrow. They like to explore and enjoy climbing. Nest-building activities often include creation of burrows where the animals can hide. Continuous chewing helps keep the incisor teeth from overgrowing.

HUSBANDRY

HOUSING

Whether housed in a research setting, in a home, or in the veterinary hospital, rats and mice should be maintained in an area that is separate from other species. Rats and mice are prey animals and must be housed away from predators to minimize stress in these animals. Rats and mice are usually housed in solid-bottomed shoebox cages with wire lids (Figure 6-3). In the research setting, suspended wire cages

are also used. When housed in shoebox cages, the animals are in direct contact with the bedding. Materials used for bedding should be soft, absorbent, dust free, and nontoxic. Soft woods such as cedar shavings should not be used for bedding materials because they contain compounds that affect hepatic enzymes and can cause respiratory problems. High-quality hardwood shavings or corn cobs are acceptable bedding materials. Environmental enrichment items can include objects to climb on, nestlets, extra bedding, tissues, hay to burrow in, and tubes or boxes to hide in. Cage toys sold for pet rodents are often unsuitable if they are painted or coated with plastic. Nearly any nontoxic item that the animals can gnaw will be a useful addition to the cage environment.

> *TECHNICIAN NOTE*   Rats and mice are usually housed in solid-bottomed shoebox cages with wire lids. Temperature should be maintained at 65° to 75° F with a relative humidity of 40% to 60%.

Low humidity predisposes rats to a condition called ringtail. Because rats are prone to audiogenic seizures, noise should be kept to a minimum. Excess noise may also cause cannibalism and a drop in reproductive rates. Fresh, potable water must be available at all times. Water consumption varies among different strains but is generally from 13 to 20 ml

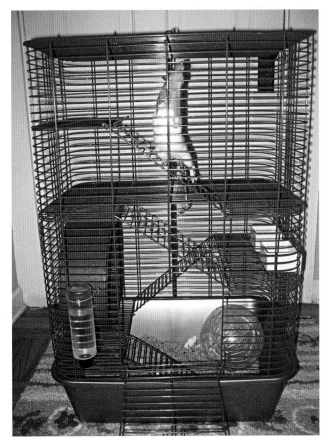

FIGURE 6-3. Solid bottom cage for pet rats. The animal should have plenty of room for exercise. (From Mitchell M, Thomas T: *Manual of exotic pet practice,* St. Louis, Saunders, 2009.)

per 100 g of body weight per day for rats and approximately 15 ml per 100 g body weight per day for mice.

New animals brought into an existing colony are usually quarantined for a period of time in order to identify any pre-existing medical problems. In the research setting, a 30-day quarantine period is common. The quarantine area is usually in an environment identical to the one where the animals will be housed.

NUTRITION

Food consumption also varies among different species and strains. Ordinarily, 5 g of food per 100 g of body weight is eaten each day per rat. The Swiss mouse normally consumes 12 to 18 g per 100 g body weight per day. Like most rodents, rats and mice are coprophagic. Most rats and mice can be fed ad libitum, but some will overeat if provided with more food than needed. They usually consume their food in several small meals throughout the day. Pregnant or lactating females require up to four times the requirements for nonpregnant, nonlactating females. Several commercial rodent chows are available and nutritionally adequate. Because mice gnaw on the relatively hard pelleted feeds, these also provide the animals with a mechanism for keeping the incisors from overgrowing.

The feed can be placed directly in the V-shaped hopper on a wire cage lid. Feed can also be provided in a food hopper that hangs inside the cage. If water bottles are placed on hangers inside the cage, avoid plastic bottles or rubber stoppers because the animals will chew on these. The shelf life of most commercial rodent chow is approximately 6 months from the milling date (Figure 6-4).

Rats and mice maintained in research colonies are not usually provided with supplemental food. Pet rats may be given small amounts of fruits, vegetables, or seeds. Raw, unwashed fruits or vegetables should never be fed to any animal. Some species of mice (e.g., spiny mice) can be maintained on seed-based diets.

> **TECHNICIAN NOTE** The shelf life of most commercial rodent chow is approximately 6 months from the milling date.

IDENTIFICATION

Methods for identification of individual animals vary in different facilities and depend in part on whether the animals are used for breeding or research. Cage cards may be used to identify an individual or group of animals. The information on the cage card may include the name of the principle investigator, date of birth and source of animals, and information regarding the research protocol for which the animals are intended or being used. Temporary identification can be made with a nontoxic colored marker on animals with light-colored hair or by shaving specific patches of hair. Recording natural markings unique to specific animals may also be used. These temporary methods are for short-term use only. Rats and mice in private veterinary hospitals are usually identified with cage cards.

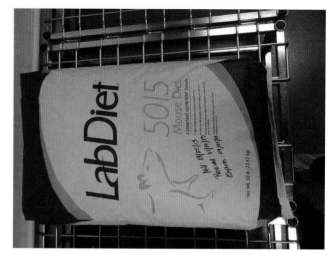

FIGURE 6-4. Rodent food should be used within 6 months of its milling date.

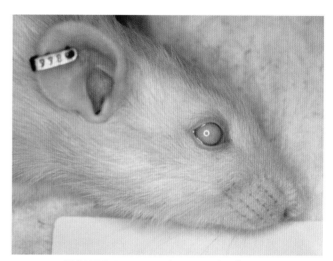

FIGURE 6-5. Rat with ear tag identification.

Permanent identification methods include tattooing the ear, tail, or toe; punching or tagging the ear (Figure 6-5); clipping the toe; or using microchips that can be read electronically. Ear punching involves placing small holes or notches at various locations on the ears. The location of the hole or notch corresponds to a specific number. For example, a hole at the top of the left ear and a notch at the top of the right ear indicate animal number 41. Figure 6-6 illustrates an ear punching code. By using just the ears, it is possible to number up to 99 animals. For colonies that have more than 99 animals, toe clipping can be combined with ear punching. Toe clipping involves removing the first bone of certain toes to correspond to a specific numbering system. The procedure for ear punching is rapid, easy, and produces little trauma to the animal. Toe clipping is more stressful, and the animals should be anesthetized for the procedure.

Tattooing of the ear, tail, or toe can be performed on neonatal animals with little difficulty. Two common types of tattoo instruments are available. One type of mechanical tattoo instrument uses metal pins contained in a holding device that is pressed against the skin on the ear (Figure 6-7).

Rodent Ear Punch Code		
	Left Ear	Right Ear	
10			1
20			2
30			3
40			4
50			5
60			6
70			7
80			8
90			9

FIGURE 6-6. Ear punch code.

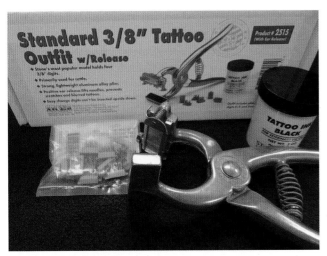

FIGURE 6-7. Pin-type tattoo instrument.

The pins may be letters, numbers, or patterns of dots. Once the instrument is applied to the ear, black tattoo ink is worked into the holes created in the subcutaneous space by the pins. A sterile needle or small brush can be used for that purpose. It is crucial that all components of the tattoo instrument be sterile and that aseptic technique is used. For tail or toe tattoo applications, a penlike instrument is used. The metal tip of the pen vibrates and creates small perforations in the dermis. The tattoo ink is worked into the perforations in much the same way as the pin-type instrument. Animals that have darker skin may be tattooed with green ink. Tattoo ink

may fade somewhat over time, and the ink-stained area may spread out as the animal grows. Tattoo procedures occasionally need to be repeated.

Microchips can also be implanted to identify individual animals. The microchip is used to identify the individual but may also contain additional information, such as the strain, source, and date of birth of the animal. Some small animal weighing scales contain built-in devices that can simultaneously read the data on the microchip and record the new weight when an animal is placed on the scale. Microchips can also be implanted in animals of any age. The procedure is relatively simple and atraumatic. The chip is implanted with a syringe into the subcutaneous space. An electronic reader is then used to read the information on the chip. Microchips have been growing in popularity in recent years because of the large number of vendors that market such products to small animal veterinary clinics. National registry services also maintain databases on animals with microchips so information can be recovered if the animal is lost or stolen.

RESTRAINT AND HANDLING

Rats and mice are easy to handle, especially when accustomed to regular manipulation. Aggressive rats usually require the use of leather or chain gloves. Because gloves reduce the sensitivity of the handler to movements of the animal, every effort should be made to acclimate them to regular, gentle handling. Specific handling and restraint techniques vary depending on the purpose of the manipulation. Latex gloves should be worn when handling rats and mice due to the possibility of transmission of *Leptospira* organisms.

> **TECHNICIAN NOTE** Latex gloves should be worn when handling rats and mice due to the possibility of transmission of *Leptospira* organisms.

Rats and mice that must be moved from one cage to another can be grasped at the base of the tail, close to the body, and moved into a new cage. This should be done relatively quickly so the body of the animal is not suspended for a prolonged period. Never pick a rat or mouse up by grasping the middle or tip of the tail. The skin on the tail can slough off, resulting in a severe degloving injury with exposed vertebrae. Very docile rats and mice can also be moved by placing a hand under their body and scooping them up. Very young pups are usually scooped up out of the cage as a group, along with a small amount of bedding. Mice can also be picked up using smooth, rubber-tipped forceps to grasp the loose skin across the back of the neck.

Restraint for technical procedures can be accomplished in several ways. The animal should first be removed from its cage and placed on a cage lid or other surface it can grasp (Figure 6-8). As the animal grasps the surface, the restrainer places the nondominant hand on the base of the tail. At that point, the restrainer may use one of two techniques to

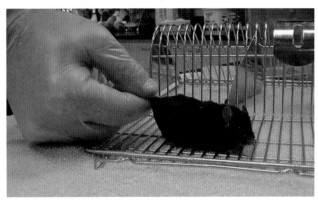

FIGURE 6-8. Proper technique for picking up a mouse. Grasp the loose skin over the back of the neck when the animal grabs the bars of the wire cage lid. (From Sirois M: *Principles and practice of veterinary technology*, ed 3, St. Louis, Mosby, 2011.)

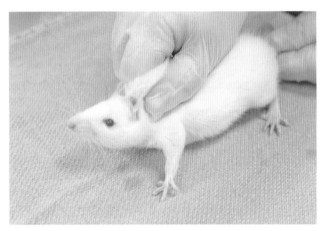

FIGURE 6-9. Restrainer grasp a large fold of skin over the head between the mandibles.

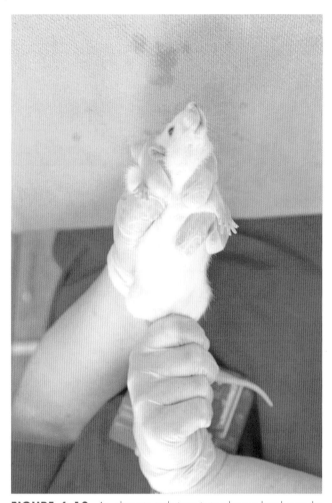

FIGURE 6-10. An alternate technique is to place a hand over the thorax directly behind the elbows and gently push the legs forward.

immobilize the animal. The first technique requires that the restrainer grasp a large fold of skin over the head between the mandibles (Figure 6-9). An alternate technique is to place a hand over the thorax directly behind the elbows and gently push the legs forward (Figure 6-10). Care must be taken to minimize pressure on the thorax to avoid impeding respiration or damaging the lungs. Regardless of the specific method chosen, the tail of the animal should also be restrained. This can be accomplished by placing the tail between the fingers of the same hand that is holding the body of the animal, thus freeing the other hand so that one person is able to perform procedures when appropriate.

A variety of restraint devices are also available for use in immobilizing rats and mice. Plastic restraint boxes contain multiple small openings and a securing block designed to allow injections and blood collection (Figure 6-11). The restraint box must be cleaned, disinfected, thoroughly rinsed, and dried between each use. The animal is picked up and its head placed in the opening of the restrainer. If the animal does not readily enter the restraint box, the box can be lifted slightly. Most animals will then walk forward into the box. The securing block is then placed behind the animal so that it cannot move or turn around. Another useful restraint device

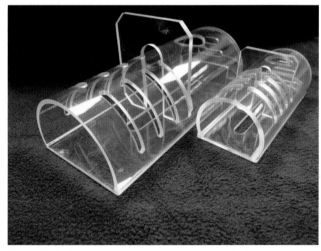

FIGURE 6-11. Plastic restraint boxes contain multiple small openings and a securing block designed to allow injections and blood collection.

is a plastic cone (Figure 6-12). These can be purchased commercially or prepared from a thick freezer bag. The device appears similar to a cake-decorating tube, with a hole in the point of the cone. The animal is lowered into the bag and then the excess material at the opening gathered together.

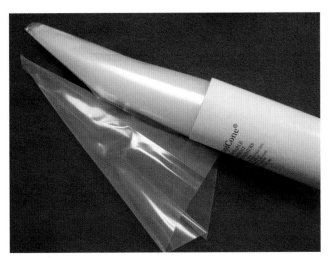

FIGURE 6-12. Commercially available cone restraint aid.

This gently pushes the animal toward the small opening at the point of the cone that allows it to breathe. Injections can be given directly through the plastic, or a small opening can be cut in the cone to allow greater access to the animal. Animals can easily overheat if held too long in a restraint cone. A type of homemade restraint device often used with pet rats is a stockinette with a small syringe case attached to one end. The syringe case allows the animal to breathe when placed in the stockinette.

CLINICAL PROCEDURES

PATIENT HISTORY AND PHYSICAL EXAMINATION

When pet rats and mice are presented to the veterinary clinic, a complete patient history must be obtained. Information regarding the source of the animal, how long the owner has had the pet, whether it has been handled regularly, and where the cage is located should be recorded. If possible, the owner should be encouraged to bring the animal in its normal primary enclosure. This will also allow for an evaluation of the husbandry conditions. If the animal is brought to the clinic in a transport cage or carrier, obtain information on the type and size of the cage, what the cage is composed of, what bedding material is used, and the types of cage furniture or other enrichment devices the animal has available. The frequency of cage cleaning, type and quantity of diet fed, frequency of water changes, and whether any supplements are given should also be recorded, as well as the presence and species of other pets in the household.

> TECHNICIAN NOTE If possible, the owner should be advised to bring the animal in its primary enclosure so husbandry conditions can be evaluated.

The complete physical examination begins with observation of the animal in its carrier or cage. Visually assess the animal's demeanor, respiratory rate and effort, attitude,

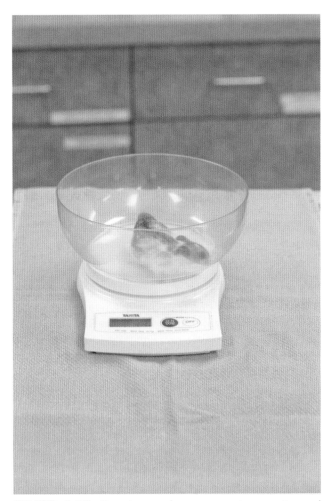

FIGURE 6-13. Place the animal in an appropriate container and obtain the weight.

posture, and activity level. Note the overall condition of the hair coat. Mice and rats are generally fastidious, and an unkempt appearance is often the first sign of disease. After the initial observation, place the animal in an appropriate container and obtain the weight (Figure 6-13). The physical exam then begins starting at the head and working toward the tail. If at any time the animal appears to be in distress, release it immediately and consider chemical restraint.

> TECHNICIAN NOTE An unkempt appearance is often the first sign of disease.

If possible, obtain the temperature, pulse, and respiration rate. Examine the eyes, ears, and nares for discharge. Use a speculum or small syringe case to open the animal's mouth. Note the color of the mucous membranes and condition of the teeth, especially the incisors. Body condition and results of palpation of the abdominal cavity are then noted.

ADMINISTRATION OF MEDICATIONS

Parenteral and oral medications can be given quite readily. Some procedures require that the animal be anesthetized.

Depending on which techniques are used, two people may be required to complete a procedure.

Injection Techniques

Injections may be given intravenously, subcutaneously, intraperitoneally, or intramuscularly. Intraosseous and intradermal administration is also possible but not commonly performed and requires that the rat be anesthetized. Although most rat and mouse injection procedures are simple to perform, proper restraint is critical to correct administration of medications. The volume of fluid that can be injected at a specific site must also be considered. Many medications used in rats and mice must be diluted to deliver the correct dose accurately. However, dilutions cannot be so great as to require excessive volumes for injection. Table 6-3 lists ideal and maximum volumes for administration of substances depending on the route of administration.

Intravenous (IV) injections may be given in the saphenous, jugular, femoral, or lateral tail veins. The animal can be restrained in a plastic restraining device or cone, or a restrainer may hold the animal while an assistant administers the medication. The most commonly used sites for small-volume injections are the lateral tail veins. These veins lie along each side of the tail and are fairly superficial.

In young albino animals, they may be easily visualized. In older rats, the skin over the tail is quite thick, making it more difficult to pass a needle through into the lumen of the vein.

To perform the procedure, restrain the animal and occlude the veins by applying pressure at the base of the tail. Clean the tail and place a syringe with an attached small-gauge needle (22 gauge or less) or butterfly catheter nearly parallel to the tail alongside the vein. Hold the tail firmly and insert the needle into the lumen of the vein at the level of the middle of the tail with a smooth motion.

Withdraw the plunger of the syringe barrel slightly to verify correct placement in the vein. Inject the medication slowly and smoothly. Withdraw the needle from the vein and apply pressure to the venipuncture site to ensure hemostasis. Administration of IV medications in the jugular, femoral, or saphenous vein is not usually practical and requires that the animal be anesthetized. Although rarely performed, a microinjection syringe may also be used to inject small volumes (less than 5 μL) into the retroorbital plexus on anesthetized rats. When repeated IV injections are needed, surgical placement of a jugular catheter can be performed.

Subcutaneous (SC or SQ) injections are administered with a 21-gauge or smaller needle. The animal can be restrained on a table for this procedure or can be placed on a wire cage top and allowed to grasp the bars on the lid. Anesthesia or sedation is not usually required. The loose skin over the nape of the neck or abdomen is gently lifted to form a tent. The needle is held at a 90-degree angle to the skin and directed into the subcutaneous space beneath the tented skin and the material injected in one smooth motion.

Intramuscular (IM) injections are complicated by the small muscle mass of rats and mice. Only small volumes can be injected by this route. Although any large muscle group can be used, those used most often are the quadriceps, gluteals, and triceps (Figure 6-14). Recommended needle gauges are 22 or less. The skin should be cleaned and the muscle stabilized and separated from underlying structures by gently pinching it between the fingers. It is extremely important to avoid blood vessels and nerves. The sciatic nerve, for example, runs along the posterior aspect of the femur. If irritating substances or excess volumes are injected near this nerve, the animal may become lame. Self-mutilation of the limb is common in those situations. Once an appropriate muscle mass has been chosen, the animal restrained, and the site cleaned, the needle should be directed at a right angle into the deepest part of the muscle. The plunger of the syringe must be slightly withdrawn to verify that the needle has not entered a blood vessel. If no blood is evident in the hub of the needle, the material can be injected in a slow, steady motion. The needle is then withdrawn and light pressure applied to the site for a few seconds.

Intraperitoneal (IP) injections are quite simple to administer and can usually be performed with one person holding the animal and administering the injection. The animal should be restrained by grasping the scruff between the mandibles or with the body restrained below the elbows. The tail is tucked between the fingers of the hand that is holding the body. The animal is held so that its head is

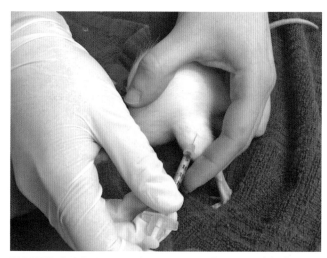

FIGURE 6-14. Intramuscular injection can be accomplished in most rodents with towel restraint and exposure of the rear leg. (From Quesenberry K, Carpenter JW: *Ferrets, rabbits, and rodents: clinical medicine and surgery*, ed 3, St. Louis, Saunders, 2012.)

TABLE 6-3	Suggested Maximum Volumes for Injection	
ROUTE	**VOLUME (RATS)**	**VOLUME (MICE)**
SQ	0.2 mL/10g	0.8 mL/10g
IP	0.2 mL/10g	0.6 mL/10g
IM	0.1 mL–0.3mL/site	0.05 mL/site
IV	0.05 mL/10g	0.1 mL/10g
ID	0.1 mL/site	0.05 mL/site

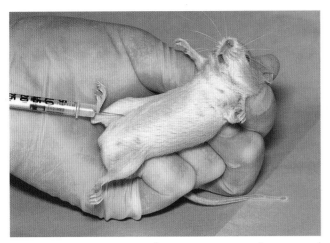

FIGURE 6-15. Intraperitoneal injection in a mouse. Intraperitoneal injection in mice is made into one posterior quadrant of the abdomen, along the line of the hindlimb. (From Thomas JA, Lerche P: *Anesthesia and analgesia for veterinary technicians*, ed 4, St. Louis, Mosby, 2011.)

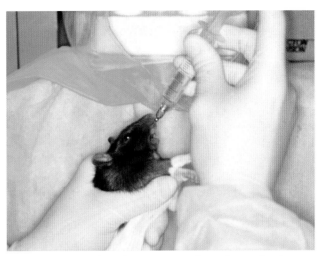

FIGURE 6-16. Place the gavage needle gently into the diastema and advance into the esophagus.

directed downward (toward the floor) at approximately a 30-degree angle. A 22-gauge or smaller needle is introduced into the lower left quadrant of the abdomen (Figure 6-15). This location is the least likely to contain internal organs, particularly the large cecum. The plunger is withdrawn to verify correct placement. If the urinary bladder, intestine, other organs, or blood vessels are punctured, fluid will enter the hub of the needle. The needle and syringe must then be discarded and the procedure started over. If no fluid is present, the material may be injected in a smooth motion and the needle withdrawn. Larger amounts of material can be administered by IP injection. However, because the material is first absorbed into the portal circulation, it may be at least partially modified by hepatocytes before reaching the systemic circulation.

Oral Administration

Medications given by mouth are similar to IP administration in that they are first absorbed into the portal circulation before moving into the systemic circulation. It is not generally advisable to place medications in the water bottle because the animal will often refuse to drink and can become quite ill. When medications must be placed into water sources for treatment of large numbers of animals, it is recommended that a small amount of sugar or syrup (5 mL/L) be added to make the solution more palatable. Medications for oral administration may also be mixed in food if the animals are being fed a powdered or meal-type diet.

> **TECHNICIAN NOTE** Gavage needles for small rodents should have a ball tip.

Gavaging the animal with a stainless steel feeding needle is the preferred method for administering oral medications to individual animals. The needle should have a ball-tip end. Feeding needle sizes appropriate for rats range from 16 to 18

gauge and from 2 to 3 inches in length. A feeding needle of 20 gauge and 1-½ inches is appropriate to use in mice. The animal must be firmly restrained, preferably with the thumb and forefinger to hold the head in place and the neck slightly extended. The needle is lubricated, usually with the material to be administered, and then placed in the diastema of the mouth. The needle is then gently advanced along the upper palate until the esophagus is reached (Figure 6-16). The needle should pass easily into the esophagus. The animal may swallow when the needle begins to move through the esophagus. Once proper placement is verified, the material can be administered by a syringe attached to the end of the needle. The needle should not be rotated once placed because the tip could rupture the esophagus. Flexible rubber catheters (8 Fr) may also be used to gavage rats and mice. However, they are likely to bite the tube, so an oral speculum must first be placed.

ANESTHESIA

One of the major responsibilities of the animal care team is to ensure that animals feel little or no pain when undergoing technical procedures. The Animal Welfare Act requires that procedures be evaluated for the potential of pain and that animals be given pain medications. Exotic animals may respond poorly to local or regional anesthesia. In particular, the loss of feeling in a limb (as in local anesthesia) or an entire section of the body (as in regional anesthesia) is a significant source of stress for animals. Exotic animals are usually administered general anesthetics. Many variables affect general anesthesia, including age of the animal, general health, species, strain or stock, and environment. Each species and individual within a species reacts differently to anesthetic agents. It is therefore necessary to understand the effects of each drug on each species. Every animal must be individually dosed with enough medication to achieve the desired result. The dose of anesthetic is always "to effect." To determine whether anesthesia is adequate, the animal's vital signs and reflexes may be monitored. The specific procedures for monitoring also vary among different species. Monitoring is aimed at characterizing the stage of anesthesia. The stages of anesthesia may be very difficult to recognize in rats and mice. The transition from one stage to another may be subtle and brief. In general, reactions of the neuromuscular system are used to determine stage of anesthesia. In rats, the toe pinch and respiratory rate are appropriate to evaluate the degree of anesthesia. Other characteristics that may be used to evaluate anesthetic depth in anesthetized rats and mice include the following:

- Movement of the whiskers and ears in response to a puff of air. This indicates minimal sedation.
- Failure to withdraw a foot or tail in response to a pinch. This indicates surgical anesthesia.
- Respiratory rate less than 60 breaths/min indicates dangerous CNS depression.
- For long procedures, the anesthetist must address the possibility of hypothermia. The use of a rectal thermometer probe is advised. A warm water bottle, electric heated

blanket, or heated table controlled by a thermostat is recommended.

General anesthetic agents are available in inhalant or injectable forms. Inhalant anesthetics used in rats and mice include isoflurane and sevoflurane. The agent can be administered by face mask that fits tightly around the muzzle through a standard anesthesia machine or by placing the animal in an induction chamber or inverting a canine face mask over the animal (Figure 6-17). Injectable agents for general anesthesia in rats and mice include barbiturates, such as pentobarbital and thiamylal, and dissociative agents, such as ketamine. Other pharmaceutical agents are also used. Table 6-4 lists some common injectable anesthetics used in rats and mice.

DIAGNOSTIC IMAGING

Rats and mice require sedation or general anesthesia in order to obtain diagnostic-quality images. Standard tabletop

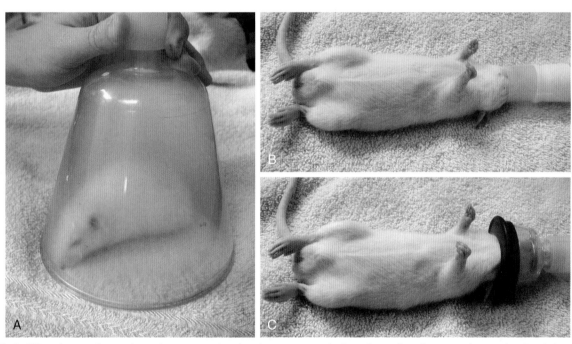

FIGURE 6-17. Induction of general anesthesia in a sedated rat by using a standard small-animal mask as an induction chamber *(A)*. Once anesthetized, anesthesia is maintained with a modified syringe case *(B)* or a commercial rodent face mask *(C)*. (From Quesenberry K, Carpenter JW: *Ferrets, rabbits, and rodents: clinical medicine and surgery,* ed 3, St. Louis, Saunders, 2012.)

TABLE 6-4	Common Anesthetic and Tranquilizing Agents Used in Rats		
DRUG	**DOSAGE (RATS)**	**DOSAGE (MICE)**	**ROUTE**
Isoflurane	1.5% to 4% induction; 0.3% maintenance to effect	1.0% to 4% induction 0.3% maintenance to effect	Inhalation
Acepromazine		2.0-5.0 mg/kg	IP
Diazepam	2.5 to 5 mg/kg	5 mg/kg	IP
Ketamine/acepromazine	75 mg/kg ketamine + 2.5 mg/kg acepromazine	100 mg/kg ketamine + 5 mg/kg acepromazine	IP
Ketamine/xylazine	40 to 80 mg/kg ketamine + 5 to 10mg/kg xylazine	80 to 100 mg/kg ketamine + 10mg/kg xylazine	IP
Propofol	10.0 to 12mg/kg	26mg/kg	IV

x-ray cassettes can be used and the animal can be taped to the x-ray cassette. Dental radiology units can also be used and provide better isolation of specific body regions and full body radiographs in extremely small patients. Mammography film often provides the best detail in these small patients. Two whole-body views are usually taken, the ventrodorsal and lateral projection.

BANDAGING AND WOUND MANAGEMENT

Wounds on mice and rats are generally not bandaged due to the animal's tendency to remove bandages and disturb the wound. Wounds must be thoroughly cleaned and the animal maintained in a clean environment. Bedding may be changed to a substance less likely to contaminate the wound, such as butcher's paper. Alternately, frequent cage cleaning can help minimize wound contamination. When deemed essential, bandages must be as unobtrusive as possible. An Elizabethan collar should also be placed. These are available commercially or can be fashioned from items such as discarded x-ray film.

DIAGNOSTIC TESTING
Blood Collection Techniques

The method used for collecting blood samples in rats and mice depends on the volume of blood needed, the age of the animal, and the skill level of the technician. The blood volume of most rodents is approximately 6% to 7% of their total body weight. No more than 10% of the blood volume should be withdrawn at one time. The total volume that may be removed from animals that are ill is usually much smaller. The lateral tail veins are the preferred site for collection of blood samples. Anesthesia is required for collection of samples from the retroorbital plexus or sinus, jugular vein, femoral vein, tail artery, cranial vena cava, or heart. For collection of small volumes of plasma, a clear-hubbed needle can be used to puncture the vessel and a heparinized capillary tube used to collect the sample from the needle hub. Hematology samples should be mixed with an appropriate amount of ethylenediamine tetraacetic acid or analyzed immediately. Blood films should always be prepared from a drop of fresh blood immediately after collection.

> *TECHNICIAN NOTE* No more than 10% of the blood volume of a healthy rat or mouse should be withdrawn at one time.

Although anesthesia is not required for collection of samples from the lateral tail vein, the animal must be firmly restrained. A plastic restraining device can be used for this procedure. However, it is often difficult to effectively restrain unanesthetized mice for blood collection even with a restraining device. The tail should be prepared by swabbing it with isopropyl alcohol and the alcohol allowed to dry. The tail can be placed in warm water for a few seconds to cause the blood vessels to dilate (Figure 6-18). Alternatively, a heat lamp may be used for a few minutes before the procedure to warm the tail and dilate the vessels. A tuberculin syringe,

1-mL syringe with a small-gauge needle, or a small-gauge butterfly catheter is required. Occlude the blood vessel by applying pressure over the vein at the base of the tail. Enter the vessel approximately one third to one half the distance of the tail from the body (Figure 6-19). Placing a few fingers or a wood block beneath the tail will help stabilize the vessel. Use a shallow angle and withdraw the sample slowly to avoid collapsing or constricting the vein. Remove the needle and apply pressure to the venipuncture site to ensure hemostasis.

> *TECHNICIAN NOTE* Blood can be collected from the cranial vena cava or lateral tail veins.

Blood collection from the tail arteries or saphenous, femoral, or jugular veins is performed in a similar matter except that the animal must be anesthetized to ensure proper restraint. Hair should be clipped from the venipuncture site before performing the procedure. Blood may also be collected from the cranial vena cava. Sedation or general anesthesia of the animal is required (Figure 6-20).

The ventral tail artery is readily accessible along the ventromedial aspect of the tail, although it is not as superficial as the tail veins. When the artery is entered, the syringe should

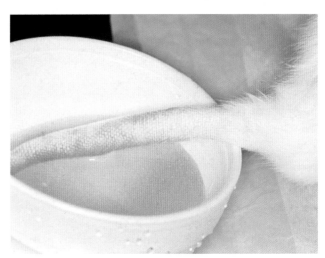

FIGURE 6-18. The tail can be placed in warm water for a few seconds to cause the blood vessels to dilate.

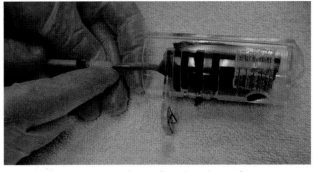

FIGURE 6-19. Blood collection from the tail vein of a mouse. (From Sheldon CC, Topel J, Sonsthagen T: *Animal restraint for veterinary professionals*, St. Louis, Mosby, 2006.)

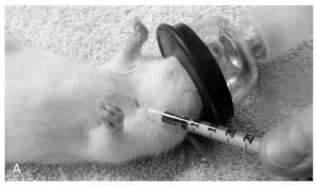

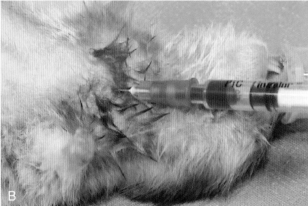

FIGURE 6-20. Blood may also be collected from the cranial vena cava. Sedation or general anesthesia of the animal is required. (From Quesenberry K, Carpenter JW: *Ferrets, rabbits, and rodents: clinical medicine and surgery,* ed 3, St. Louis, Saunders, 2012.)

immediately fill with blood. Hemostasis by using digital pressure may take slightly longer than for hemostasis of the tail veins.

> **TECHNICIAN NOTE** Blood collection from the medial canthus of the eye should not be performed in the presence of pet owners.

Blood collection from the retroorbital plexus or sinus must be performed under anesthesia. It may be helpful to apply a small amount of ophthalmic lubricant to prevent corneal desiccation. Hold the upper and lower eyelids open with one hand. Using a dorsolateral approach, place a Pasteur pipette or capillary tube into the orbit at the site slightly dorsal to the medial canthus. The pipette or tube should be sliding along the side and back of the globe. Gently rotate and advance the pipette or tube through the conjunctival membrane. Blood should then flow into the tube. If blood does not flow freely, it may be necessary to slightly withdraw the tube. Once the sample is collected, withdraw the tube, hold the eye closed, and apply slight pressure with a gauze square. Although this procedure is relatively painless and atraumatic, for aesthetic reasons it should probably not be performed on pets in front of clients.

Cardiocentesis must be performed with the animal under anesthesia. Because of the relatively high probability of

cardiac damage and other complications, collection of blood from the heart is normally only performed as a terminal procedure on animals in biomedical research. The procedure can be performed with the animal in either lateral or dorsal recumbency. For lateral recumbency, the heart can be entered just caudal to the elbow. The procedure for intracardiac blood collection by dorsal recumbency involves inserting the needle through the abdomen, just lateral to the xiphoid process and directed cranially into the heart. A tail clip or toenail can be performed readily but are unsuitable for repeated collection and samples are rarely of diagnostic quality.

COMMON DISEASES OF RATS AND MICE

Much of the job of the veterinary technician in exotic and laboratory animal medicine is focused on preventing disease in the animal colonies. A number of diseases can be caused or worsened when animal husbandry practices are poor or inappropriate for the species. The veterinary technician should ensure that the pet rat or mouse owner is knowledgeable about proper housing, environment, nutritional needs, and signs of common diseases.

Rats and mice are primarily nocturnal animals. When examining a rat or mouse or performing diagnostic testing when the animal is irritable or drowsy, it may not respond as it would if fully awake. Clients with pet rats or mice should be advised to bring their pet in to the clinic as late in the day as possible. In addition, always request that the owner bring the animal to the clinic in its own cage. This allows the technician to identify any possible housing or care-related problems that may exist as well as evaluate the overall sanitation of the environment in which the animal is housed.

Rats and mice are susceptible to infectious diseases caused by bacteria, viruses, parasites, and mycotic agents. Noninfectious diseases seen in rats and mice include those related to nutrition, genetics, environmental conditions, and age. A complete review of all possible diseases is beyond the scope of this text. The most common diseases are summarized in the following section.

> **TECHNICIAN NOTE** Noninfectious diseases seen in rats and mice include those related to nutrition, genetics, environmental conditions, and age.

INFECTIOUS DISEASES

Definitive diagnosis of infectious diseases of rats and mice is especially important because some have zoonotic potential. Diagnosis of bacterial diseases can be done with microbiologic cultures. Viral diseases are often diagnosed on the basis of clinical signs. Parasitic diseases can be diagnosed with fecal or urine examinations.

Bacterial Diseases
Tyzzer's Disease. Tyzzer's disease has been reported in nearly all species of laboratory animals and is found throughout the world. The causative agent is the gram-negative,

spore-forming, flagellated bacterium *Clostridium piliforme* (formerly *Bacillus piliformis*). The bacterium is difficult to culture, and definitive diagnosis often requires histologic examination of tissues from suspected infected animals. A polymerase chain reaction test is available to detect antibodies in rats and mice. The organism is transmitted by the fecal-oral route. Rats and mice may harbor the organism without clinical signs. Poor sanitation and overcrowding predispose animals to this disease. Clinical signs are variable with different species but usually include diarrhea and anorexia. Gray foci throughout the liver, sometimes on the spleen or heart, develop in affected animals. Hepatic necrosis and myocardial degeneration may occur. Antibiotics can be used to treat infected animals, but infection is often fatal. Careful attention to proper sanitation and reduction of stress aids in preventing this disease. The organism is difficult to eradicate from an animal facility because of resistant spores produced by the bacterium.

> TECHNICIAN NOTE The causative agent of Tyzzer's disease is *Clostridium piliforme.*

Murine Respiratory Mycoplasmosis. This relatively common chronic bacterial infection presents the greatest negative impact on scientific studies. The causative agent, *Mycoplasma pulmonis*, is pleomorphic and one of the smallest free-living organisms containing both DNA and RNA. The organism can pass through small-pore filters. Other organisms, particularly *Pasteurella pneumotropica, Corynebacterium kutscheri, Bordetella bronchiseptica*, cilia-associated respiratory bacilli, streptococci, and viruses, may act synergistically and worsen the symptoms. Clinical signs include mucopurulent oculonasal discharge, sneezing, snuffling, rales, and dyspnea. Otitis media often occurs, and affected animals may demonstrate head tilt, incoordination, and circling. Transmission is by direct contact, aerosol, and fomites. Prevention of outbreaks is accomplished by maintaining an infection-free colony in a barrier facility. Oxytetracycline in the drinking water may be used to control outbreaks but does not eliminate the organism.

Pasteurellosis. Infections with *Pasteurella pneumotropica* and *P. multocida* may be fatal in athymic mice or those that are immunocompromised in any way. The organisms can colonize automatic watering systems when the systems are not properly flushed. Many healthy rats harbor the gram-negative bacteria *Pasteurella pneumotropica* and *Pasteurella multocida* in the upper respiratory tract. In rats, the organisms are opportunistic pathogens and act synergistically with other infectious agents, such as *Mycoplasma* and Sendai virus. Clinical signs are those related to upper respiratory infection or pneumonia. However, abscesses may occur in skin, lymph nodes, uterus, and the urinary system.

> TECHNICIAN NOTE A variety of bacterial agents may cause respiratory disease in rats and mice.

Streptococcosis. Infections with the bacterium *Streptococcus pneumoniae* are rare in well-managed animal facilities. Mice infected with Streptococcus species usually have signs of dermatitis, although a variety of other disease processes can also result from infections with this organism. Like *Pasteurella*, rats often harbor this bacterium in the upper respiratory tract, and opportunistic infection can occur when animals are under stress. Young rats are particularly susceptible. Infections are spread by aerosol transmission. Clinical signs include chromodacryorrhea, inflammation of the nasopharynx, pleuritis, meningitis, bronchopneumonia, and consequently pulmonary consolidation and death.

Streptobacillosis. *Streptobacillus moniliformis* is present in the nasopharynx of healthy rats and is not considered a disease-causing organism in this species. *S. moniliformis* infections are uncommon in mice. However, other rodents and human beings are susceptible to infection. In human beings, infection with this organism is commonly referred to as rat bite fever or Haverhill fever.

Miscellaneous Bacterial Infections. Infections with *Leptospira* are usually inapparent but the organism has zoonotic potential. The organism is transmitted in the urine. Rats and mice with chronic respiratory disease may be infected with the cilia-associated respiratory bacillus. This organism is an opportunistic pathogen of the respiratory system and concurrent infection with *Mycoplasma* is common.

Pseudomonas species are normal inhabitants of the intestinal tract of rodents. Clinical illness from infection with *Pseudomonas aeruginosa* is rare unless the animal is immunocompromised.

Bordetella bronchiseptica is a common inhabitant of the respiratory tract of rats. The organism is transmitted through direct contact, through fomites, and by aerosol contamination. Rats rarely develop clinical infections with this organism but serve as carriers. Clinical infection, usually with pneumonia, can occur in rats that are under stress. The primary concern with this disease is its pathogenicity in other laboratory animals, particularly guinea pigs.

> TECHNICAN NOTE *Pseudomonas* and *Bordetella* are normal inhabitants of the respiratory tract of rodents.

Infections with the opportunistic bacteria *Corynebacterium kutscheri* are usually subclinical but may cause clinical infection in immunocompromised mice. The organism is a gram-positive, nonmotile bacillus that causes a disease known as pseudotuberculosis. Symptoms usually include nasal and ocular discharge, dyspnea, arthritis, or skin abscesses. Focal abscesses in liver, kidney, lungs, and lymph nodes may be evident. Diagnosis is made on the basis of these lesions at necropsy, isolation of the organism through bacterial culture, or serologic testing.

Viral Disease

Sialodacryoadenitis.
The sialodacryoadenitis virus is the most significant viral disease of rats, although infections are usually self-limiting. The organism is highly contagious, with a short incubation period (2 days). Transmission is by respiratory aerosol and direct contact with respiratory secretions. Diagnosis is made on the basis of clinical signs or serologic testing. Necrosis of the salivary and nasolacrimal glands occurs, especially in young rats. Clinical signs include rhinitis, swollen salivary and harderian glands, cervical edema, photophobia, and chromodacryorrhea. Corneal desiccation and secondary ocular lesions are common. Treatment is symptomatic and focused on minimizing secondary ocular infection. Isolation of infected animals for 6 to 8 weeks may be required. Recovered animals retain long-lasting immunity from reinfection.

Sendai Virus.
Sendai virus is the primary causative agent of viral respiratory disease in mice. It usually remains subclinical in rats but is highly contagious. The disease causes serious epidemics and high mortality rates among neonates and weanlings in mouse colonies. Clinical signs include weight loss, dyspnea, and chattering. The virus is pneumotropic, and diagnosis is made on the basis of serologic testing or the presence of characteristic lesions, such as interstitial pneumonitis, and alveolar bronchiolization with focal collections of macrophages. Concurrent infection with various bacterial organisms, especially *Mycoplasma pulmonis*, is common and increases mortality. Outbreaks in animal colonies are usually controlled by excluding all young and weanling animals from the colony for several months.

Mousepox (Ectromelia).
This disease is relatively uncommon in the United States. The only known natural host for the virus is mice. Very young and very old mice have the highest susceptibility. There is also a significant difference in susceptibility to this virus among different strains of mice. The disease is highly contagious, with high rates of morbidity and mortality. Mice imported from other countries or the use of tissues and other biologic materials imported from other countries appears to be the primary source of infection. Serologic testing and quarantine of imported animals are crucial to prevent devastating outbreaks.

Lymphocytic Choriomeningitis.
In addition to mice, the lymphocytic choriomeningitis virus can infect guinea pigs, chinchillas, hamsters, canines, and primates, including humans. Natural infection is nearly 100% in wild mouse populations. Transmission occurs by aerosol contamination, bite wounds, and transplacentally. Transmission by arthropod vectors may also occur. Mice infected in utero often have no circulating antibody to the virus and are asymptomatic carriers. Clinical signs vary depending on the specific strain of the virus. Lymphocytic infiltration of a variety of organs can occur, and immune complexes associated with the virus can cause glomerulonephritis. The cerebral form, a result of lymphocytic infiltration of the meninges, is characterized by convulsions, photophobia, and weakness. Hamsters rarely have clinical signs of disease and can serve as reservoirs for infection in a research facility. The virus is transmissible to human beings and can cause flulike symptoms. Prevention of this viral disease requires exclusion of wild rodents from the population and assurances that animal feed is not contaminated from wild rodents or arthropod vectors. Because of the high prevalence of mice infected in utero and the zoonotic potential of this virus, treatment is usually not attempted and infected animals must be eliminated from the colony.

Mouse Hepatitis Virus.
This common coronavirus is highly contagious and widespread. Latent infections in a colony are typical and very difficult to control. Transmission occurs by the oral-nasal route, direct contact, fomites, and transplacentally. Although enteric strains are most common, respiratory strains of the virus exist; a wide variety of disease syndromes are therefore possible. Clinical signs include diarrhea, jaundice, and tremors. Suckling mice are often fatally infected. The virus can be eliminated from a colony by isolating the colony for 4 weeks while preventing breeding of the animals. This allows infected animals to clear the infection. The use of cesarean-derived or barrier-reared mice and placement of microisolator tops on cages may aid in preventing spread of this significantly infectious virus.

Other Viral Diseases.
Mice may become infected with a variety of viral agents such as K-virus, the epizootic diarrhea of infant mice rotavirus, and mouse parvovirus. Mice also harbor murine mammary tumor virus, which is also referred to as the Bittner agent. Other viruses of mice include murine leukemia virus and mouse adenovirus.

A large number of viruses occur naturally in the rat. These include hantaviruses, rat coronavirus, adenovirus, and cytomegalovirus. Clinical disease usually does not develop in rats unless the viruses are activated by stress or concurrent disease. A rotavirus of rats may cause infectious diarrhea in suckling rats. Infected animals are identified by the presence of soft, yellow diarrhea that stains the perineum. Treatment involves supportive care. Infections are self-limiting, but the rat often demonstrates stunted growth.

Mycotic Disease
Systemic mycotic infections are extremely rare in rats and mice. Infection with *Trichophyton mentagrophytes* can occur. The clinical disease is referred to as ringworm and is characterized by crusty skin lesions and alopecia. Asymptomatic carriers may be present. The organism is easily transmitted by direct contact and poses a significant zoonotic potential. Culture with dermatophyte test medium of hair shafts and skin debris may demonstrate the organism. Microscopic examination is necessary to confirm the diagnosis. Mice that are kept in proximity to certain species of birds or exposed to items contaminated with avian feces may acquire infection with *Histoplasma capsulatum*.

Parasitic Disease

Rats and mice may be infected with a number of external parasites (mites, lice) as well as parasites of the gastrointestinal system, urinary system, and blood. Animals obtained from reputable breeders rarely harbor these organisms; however, infections may be latent unless certain stress factors are present.

Endoparasites. Protozoal parasites include *Pneumocystis carinii*, *Cryptosporidium*, *Eimeria*, *Toxoplasma*, *Spironucleus*, and *Giardia*. Rats and mice may harbor the cestode parasites *Vampirolepis* (also *Hymenolepis* or *Rodentolepis*) *nana* (Figure 6-21), *Hymenolepis diminuta*, and some life stages of Taenia species *V. nana* are capable of infecting humans. Rats and mice may also be infected by blood parasites from a variety of phyla. Blood parasites that may occur in rats include *Plasmodium berghei* and *vinckei*, *Trypanosoma lewisi*, *T. cruzi*, *Hepatozoon muris*, *Babesia muris*, and *Mycoplasma* (formerly *Haemobartonella*) *muris*. These organisms are primarily transmitted by the bite of an ectoparasite. Clinical disease may not be apparent unless the animals are under stress. Blood parasites of mice are rare but infection with *Eperythrozoon coccoides* is possible. Infections with these parasites are almost never seen in mice acquired from reputable breeders.

Nematodes that may infect mice include the pinworms in the *Syphacia obvelata* and *Aspicularis tetraptera*. *Heterakis spumosa* is a nematode parasite found in the cecum and colon of rats and mice. Infections do not normally cause clinical signs but impaction, colonic intussusception, or rectal prolapse can occur. *Nippostrongylus muris* is a nematode parasite of the small intestine. The larvae of this parasite migrate through the lungs and can cause dyspnea and pulmonary hemorrhage. Diarrhea and generalized unthriftiness may also be evident. Other nematode parasites include *Gongylonema neoplasticum*, *Trichinella spiralis*, *Capillaria hepatica*, and *Trichosomoides crassicauda*.

At least four species of *Eimeria* are capable of infecting the intestine of rats and mice. *Cryptosporidium muris* is found in the stomach. Diagnosis is made by identifying oocysts after fecal flotation or by finding organisms in the epithelial cells of the intestinal tract. The rat can also serve as an intermediate host of *Toxoplasma gondii*. Infection with *Spironucleus (Hexamita) muris*, a flagellated protozoan found in the duodenum, may cause diarrhea and weight loss.

Ectoparasites. Lice, mites, and fleas can infest rats and mice. Diagnosis of ectoparasite infestation can be accomplished with a magnifying glass to identify the adult stage of the parasite or with a cellophane tape preparation of hair. Species that burrow into the dermis require skin scraping for identification. Infestation with the louse species *Polyplax spinulosa* (Figure 6-22) and *P. serrata* may occur and can cause hair loss and pruritus. Other ectoparasites include *Laelaps echidninus*, *Radfordia ensifera*, and *Notoedres muris*. *Myobia musculi* is an important fur mite of mice. Flea infestation is uncommon in mice and rats. Ectoparasites are difficult to eliminate from colonies. Anthelmintic medications and insecticides may be placed on cage tops to aid in treating infested animals. In some cases, bedding materials may be dusted with insecticide powders. Ivermectin administered orally may also be beneficial.

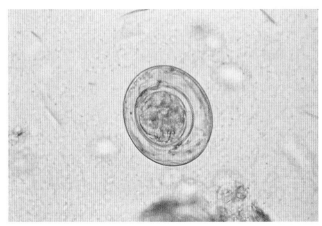

FIGURE 6-21. Egg of *Rodentolepis nana.* (Image courtesy of CDC/Dr. Moore.)

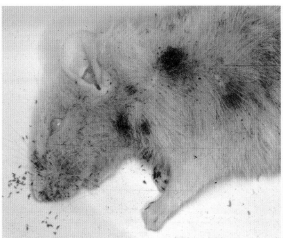
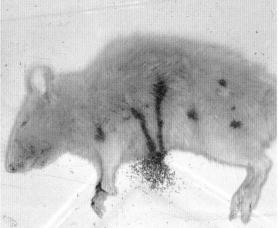

FIGURE 6-22. Polyplax spinulosa leaving a rat that died of the effects of its louse population. (From Bowman D: *Georgis' parasitology for veterinarians,* ed 10, St. Louis, Saunders, 2014.)

NONINFECTIOUS DISEASES

Neoplasia

The incidence of spontaneous tumor development in rats and mice can be as much as 87% in animals older than 2 years. In some cases, tumors once designated as spontaneous have been studied sufficiently to identify a dietary, hormonal, environmental, microbiologic, or genetic causative agent. In random-bred mice, pulmonary tumors are most common. In inbred mice, the incidence of neoplasia is often related to infection with one of the several oncogenic viruses. These include mouse mammary tumor virus, mouse leukemia virus, and mouse sarcoma virus. The murine oncogenic viruses are primarily transmitted by the placenta to the fetus or in the milk to suckling mice. Specific development of tumors varies with sex, age, and strain of the animal.

The most common neoplasia of rats is mammary fibroadenoma (Figure 6-23). The mammary tissue of rats has a wide distribution in the animal, and these tumors can occur almost anywhere on the body. The tumors are usually benign, well encapsulated, and can be surgically removed. Pituitary adenomas may also occur, especially in older rats. These tend to grow rapidly and become large enough to compress adjacent nervous tissue, resulting in depression, incoordination, and death. Fisher 344 rats are particularly prone to lymphocytic leukemia; affected animals will show evidence of splenomegaly, hepatomegaly, and lymphadenopathy. Anemia, jaundice, and depression are common findings. Other tumors of rats include keratoacanthoma (a benign skin tumor), uterine endometrial polyps, testicular interstitial cell tumors, thyroid adenomas, pancreatic islet cell tumors, and pheochromocytomas of the adrenal gland.

Age-Associated Diseases

Age-related changes in rats and mice vary with different strains and stocks. Environmental factors play a significant role in influencing life span. Certain inbred strains of mice are more susceptible to disease than random-bred animals. Amyloidosis can occur in older mice. Amyloid deposition can be found in a variety of organs, including the liver, kidneys, and intestinal tract. Progressive changes in the myocardium, particularly the left atrial tissue, also occur in older mice. Acute death is a common outcome. Numerous neoplastic diseases of mice are also common in older animals, particularly inbred strains.

Age-related, nonneoplastic diseases of rats include chronic glomerulonephropathy, polyarteritis nodosa, myocardial degeneration, and radiculoneuropathy. Chronic glomerulonephropathy is a progressive disease that is widespread in older Sprague-Dawley rats. Acute death from renal failure is common. Sprague-Dawley and SHR rats are also particularly prone to polyarteritis nodosa. Thickening of the medium-sized arteries is evident on necropsy. Radiculoneuropathy is a degenerative disease that affects spinal roots and results in muscular atrophy in the lumbar region and hind limbs.

Husbandry-Related Diseases

Trauma. Trauma from fighting is often a significant cause of morbidity and mortality in male rats, with a predisposition in particular strains. Fighting usually occurs at night and results in bite and scratch wounds over the head, perineum, and lumbosacral skin. These lesions frequently become infected. A high incidence of secondary amyloidosis has been reported in animals that have chronic lesions stemming from fighting. Fighting can be prevented by separating males or, preferably, by grouping males at weaning rather than at a later time. Trauma from fighting is not as common in mice as it is in rats. Male mice housed together fight more commonly than females. Fighting usually occurs at night and results in bite and scratch wounds over the head, perineum, and lumbosacral skin (Figure 6-24). These lesions frequently become infected with *Staphylococcus aureus* and treatment is generally not effective. Pet rats and mice may also suffer from traumatic injury. This is a particular problem when owners (and

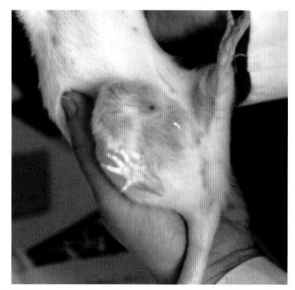

FIGURE 6-23. Mammary fibroadenoma in the inguinal region of a 355-g female rat. The excised tumor weighed 40 g and represented 11% of the rat's body weight. (From Quesenberry K, Carpenter JW: *Ferrets, rabbits, and rodents: clinical medicine and surgery,* ed 3, St. Louis, Saunders, 2012.)

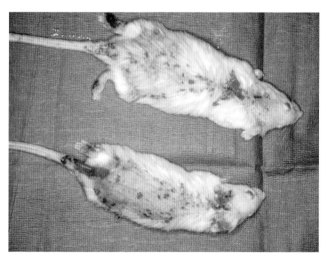

FIGURE 6-24. Severe wounds caused by fighting with cagemates.

their young children) are not accustomed to proper handling and drop the animal.

Barbering. In the absence of pruritus, rats with evidence of alopecia are most likely suffering from **barbering**. This condition results from chewing of hair by cagemates. Alopecia is often restricted to the muzzle, head, and middorsal region of the trunk. Removal of the animal that has no evidence of hair chewing usually resolves the problem.

Nutritional Diseases. Rats and mice that are provided with an adequate fresh supply of commercially available rodent food rarely develop nutritional problems. The food must be stored properly to prevent contamination and should be fed within 6 months of the milling date. Most rats and mice will eat only to their caloric requirements. However, some rats fed ad lib will become obese and have an increased incidence or severity of age-associated changes. Rats and mice should not be fed fresh vegetables because they may be contaminated with *Salmonella* species, *Yersinia* species, or *Bacillus piliformis.* Certain strains of rats have been bred specifically for their predisposition to obesity and other nutrition-related problems.

Ringtail. This disease is prevalent in young rats kept in low-humidity environments. Affected animals have annular constrictions of the tail. Edema, necrosis, and sloughing of the tail distal to the constrictions follows. Ringtail can be prevented by providing an environment with a relative humidity of 50% or greater and by housing young rats in shoebox cages with deep bedding.

Malocclusion. The incisor teeth of rats grow continuously throughout life. If the jaw occlusion is abnormal or the animal is fed soft diets, the incisors may overgrow (Figure 6-25). If incisors are not clipped back or worn down with chewing, the animal will be unable to eat. Incisors can be clipped with toenail clippers. The procedure is painless and requires minimal restraint. Dental burs or grinding tools can also be used to file the incisors to an acceptable length.

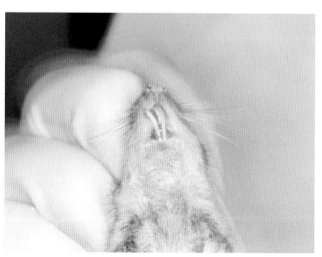

FIGURE 6-25. Malocclusion in a mouse.

EUTHANASIA

Animals maintained in biomedical research facilities may be euthanized at the end of a research study to collect tissue samples for further analysis. Pet animals that are suffering are often humanely euthanized rather than allowing the animal to live its final days in pain. Methods of euthanasia vary depending on the species and on whether tissues must be harvested from the animal without contamination from chemical agents. The American Veterinary Medical Association (AVMA) publishes the *American Veterinary Medical Association Guidelines for the Euthanasia of Animals.* The AVMA report discusses only methods and agents for euthanasia supported by data from scientific studies. It emphasizes professional judgment, technical proficiency, and humane handling of the animals. Euthanasia should never be performed in the same room where other animals are housed because this causes unnecessary stress in the other animals.

Acceptable methods of euthanasia for rats include injectable or inhalant anesthetic overdose and barbiturate overdose. Only specific agents are approved, such as isoflurane. Carbon dioxide chamber asphyxiation can only be used under specific conditions. Carbon dioxide is administered by gradual displacement. The carbon dioxide can be supplied as a humidified compressed gas or by a dry ice pack. The animals must not be permitted to come into contact with the dry ice container. Avoid placing large groups of animals in the carbon dioxide chamber simultaneously because this stresses the animals and reduces the effectiveness of the inhalation agent. Animals should be left in the carbon dioxide chamber for at least 5 minutes after obvious respiratory motions have ceased. These procedures are often followed by thoracic incision to ensure that the animal will not recover in the event that assessment of death was in error. In rare instances, decapitation or exsanguination under anesthesia may be permitted, but the need to avoid administration of drugs must be justified by the investigator and be approved by the institutional animal care and use committee.

Barbiturate overdose is usually administered by IP injection. If the animal is sedated, rapid IV injection can also be used. The use of decapitation is allowed only in instances in which tissues and body fluids must be uncontaminated to yield valid results. The animal is normally sedated or lightly anesthetized before performing the procedure. Commercially available guillotines are available for this purpose. The specific procedure for euthanasia by exsanguination varies somewhat depending on whether the blood is to be retained for study. A common method involves placing the animal under anesthesia and incising the jugular vein and carotid artery. This method may also be used to confirm death when euthanasia was performed by other means. When sterile blood is to be collected for study, a cannula may be placed in the carotid or femoral artery of the anesthetized animal. Animals that are also being preserved for tissue analysis may have simultaneous infusion of fixative solutions into the left ventricle of the heart.

KEY POINTS

- The scientific names for the commonly used laboratory rat and mouse are *Rattus norvegicus* and *Mus musculus,* respectively.
- Unique anatomic and physiologic features of rats include the presence of a harderian gland and the lack of a gallbladder. Mice also possess harderian glands.
- Mice are useful animal models because of their small size, low cost, ease of maintenance, and high reproductive rate.
- Rats are used in biomedical research studies of dental disease, toxicology, audiology, and obesity.
- Rat-breeding programs produce stocks and strains that are susceptible to a number of human diseases, including diabetes insipidus, hypertension, and cataracts.
- The gender of mice and rats can be determined by observation of anogenital distance.
- Rat and mouse breeding systems include intensive and nonintensive systems.
- Rats and mice are usually housed in shoebox cages with feeding devices integrated into the cage lid.
- Restraint of rats and mice for technical procedures can be done manually or by using specially designed restraint devices.
- Methods of permanent identification include tattooing the ear, tail, or toe; punching or tagging the ear, clipping the toe, or using implants that can be read electronically.
- Injections are usually given intravenously, subcutaneously, intraperitoneally, or intramuscularly.
- Blood is usually collected from the lateral tail veins or the retroorbital plexus or sinus.
- Common bacterial diseases of rats include murine respiratory mycoplasmosis and Tyzzer's disease.
- Common infections of mice include *Mycoplasma pulmonis,* Sendai virus, mouse hepatitis virus, and Tyzzer's disease.
- A variety of viral and parasitic agents may infect rats and mice, but clinical disease usually does not occur.

REVIEW QUESTIONS

1. The scientific name of the most common species of laboratory rat is _____ _____.

2. In rats, secretions from the harderian gland are commonly referred to as _____ _____.

3. What physiologic feature makes the rat useful as a model for toxicology studies?

4. Rats have been _____ to be susceptible to specific diseases.

5. Animals that are produced as a result of random matings are referred to as _____.

6. When 20 or more generations of brother-sister or parent-offspring mating have occurred, the offspring are referred to as _____.

7. An animal with a hole punch at the middle of the left ear and a notch at the bottom of the right ear is designated with the number _____.

8. An appropriately sized needle to use for collection of blood from the lateral tail vein of a rat is _____.

9. List the techniques that may be used to evaluate the level of anesthesia in rats.

10. The small muscle mass of rats complicates _____ injections.

11. Tyzzer's disease is caused by _____ _____.

12. The most common respiratory disease of rats is _____ _____ _____.

13. The most significant but self-limiting viral disease in rats is _____.

14. A parasite of rats that has significant zoonotic potential is _____ _____.

15. The incidence of spontaneous tumor development can be as high as _____% in animals over 2 years of age.

7 The Rabbit

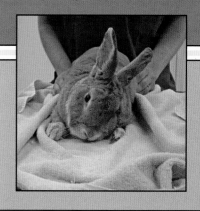

OUTLINE

KEY TERMS

Buphthalmia
Cecotrophs
Dewlap
Hypsodontic
Kindling
Lagomorph
Malocclusion
Pododermatitis
Posterior paralysis
Pseudopregnancy
Rabbit fever
Sacculus rotundus
Slobbers
Snuffles
Splay leg
Torticollis
Trichobezoars
Wolf teeth
Wry neck

LEARNING OBJECTIVES

After studying this chapter, you will be able to:

- Identify unique anatomic and physiologic characteristics of rabbits.
- Describe breeding systems used for rabbits.
- Identify unique aspects of rabbit behavior.
- Explain routine procedures for husbandry, housing, and nutrition of rabbits.
- Describe various restraint and handling procedures used on rabbits.
- Describe methods of administering medication and collecting blood samples.
- List and describe common diseases of rabbits.
- Describe appropriate methods of euthanasia that may be used on rabbits.

Rabbits are popular game animals, especially in Europe. They are also raised commercially for meat, skins, and fur. Rabbits are popular as pets and are used extensively in biomedical research and consumer product safety testing.

TAXONOMY

Rabbits and hares were originally classified as a suborder within the order Rodentia. Because they possess two pairs of upper incisors, they were eventually reclassified into the order Lagomorpha. There are 80 recognized species of **lagomorphs**, placed in 2 families containing 13 genera. The family Leporidae contains the genera *Oryctolagus* and *Sylvilagus*, which are the rabbits and hares. The domestic rabbit is the only member of the genus *Oryctolagus* and is referred to as the scientific name *Oryctolagus cuniculus*. This species is thought to have originated on the Iberian Peninsula and then spread to Mediterranean countries.

Romans were the first to domesticate the rabbit. Rabbits were carried on sailing ships and placed on hundreds of islands to be used as a food source on future voyages. The European rabbit was later introduced to many other countries, including New Zealand and Australia. One pair of rabbits was released in Victoria (Australia) in 1859. Thirty-one years later, the rabbit population was estimated at 20 million. The introduction of *O. cuniculus* into Australia resulted in a significant alteration in the economic and ecologic health of the region. Agriculture continues to be seriously threatened. The use of poison baits in an effort to control the population resulted in secondary poisoning of natural predators. The use of introduced predators as a population control measure has also had a detrimental effect on the native flora and fauna. Plant communities have been destroyed by the ravenous feeding habits of rabbits. The resulting bare landscape is prone to increased erosion and subsequent habitat destruction. In the 1950s, another control measure was tried. The introduction of the disease myxomatosis was designed as a control measure for European rabbits. The disease is caused by a virus that is native to South American rabbits, who are resistant to its effects. When first introduced, the virus decimated the European rabbit population. Initially, the disease greatly reduced the numbers of European rabbits. However, those rabbits that survived were highly resistant to the virus.

Two additional genera of lagomorphs are the *Sylvilagus* and *Lepus*. The genus *Lepus* contains the hares and *Sylvilagus* consists of cottontail rabbits. Rabbit genera do not interbreed. Cottontail rabbits or hares may be seen rarely as pet animals, although like most wild animals, they do not do well in captivity. The species of domestic rabbit kept as pets and used in biomedical research is *Oryctolagus cuniculus*.

UNIQUE ANATOMIC AND PHYSIOLOGIC FEATURES

GENERAL CHARACTERISTICS

In addition to the presence of a second pair of upper incisors, rabbits have a number of characteristics that distinguish them from rodents. Table 7-1 contains a summary of unique physiologic data. Rabbits have a high muscle/bone ratio and large body fat reserves. These factors account for their relatively light weight compared with their size. Females tend to be larger than males. The limbs are long, with the hindlimbs longer than forelimbs to make them well adapted for running. There are no footpads, and the soles of the hind feet are covered with fur. The toes terminate in long, nearly straight claws. The tail is short and sometimes conspicuously marked. Leporidae have a small, rudimentary clavicle. Domestic rabbits have smaller ears and shorter, less powerful legs than the hares. Wild rabbits tend to be somewhat smaller than their domestic cousins. Rabbits are well haired except for the tip of the nose and scrotum of males. Their fur is thick and soft and ranges in color from white to dark brown. Northern species may undergo a seasonal molt from a summer brown pelage to a winter white. Domesticated *O. cuniculus* vary tremendously in size, fur type, coloration, and general appearance. There are hundreds of different rabbit breeds, classified as either fancy breeds or fur breeds. Fur breeds include rex, Angoras, and satin rabbits.

TABLE 7-1	Normal Physiologic Values for Rabbits	
Body Weight		
Adult buck (male)		2-5 kg
Adult doe (female)		2-6 kg
Birth weight (kit)		30-80 g
Clinical Examination*		
Rectal body temperature		38.5°-40.0° C (101.3°-104.0° F)
Normal heart rate		180-250 beats/min
Normal respiratory rate		30-60 breaths/min
Blood		
Whole blood volume		55-70 ml/kg
Plasma volume		28-51 ml/kg
Amounts of Food and Water		
Daily food consumption (rabbit pellets)†		50 g/kg
Gastrointestinal transit time for hard feces		4-5 hours after eating
Gastrointestinal transit time for cecotropes		8-9 hours after eating
Daily hard feces excretion		5-18 g/kg
Daily water consumption‡		50-150 ml/kg
Daily urine excretion		10-35 ml/kg
Age at Onset of Puberty and Breeding Life		
Sexual maturity, male		22-52 weeks
Sexual maturity, female		22-52 weeks
Breeding life, male		60-72 months
Breeding life, female		24-36 months
Female Reproductive Cycle		
Estrous cycle		Induced ovulators
Estrus duration		Prolonged
Ovulation rate		6-10 eggs
Pseudopregnancy		16-17 days
Gestation length		30-33 days
Litter size		4-12 kits
Male Copulatory Patterns		
Mounting time		2 seconds
Preejaculatory intromissions		1
Ejaculations per mating		1-3

(From Hillyer EV, Quesenberry KE: *Ferrets, rabbits, and rodents: clinical medicine and surgery,* St Louis, 1997, Mosby.)

Data listed are ranges for healthy 2.5- to 3.0-kg New Zealand white rabbits. Generally, New Zealand white rabbits reach this weight at approximately 18 weeks of age. The data should be used as a guide only; these ranges are approximations, and actual values may vary depending on the sex, age, and supplier of the rabbit.

*Lower values are expected in rabbits acclimatized to handling.

†Food consumption is greater in growing, pregnant, and lactating animals.

‡The amount of water required is influenced by food intake, feed composition, and environmental temperature. These values are for a normal rabbit fed standard rabbit pellets.

Fancy breeds include the Belgian hare, and lop and dwarf rabbits. The breed used in biomedical research is the New Zealand white. Other common pet breeds include the Dutch belted, Flemish giant, Polish, and chinchilla.

THE HEAD AND NECK

As mentioned previously, the second pair of incisors is one of the distinguishing features of the rabbit. This second pair of upper incisors are referred to as peg teeth or **wolf teeth** and are located just posterior to the first incisors (Figure 7-1). Like rodents, a diastema exists between the incisors and premolars.

The teeth of rabbits are **hypsodontic. Malocclusion** can result in overgrown incisors if untreated and lead to anorexia and weight loss (Figure 7-2). Rabbits also have a large, fleshy tongue with a small elevation in the posterior portion. This

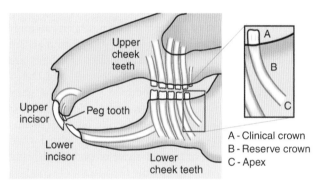

FIGURE 7-1. Cross-section schematic of a rabbit skull showing dentition of mandible and maxilla and of an individual tooth. (From Quesenberry K, Carpenter JW: *Ferrets, rabbits, and rodents: clinical medicine and surgery,* ed 3, St. Louis, 2012, Saunders.)

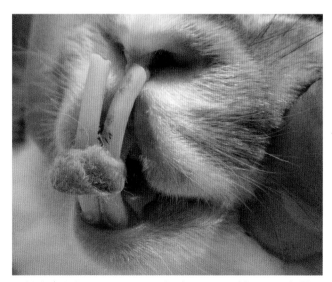

FIGURE 7-2. Severe incisor malocclusion in a rabbit. A wad of hair has become entrapped in the lower incisors. (From Mayer J, Donnelly TM: *Clinical veterinary advisor: birds and exotic pets,* St. Louis, 2013, Elsevier.)

makes endotracheal intubation especially challenging. The ear pinnae of leporidae are generally longer than they are wide. The ears are highly vascular and serve as a thermoregulatory organ. Female rabbits have prominent skin folds on the underside of the neck, referred to as the **dewlap.** Persistent wetness of this area can result in significant dermatitis.

THORAX

The heart is relatively small compared with other species of similar size. The respiratory system includes a large right lung divided into three lobes. The left lung is much smaller and contains two lobes. Rabbit neutrophils have a predominant granule type that stains red and appears similar to the eosinophil of other mammals. This cell is often referred to as a pseudoeosinophil or heterophil.

ABDOMEN

Like the rat and horse, rabbits cannot vomit. The stomach is large, thin walled, and not compartmentalized. The terminal portion of the ileum consists of the **sacculus rotundus.** This is a round, expanded, muscular sac with attached lymphoid tissue. A very large cecum is also present. The colon is divided into proximal and distal portions and is separated by fusus coli. This structure plays a role in production of **cecotrophs,** also referred to as soft feces. Cecotrophs are composed of water, nitrogen, electrolytes, and vitamins. They are normally ingested directly from the anus in the evening and are also referred to as "night feces."

GENITOURINARY SYSTEM

Rabbit urine is thick and creamy, and albuminuria or proteinuria is common. Ammonium magnesium phosphate and calcium carbonate crystals are also commonly found. Rabbit urine tends to be highly alkaline, often with a pH greater than 8.0. Urine color varies from dark brown to yellow. Younger rabbits tend to have less opaque urine with no significant crystalluria. Urine consistency varies considerably with diet.

The uterus is duplex, with two cervixes and two cervical orifices. There is no uterine body: the cervices open directly into the vagina. In males, the scrotum is anterior to the penis.

ANIMAL MODELS

The domestic rabbit was the first animal model of atherosclerosis. Rabbits have been used in many studies of diet-induced atherosclerosis. Feeding a high-cholesterol and high-fat diet will cause lesions similar to those seen in human atherosclerosis. In 1973, a Japanese veterinarian, Yoshio Watanabe, was collecting serum from the group of rabbits and discovered that one rabbit consistently had hypercholesterolemia. He started a breeding program to develop this condition in a colony of rabbits. Several of these colonies now exist in the United States. Their ease of handling and large, readily accessible ear veins also make rabbits useful in antibody production and other studies for which large volumes of blood must be collected. Rabbits are also used in eye irritancy evaluations. The eye irritancy test has been greatly refined since its initial development to allow researchers to anesthetize the animal's eyes before performing the evaluation. This has also improved the validity of the test results by removing a significant potential source of pain and distress in the animals.

REPRODUCTION

Determination of gender in rabbits can be accomplished by applying gentle digital pressure along the genital opening. Females, referred to as does, have a slitlike opening (Figure 7-3). Digital pressure exposes the mucosal surface of the vulva. Males, referred to as bucks, have a rounded urethral opening. Digital pressure will extrude the penis from the rounded penile sheath. The onset of puberty varies greatly in different breeds of animals. Smaller breeds, such as the Dutch and Polish, develop more rapidly. Does mature earlier than bucks. Female New Zealand white rabbits generally mature at approximately 5 months of age, whereas males reach puberty by 6 to 7 months. Breeding colonies usually consist of 1 buck for 10 to 20 does. The doe is taken to the buck's cage for breeding. Does do not have a typical estrous cycle; they are induced ovulators and show seasonal variation in receptivity. Ovulation occurs approximately 10 hours after coitus. The length of the gestation period is 29 to 35 days. The doe will often begin nest building a few hours or days before delivery. The doe plucks fur from her abdomen, sides, and dewlap to line the nest. Ideally, nesting boxes are provided that also allow the doe to keep the neonates, referred to as kits,

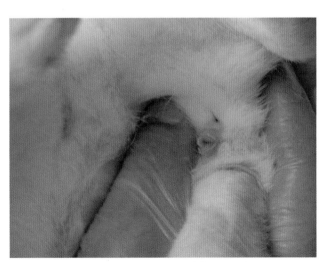

FIGURE 7-3. Female rabbits have a slitlike genital opening. (From Sheldon CC, Topel J, Sonsthagen T: *Animal restraint for veterinary professionals*, St. Louis, 2006, Mosby.)

in a single location. Parturition, referred to as **kindling**, usually occurs in the morning hours. Litter size is 4 to 12 kits, depending on the breed. Kits are born blind, hairless, and helpless. The doe will usually exhibit a period of postpartum receptivity, although most breeding programs do not rebreed the animal until after the kits are weaned. The doe nurses for only a few minutes each day, but the milk is highly enriched and kits can consume as much as 20% of their own body weight in just a few minutes. Weaning occurs between 5 and 8 weeks of age.

> **TECHNICIAN NOTE**   Female rabbits are induced ovulators.

Pseudopregnancy is common in does and can result from mounting by other does or stimulation of a nearby male. Pseudopregnancy generally lasts from 15 to 17 days, during which the doe will often exhibit mammary development and typical nest-building behavior.

GENETICS AND NOMENCLATURE

The term stock refers to an animal that has been randomly bred or, more specifically, not inbred. These animals are also referred to as outbred. Outbred stocks of rabbits are available in the New Zealand white, California, and Dutch belted breeds. As with rodents, outbred stocks are usually described according to their source, with a colon separating the source and stock name. The term strain refers to an animal that has been inbred. A strain is considered inbred when at least 20 generations of brother-sister or parent-offspring mating have occurred. A commonly used strain of rabbits is the Watanabe hyperlipidemic strain, mentioned previously. Hybrid animals are the result of a single mating between two different inbred strains. These animals are identified with the name of the originating strains followed by the designation F1. Frequently, rabbits used in biomedical research are designated SPF (specific pathogen free). This is especially common in rabbits because they can harbor a number of bacterial and viral agents and be asymptomatic unless subjected to stressful conditions. Researchers must use animals that are free of specific bacterial and viral agents to avoid introducing variables into their studies.

BEHAVIOR

Rabbits make excellent pets and rarely bite. They can be easily trained to use a litter box. Rabbits housed in groups may develop aggressive tendencies, especially among males. Females will also fight unless raised together from a young age. Feral and wild *O. cuniculus* are likely to live in groups of roughly a dozen animals of both sexes. Rabbits tend to develop specific dominance hierarchies. During the breeding season, males display distinct territorial characteristics. Rabbits are generally nocturnal, often spending the evening and early morning hours foraging for food. Pet rabbits do not usually exhibit strong nocturnal tendencies.

Although not particularly vocal, rabbits may squeal loudly when frightened or injured. They communicate with each other through scent cues and touch and thump their hindlimbs on the ground to warn of danger.

HUSBANDRY, HOUSING, AND NUTRITION

Rabbits maintained in biomedical research facilities are usually housed in stainless steel or plastic cages with mesh floors. These cages open at the front, may be placed on hanging cage racks, and contain a tray underneath to catch waste materials. Food and water are provided by a hanging feed hopper and water bottles attached to the front of the cage. Daily cleaning of the trays is essential to keep ammonia levels and odors to a minimum. The high crystalline content of rabbit urine forms a precipitate on the trays that requires an acidic cleaner to remove. Rabbits may be given a litter box containing shredded paper bedding. Clay cat litter or wood shavings should be avoided because the animals tend to eat these products. Outdoor rabbit hutches are available for housing pet rabbits. These should be made of nonporous materials to allow for proper disinfection. Pet rabbits can be maintained indoors in a solid bottom cage with a wire top.

Rabbits tolerate cool temperatures better than warmer temperatures. Indoor housing should be maintained at a temperature range of approximately 62° to 70° F with a relative humidity between 30% and 70%. Rabbits exposed to excessive temperature fluctuations or temperatures greater than 85° F require additional ventilation and should be closely monitored for signs of heat stress. Ventilation requirements are 10 to 15 room air changes per hour.

Rabbits are herbivorous and coprophagic. Wild and feral rabbits consume a diverse diet of grasses, leaves, buds, tree bark, and roots. They are notorious for consuming lettuce, cabbage, root vegetables, and grains from gardens and farm fields. Commercial rabbit feed contains approximately 15% protein and 10% fiber. The specific requirements for nutrients vary somewhat with different species and at different life cycle stages. Higher-fiber diets are given as needed to prevent the formation of hairballs and minimize the tendency toward obesity. The addition of proteolytic enzymes, such as in papaya juice, may also aid in prevention of hairball formation. One technique to provide this involves soaking a small amount of timothy hay in unpasteurized pineapple or papaya juice and then feeding the hay to the rabbits several times a week.

Rabbits fed ad libitum usually become obese. Rabbits can be provided with supplemental foods, such as clean, raw carrots and other vegetables. These should not be given more than a few times per week because the nutritional value of these foods is low. Some rabbits will develop diarrhea when overfed supplemental foods.

TECHNICIAN NOTE Rabbits fed ad libitum usually become obese.

RESTRAINT AND HANDLING

A slow, soft-spoken approach is necessary when handling rabbits. They tend to become easily frightened and will vocalize or try to escape when scared. Rabbits are removed from the cage by grasping the loose skin over the back (scruff) of the neck. The hindlimbs must be supported to minimize injury to both the handler and the animal. Rabbits are known to kick with the hind legs and can inflict deep scratch wounds on the handler. In addition, if the hindlimbs are not well supported, the rabbit can easily injure its spinal cord. This condition, referred to as **posterior paralysis**, is a common problem when rabbits are not handled properly. When the animal tries to kick, its heavy hindquarters twist and fracture occurs, usually at the seventh lumbar vertebrae. This condition is not treatable and the animal must be euthanized.

To remove a rabbit from its cage or transport it, grasp the animal by the scruff, support the hindquarters with the other hand, and tuck its head in the bend of the elbow (Figure 7-4). The body of the rabbit should be draped along the forearm. When placing the animal on a table, especially a stainless steel table, it is helpful to place a towel or other covering around or under the rabbit. This will make the rabbit less likely to slip and struggle. When returning a rabbit to its cage, it is best to turn the animal so that it is facing outwards before releasing it. This will ensure that the rabbit does not scratch the handler by kicking the handler's arm.

TECHNICIAN NOTE Posterior paralysis is a common problem when rabbits are not handled properly.

Rabbits can be manually restrained for most technical procedures. Some rabbits respond extremely well to relaxation techniques. This involves placing the rabbit on its back,

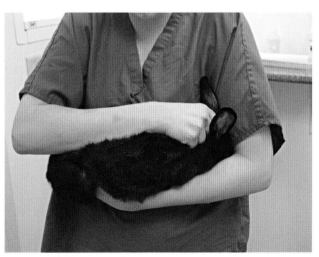

FIGURE 7-4. Proper restraint while transporting a rabbit. Notice the head is tucked in the crook of the elbow and the dorsum and feet are supported. (From Mitchell M, Thomas T: *Manual of exotic pet practice*, St. Louis, 2009, Saunders.)

usually in a V-trough, and gently stroking the animal in a downward direction on its abdomen (Figure 7-5). Light massage of the masseter muscles is also beneficial. It is helpful to dim the room lights or cover the rabbit's eyes. Many rabbits respond to this type of handling by becoming immobile. The rabbit's respiratory rate becomes significantly lower and the animal appears to be in a state of hypnosis. Nearly all noninvasive procedures can be performed with this restraint method in responsive animals.

For more invasive procedures, firmer manual restraint or the use of a restraint box is needed. Manual restraint for technical procedures can be performed by wrapping the rabbit snugly in a towel (Figure 7-6). A hindlimb can be removed from the towel for injection of medications. For procedures that require access to the head, the rabbit can be restrained with a handler gently holding the animal up against the body while a second person performs the

procedure. Technical procedures that are more invasive or potentially painful, such as blood collection, are usually best performed by placing the animal in a restraint box. There are many types of restraint boxes available (Figure 7-7). The most common of these is a polycarbonate container that immobilizes the rabbit while still allowing access to the limbs and head. A cat restraint bag may also be used to restrain rabbits.

IDENTIFICATION

Cage cards or descriptions of a particular animal's color patterns can be used for identification purposes. Ear tags, tattoos, and implanted microchips are also used for permanent identification. Rabbits raised by commercial breeders are often supplied with microchips already implanted. Temporary identification can be accomplished with markers or dyes. For permanent identification the most commonly used method is ear tattooing. The tattoo is applied on the nonvascular space of the ear pinna between the auricular artery and the marginal vein (Figure 7-8). In show rabbits, the right ear is reserved for registration marks applied by registrars of the American Rabbit Breeders Association.

CLINICAL PROCEDURES

ADMINISTRATION OF MEDICATION

Medications can be administered orally or by subcutaneous, intravenous, intramuscular, or intradermal injection. Intranasal administration can also be useful for some anesthetic agents. Intravenous catheterization and nasogastric intubation are also used for medical treatment of rabbits. Medication dosages for rabbits tend to be quite variable and differ by breed, strain, age, and sex. Obtaining an accurate weight before calculating any medication dosage is especially important because body weight estimates are unreliable in this species. In addition, overestimation of body weight is common considering the large volume of material that can be present in the intestinal tract, particularly the cecum.

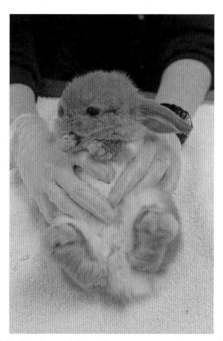

FIGURE 7-5. Many rabbits will enter a trance-like state when placed in dorsal recumbency.

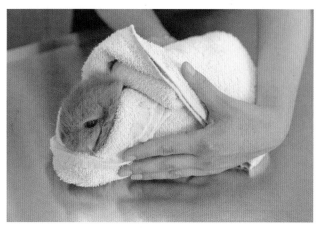

FIGURE 7-6. Rabbits can be wrapped firmly in a towel making a "bunny burrito."

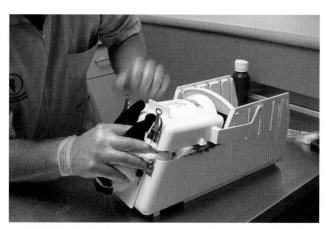

FIGURE 7-7. Rabbit in restraining box. (From Sheldon CC, Topel J, Sonsthagen T: *Animal restraint for veterinary professionals*, St. Louis, 2006, Mosby.)

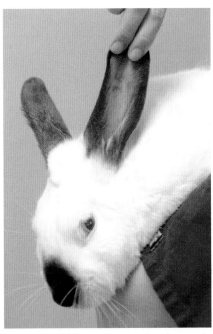

FIGURE 7-8. Tattoo on rabbit ear pinna made with a punch-type tattooer.

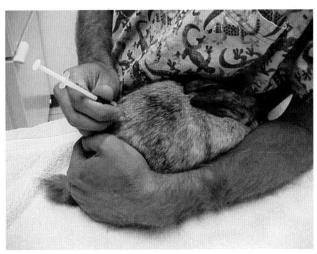

FIGURE 7-10. Intramuscular injection into the large lumbar muscles on either side of the rabbit's spine, just cranial to the pelvis. (From Quesenberry K, Carpenter JW: *Ferrets, rabbits, and rodents: clinical medicine and surgery*, ed 3, St. Louis, 2012, Saunders.)

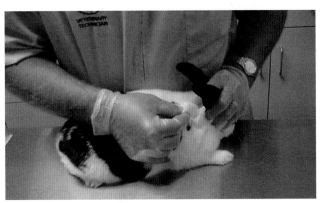

FIGURE 7-9. Subcutaneous injection in a rabbit. (From Sheldon CC, Topel J, Sonsthagen T: *Animal restraint for veterinary professionals*, St. Louis, 2006, Mosby.)

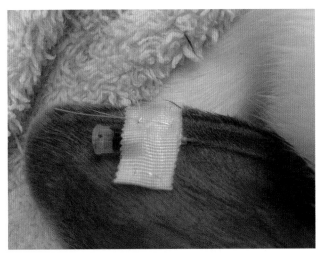

FIGURE 7-11. Correct placement of a catheter into the marginal auricular vein. (From Jepson L: *Exotic animal medicine*, St. Louis, 2009, Saunders.)

INJECTION TECHNIQUES

Injections are routinely given by the subcutaneous route. Intravenous and intramuscular injections are also used. In biomedical research, intradermal injections are used when animals are involved in antibody production protocols. Regardless of the route used, the rabbit must be firmly but gently restrained. It may also be helpful to squeeze the rabbit gently before introducing the needle through the skin to prevent the animal from jumping if startled.

> **TECHNICIAN NOTE** Injections in rabbits are routinely given by subcutaneous, intravenous, and intramuscular routes.

Subcutaneous injections are usually given in the loose skin over the back (scruff) of the neck (Figure 7-9). The rabbit may be restrained in a towel or restraint box. Subcutaneous

injections can also be administered at the lateral space just cranial to the pelvis. Depending on the site chosen, as much as 100 ml can be administered subcutaneously. Intramuscular injections may be given in the large epaxial (lumbar) muscles, the quadriceps, or the thigh muscles (Figure 7-10). In general, a maximum volume of 1.5 ml can be administered intramuscularly. When injecting into the quadriceps or thigh muscles, care must be taken to avoid the sciatic nerve, which is located behind the femur just caudal to the quadriceps muscle group. The marginal ear vein is also used as a site for intravenous injection. A small-gauge butterfly-type catheter is ideal for this procedure to minimize possible laceration to the vessel if the animal moves during the procedure. A small amount of topical local anesthetic can be applied to the ear to reduce the sensation of pain in the animal. An intravenous catheter can be placed in the vessel for administration of fluids (Figure 7-11). However, these vessels are delicate and easily damaged by mechanical irritation from the catheter or chemical irritation from the infused substances, so only isotonic fluids should be administered. Intravenous catheters can also be placed in the jugular, cephalic, or saphenous veins (Figure 7-12). Intraosseous infusions can also be used.

Intradermal injections can be given in numerous locations, but the most common sites are along the back just lateral to the spinal cord. The fur should be clipped or plucked from the site and the site cleaned with alcohol before performing the procedure. The alcohol must be allowed to dry thoroughly before proceeding. The volume given by intradermal injection is usually 0.1 mL or less. A small, raised bleb (wheal) should be evident at the injection site. If no wheal is evident, it is likely that the injection passed into the subcutaneous space.

ORAL ADMINISTRATION

Medications requiring oral administration can be added to the drinking water. However, some animals may refuse to drink, especially if the medication is unpalatable. A small amount of sugar or syrup can be added to the medication to increase palatability. Solid medications (pills, tablets) can be administered by inserting the medication through the diastema into the mouth. Some rabbits will readily chew and swallow tablets. Alternately, a solid medication can be crushed and added to a small amount of paste nutritional supplement or other palatable substance and added to the rabbit's food. Oral medications can also be administered through a feeding tube, with a syringe, or with a stainless steel feeding needle (Figure 7-13). A small mouth speculum is necessary to keep the animal from chewing on the feeding tube. A syringe casing works well for this purpose. Nasogastric tubes can be placed in anorectic animals with the same technique used for cats (Figure 7-14). The rabbit should have an Elizabethan collar applied to prevent it from removing the tube.

> **TECHNICIAN NOTE** Oral medications can be administered through a feeding tube, with a syringe, or with a stainless steel feeding needle.

ANESTHESIA

Rabbits present a somewhat greater anesthetic risk than other laboratory animals. Rabbits are easily stressed by anesthesia, are difficult to intubate, and have highly variable responses to anesthetic agents. In addition, preanesthetic regimens that include atropine are often ineffective because 30% to 40% of rabbits have a serum enzyme called atropine esterase, which hydrolyzes atropine. Their respiratory center is very sensitive to anesthetics, and their high reserves of body fat complicate barbiturate anesthesia. Because rabbits cannot vomit, preanesthetic fasting is not necessary. However, a few hours of fasting before administration of anesthesia aids in obtaining a more accurate weight by allowing some of the

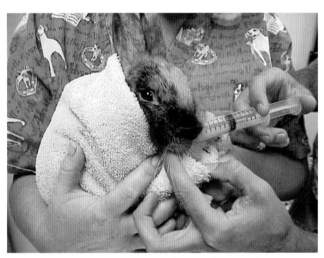

FIGURE 7-13. Oral medication being administered to a rabbit. (From Quesenberry K, Carpenter JW: *Ferrets, rabbits, and rodents: clinical medicine and surgery*, ed 3, St. Louis, 2012, Saunders.)

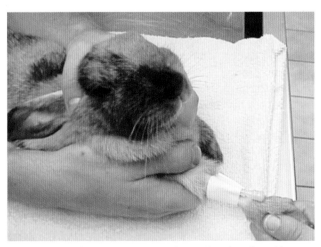

FIGURE 7-12. An intravenous catheter placed in the rabbit's cephalic vein. (From Quesenberry K, Carpenter JW: *Ferrets, rabbits, and rodents: clinical medicine and surgery*, ed 3, St. Louis, 2012, Saunders.)

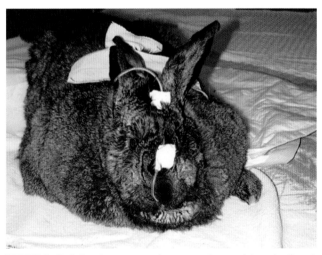

FIGURE 7-14. Nasogastric tube in an obese adult male Flemish giant rabbit. (From Quesenberry K, Carpenter JW: *Ferrets, rabbits, and rodents: clinical medicine and surgery*, ed 3, St. Louis, 2012, Saunders.)

intestinal contents to be eliminated. Care must be taken to keep the fasting period to a minimum because rabbits have a high metabolic rate and prolonged fasting can lead to hypoglycemia and alteration in acid-base balance.

Rabbits can be anesthetized using a combination of preanesthetic agents and mask or chamber induction (Table 7-2). Long procedures necessitate the placement of an endotracheal tube. Endotracheal intubation can be challenging in the rabbit due to the small size of the oral cavity, difficulty in visualizing the larynx, and the rabbit's tendency for laryngospasms. Topical lidocaine on the epiglottis may facilitate passage of the endotracheal tube. Once the animal has received appropriate preanesthetics or has been mask induced, the rabbit can be intubated using a blind technique. The head must be extended so that the passage of the endotracheal tube is essentially in a straight line. Place the tube in the oral cavity over the tongue. When the rabbit exhales, condensation should be visible in the tube. Exhalation may also be confirmed by listening for breath sounds at the end of the tube. During exhalation, advance the tube firmly with slight rotation so that it enters the trachea.

> **TECHNICIAN NOTE** Rabbits can be anesthetized using a combination of injectable agents and mask or chamber induction.

Rabbit skin is rather thin and delicate. Care must be taken when preparing the animal for surgery to avoid tearing the skin when clipping hair. During surgery, the animal should be closely monitored. Heart rate and blood pressure should be recorded every 5 minutes. Capnography and pulse oximetry may also be useful.

BLOOD COLLECTION TECHNIQUES

Blood samples can be easily collected from the marginal ear vein or central auricular artery. The jugular, cephalic, or lateral saphenous veins can also be used for blood collection. Blood collection by cardiocentesis must be performed under anesthesia and is usually followed by euthanasia because of the high probability of painful complications. All techniques require that the fur over the venipuncture site be shaved or plucked. The site is cleaned with alcohol and the alcohol allowed to thoroughly dry before proceeding.

For collections from the vessels of the ear, warm the vessel by holding the ear against your hand or applying a warm, moist cloth. Application of a small amount of topical local anesthetic will minimize the sensation of pain on venipuncture. A small-gauge needle (25 to 27 gauge) can then be introduced into the vessel (Figure 7-15). When small volumes are needed, the blood can be collected directly from the hub of the needle. Use of syringes or large Vacutainer tubes can collapse these vessels, especially in small rabbit breeds.

In some breeds, particularly the small breeds, the cephalic vein is not readily visible. In larger breeds, this vessel can be used for blood collection. The lateral saphenous vein is also commonly used (Figure 7-16). For either vessel, the rabbit should be restrained on its side by a handler who also compresses the vessel. Blood collection from the jugular vein usually requires that the rabbit be sedated or lightly anesthetized. The rabbit is held in dorsal recumbency with its head over the edge of a table and its forelimbs directed caudally under the animal. The neck is then gently tipped back to allow for visualization of the paired jugular veins (Figure 7-17). Alternately, the rabbit can be restrained with its forelimbs held over the edge of a table. Either technique can be difficult in does with large dewlaps.

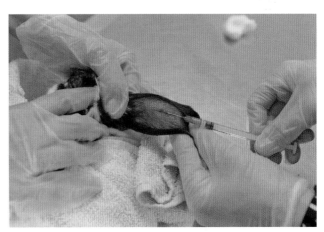

FIGURE 7-15. Blood collection from the ear vein.

TABLE 7-2	Selected Preanesthetic and Anesthetic Agents Used in Rabbits		
DRUG	**DOSAGE**	**ROUTE**	**INDICATION**
Acepromazine	0.5-1 mg/kg	IM, SC	Premedication
Acepromazine + butorphanol	0.5 mg/kg + 0.5 mg/kg	SC, IM	Sedation
Diazepam	1-2 mg/kg	IV, IM	Sedation
Fentanyl/fluanisone	0.2-0.5 mL/kg	IM	Premedication
Ketamine + xylazine	35 mg/kg + 5 mg/kg	IM	Anesthesia
Medetomidine	0.1-0.5 mg/kg	IM	Premedication or sedation
Midazolam	0.5-2 mg/kg	IV, IM, IP	Tranquillizer
Propofol	7.5-15 mg/kg	IV	Anesthesia
Isoflurane	1.5%-5% to effect	Inhalation	Anesthesia

DIAGNOSTIC IMAGING

When diagnostic imaging is indicated, two views are routinely taken, a dorsoventral or ventrodorsal and a lateral. Most imaging studies do not require that the patient be anesthetized. Skull radiographs can be used to evaluate the teeth and identify malocclusion. Abdominal radiographs can identify the presence of **trichobezoars**.

COMMON DISEASES

Rabbits are prone to a number of gastrointestinal, respiratory, reproductive, and dermatologic diseases. As with most other small mammals, diet and housing play a significant role in maintaining the health of the animals. Diseases are genetic in origin or result from infection with a number of viral and bacterial agents.

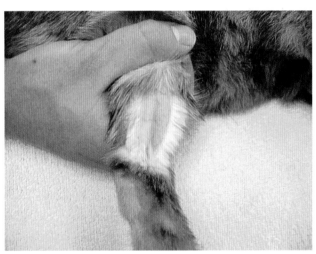

FIGURE 7-16. The rabbit's lateral saphenous vein. (From Quesenberry K, Carpenter JW: *Ferrets, rabbits, and rodents: clinical medicine and surgery*, ed 3, St. Louis, 2012, Saunders.)

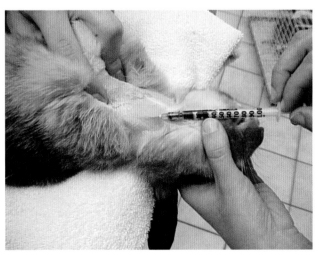

FIGURE 7-17. Jugular venipuncture. (From Quesenberry K, Carpenter JW: *Ferrets, rabbits, and rodents: clinical medicine and surgery*, ed 3, St. Louis, 2012, Saunders.)

INFECTIOUS DISEASES

Infectious diseases result from a number of bacterial, viral, fungal, and parasitic agents. In some cases, these organisms are present as normal flora and fauna and do not cause disease unless the animals are under stress. Careful attention to appropriate husbandry procedures minimizes the susceptibility of this species to disease.

BACTERIAL DISEASE

Bacterial infections of the respiratory and gastrointestinal systems are leading causes of morbidity and mortality in pet and laboratory rabbits. The organisms that cause these diseases are present in many asymptomatic animals. In some cases, different variants of the organisms exist that range in virulence.

Pasteurellosis

Pasteurellosis is the most common bacterial infection of rabbits. The causative agent, *Pasteurella multocida*, is a small gram-negative coccobacillus. Many asymptomatic rabbits harbor this organism in the upper respiratory tract. The organism can spread to multiple locations and cause a variety of disease syndromes. The upper respiratory form of the disease is commonly referred to as **snuffles**. Clinical signs of this syndrome include sneezing and the presence of a serous to mucopurulent discharge from the nares. Other bacterial agents have also been implicated in the development of this syndrome. Many rabbits wipe the discharge with their forelimbs, so the feet will show evidence of the discharge. This disease can become chronic; with some strains of the organism, affected animals will develop a fatal septicemia. Because the organism can easily spread throughout the body, infections may be evident as conjunctivitis, bronchopneumonia, pyometra, and orchitis. Multiple, large, creamy abscesses may occur on the neck area and mammary glands. **Torticollis** (head tilt) can be seen in animals with otitis media or otitis interna. The common name for this condition is **wry neck**. The accumulation of pus and fluid in the inner ear causes the torticollis. In addition to *P. multocida*, *Encephalitozoon cuniculi* may also be involved (Figure 7-18). Rabbits with *P. multocida* infection can die from acute bronchopneumonia.

Transmission of infection is by direct contact or aerosol contamination. Neonates are infected shortly after birth. A number of factors can predispose an animal to develop disease (Figure 7-19). In rabbit colonies, infected animals must be quarantined or removed from the colony. Antibiotics may be helpful but should be used with caution because prolonged use can cause a fatal diarrhea. Effective antibiotics include penicillin, chloramphenicol, and enrofloxacin. Antibiotic therapy can produce remission but reinfection is common. Cesarean derivation is required for complete elimination of the organism from breeding stock. Immunologic tests are available that use indirect fluorescent antibody or enzyme-linked immunosorbent assay techniques to identify carrier animals.

Pneumonia

In addition to the bronchopneumonia that can result from *P. multocida* infection, rabbits are susceptible to infection with *Bordetella bronchiseptica* and cilia-associated respiratory bacilli. *Pseudomonas, Klebsiella pneumoniae, Staphylococcus, Streptococcus,* and *Pneumococci* are also suspected of causing respiratory disease in rabbits. The organisms can be transmitted by direct contact, aerosol, and fomites. Clinically normal rabbits harbor these organisms, and infections are usually asymptomatic except in weanlings and animals under stress. However, these organisms can cause significant mortality rates in guinea pigs and other rodents. For this reason, rabbits should never be housed in close proximity to guinea pigs and other rodents.

Enterotoxemia and Mucoid Enteropathy

The term mucoid enteropathy encompasses a clinical complex primarily of concern in young rabbits (usually 7 to 10 weeks old), although it may occur in adults. Clinical signs vary from constipation with mucous hypersecretion to profuse watery diarrhea. Impaction of the colon from constipation is a common finding. Definitive diagnosis is difficult but the presence of mucus-covered or gelatinous feces is considered pathognomonic. Infected animals also exhibit hypothermia. The animals appear depressed, with a crouched posture and rough hair coat. The stomach is usually distended with fluids and gas, the duodenum and jejunum are filled with watery bile-stained contents, and petechial hemorrhage is present on the mucosa of the small and large intestines.

A number of infectious entities can cause this syndrome. The etiology is unknown, but an enterotoxin-induced secretory diarrhea caused by *E. coli* or *Clostridium spiroforme* is suspected. Transmission mechanisms are unclear. The causative agents may be part of the normal flora, usually present in small numbers. In addition, antibiotic-induced enterotoxemia

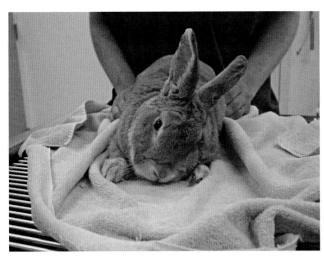

FIGURE 7-18. Head tilt in rabbit caused by *E. cuniculi.* (From Mitchell M, Thomas T: *Manual of exotic pet practice,* St. Louis, 2009, Saunders.)

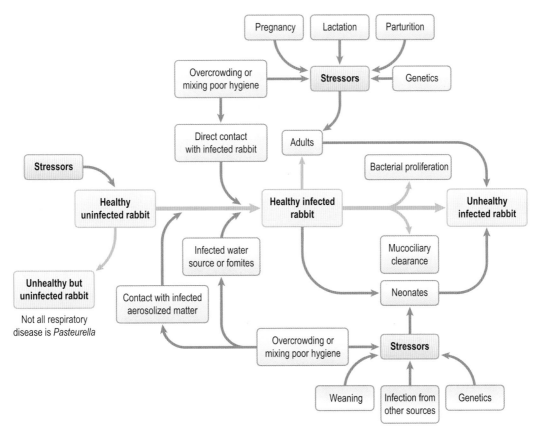

FIGURE 7-19. Factors that affect the expression of *Pasteurella* infection in rabbits. (From Varga M: *Textbook of rabbit medicine,* Oxford, 2014, Butterworth-Heinemann.)

can be a factor, especially with administration of lincomycin, clindamycin, or erythromycin.

Mucoid enteropathy can occur in combination with Tyzzer's disease, salmonellosis, or coccidiosis. A relation between mucoid enteropathy and dietary fiber content is suspected. Higher-fiber diets are thought to provide a measure of protection from this syndrome. Treatment is not usually successful, and infected animals often die within a week. Measures to reduce stress must also be addressed.

Listeriosis

Listeriosis is characterized by sudden death or abortion and is most often seen in does in the late stages of pregnancy. The causative agent is *Listeria monocytogenes*. The organism spreads by the blood to the liver, spleen, and gravid uterus. Clinical signs include anorexia, depression, and weight loss. *L. monocytogenes* is a zoonotic disease and treatment is rarely attempted.

Tyzzer's Disease

As discussed in Chapter 6 Tyzzer's disease has been reported in nearly all species of laboratory animals and is found throughout the world. The causative agent is the gram-negative, spore-forming, flagellated bacterium *Clostridium piliforme*. Definitive diagnosis requires histologic examination of tissues from suspected infected animals. Poor sanitation and overcrowding predispose animals to this disease. Weanling and immunocompromised animals are most severely infected. Clinical signs include diarrhea, dehydration, and anorexia. Careful attention to proper sanitation and reduction of stress aids in preventing this disease. The organism is difficult to eradicate from an animal facility because of the ongoing presence of resistant spores.

Mastitis

Mastitis is not common except in colonies maintained in commercial rabbit-breeding facilities. Like many bacterial diseases of laboratory animals, poor sanitation contributes to the incidence and spread of this disease. Mastitis can develop into a generalized septicemia and is usually fatal under those conditions. Staphylococcus is the most commonly isolated causative agent, but other bacterial agents have also been implicated. Infected does have inflamed mammary glands. The initial red, swollen appearance of the mammae can progress to cyanosis. The disease is sometimes referred to as "blue bag" for this reason. The doe is usually anorectic and febrile and may manifest polydipsia. Care must be taken in treating this condition because antibiotics can lead to diarrhea from microbial imbalance in the gastrointestinal system. During treatment a high-fiber diet is indicated to minimize the possibility of diarrhea. Kits from infected does should not be fostered to another doe because they will spread the infection to the foster mother.

Treponematosis

Treponematosis, also referred to as vent disease or spirochetosis, is caused by the spirochete *Treponema cuniculi*. It occurs in both does and bucks and is transmitted venereally and transplacentally. The incubation period is 3 to 6 weeks. Infected animals develop lesions of the genital region that initially appear as small ulcers and eventually become covered with thick scabs. Definitive diagnosis is based on clinical signs and observation of the spirochete by dark-field microscopy or serologic testing. Infected rabbits are treated with penicillin, given by parenteral injection once a week for 3 weeks. A high-fiber diet and administration of antidiarrheals may be needed to avoid potential complications of antibiotic therapy. If rabbits are maintained in a herd for commercial breeding, all rabbits in the herd must be treated and not bred until the organism is eliminated from the colony.

Tularemia

Infections with the gram-negative organism *Francisella tularensis* are commonly referred to as **rabbit fever**. Numerous species can become infected with this organism, but it is primarily a disease of wild rabbits (*Sylvilagus* specie) and hares (*Lepus* species). The organism is usually transmitted by direct contact or by a bite wound, but inhalation, ingestion, and transmission by arthropod vectors have also been implicated as mechanisms of infection. Affected animals often die before clinical signs are evident. In human beings, the organism can cause fever and lymphadenopathy and may be fatal if not treated.

Miscellaneous Bacterial Diseases

A number of additional diseases of bacterial origin can occur in rabbits, although many of these are quite rare. Reports of salmonellosis have been increasing in recent years. The disease has primarily been reported in young rabbits and pregnant females. The causative agents are *Salmonella typhimurium* and *S. enteriditis*, and transmission is by direct contact or fecal contamination of food and water. Like many diseases of laboratory animals, poor sanitation and stress are contributing factors. Clinical signs include anorexia, fever, and occasionally diarrhea. Affected animals may exhibit signs of septicemia, and death is usually rapid. Because the organism has significant zoonotic potential, it can spread to many other species, and treated rabbits are prone to becoming carriers of disease. Treatment is not usually attempted.

Colibacillosis is caused by certain serotypes of *Escherichia coli*. The disease is not common in North America but is fairly common in Europe. *E. coli* is not normally present in the rabbit gastrointestinal tract but can colonize under certain conditions. Clinical signs vary depending on the age and immune status of the rabbit. Diagnosis requires isolation and demonstration of the organism by standard microbiologic techniques. Neonates often develop severe diarrhea, and death is common. In many cases the entire litter will become infected and die. In weanlings, a disease syndrome similar to that described for mucoid enteropathy is seen. Death usually occurs within a week. Survivors have stunted growth and appear generally unthrifty. Rabbits with severe infections rarely respond to treatment and should be culled from the colony. Mild cases may respond to antibiotic therapy. High-fiber diets can help prevent disease or minimize symptoms in weanlings.

VIRAL DISEASE

Most viral diseases that can infect rabbits are not routinely found in the United States, although they are common in many other parts of the world. Viral diseases of rabbits include the infectious fibromas, papillomatosis, rabbit pox, herpesvirus III infections, myxomatosis, and infectious rotaviral enteritis. Viral hemorrhagic disease is not seen in the United States but is found in nearly every country where rabbits are raised. Although domestic rabbits can be infected experimentally with the Shope fibroma virus, the normal host is the cottontail rabbit. The virus is a type of poxvirus and causes subcutaneous tumors. In areas where Shope fibroma occurs in the wild rabbit population, it is possible for domestic rabbits to become infected, especially when husbandry practices are poor.

Papilloma Virus

Papilloma viruses that may infect domestic rabbits include the oral papilloma virus and the cutaneous papilloma virus. The oral papilloma type is more common than the cutaneous type and is characterized by small, grayish nodules located on the floor of the mouth or underneath the tongue. Cutaneous papilloma virus usually only infects cottontails and is characterized by thick, wartlike lumps on the neck, shoulders, and ears. Infections with either papilloma virus are usually self-limiting.

Rabbit Pox

Rabbits can become infected with rabbit pox. This disease is highly contagious and has a high mortality rate but can be prevented by administering a smallpox vaccine. Infected rabbits have fever, skin rash, and lacrimal and nasal discharge.

Myxomatosis

Myxomatosis, mentioned previously, is a viral infection that causes a high mortality rate in domestic rabbits. The virus is transmitted by insect vectors and direct contact. The reservoir for infection in the United States is the California brush rabbit. As a result, the disease occurs naturally in that species' normal habitat range, the Western United States, particularly the coastal areas of California and Oregon. Clinical infection normally does not occur in rabbits younger than 2 months of age. Signs of infection begin with conjunctivitis and rapidly progress to pyrexia, anorexia, and lethargy. Death can occur within 2 days, or the disease may progress through several stages before fatality occurs at approximately 2 weeks after initial signs develop. Treatment is not effective, and infected rabbits must be culled from the colony.

Rotavirus

Rotavirus type A has been found in clinically normal rabbits, and infections are generally self-limiting. The virus is transmitted by the fecal-oral route, and young rabbits may exhibit a severe watery diarrhea. Anorexia and dehydration are common signs. The mortality rate can be as high as 80% in rabbits younger than 6 months. The disease can be complicated by secondary infection with *Clostridium* species or *E. coli,* resulting in a much higher mortality rate. There is no effective treatment, but recovery provides a degree of immunity, although the animals remain seropositive for the virus.

MYCOTIC DISEASE

Ringworm is the only significant mycotic disease of domestic rabbits. Etiology, transmission, and clinical signs are much the same as for other mammals.

In domestic rabbits, ringworm infection is more common in Europe than in the United States. Poor husbandry practices contribute to the incidence of infection. The lesions usually appear on the head and can spread to any area of the skin. As in other mammals, lesions appear circular, raised, reddened, and may be covered with a white, flaky material. *Trichophyton mentagrophytes* is the most common causative agent, although *Microsporum canis* has also been implicated. Infections have a high zoonotic potential and can also be transmitted to other animals. Infected animals must be isolated or culled from the colony. Topical treatment of lesions can be effective.

PARASITIC DISEASE

Parasitic infections of domestic rabbits are rarely a problem in well-managed facilities. Most clinically important parasite infections are caused by ectoparasites. A number of endoparasites can also infect rabbits.

Endoparasites

Parasites of the gastrointestinal system include nematodes, cestodes, and protozoans. Of these, the protozoal parasites in the coccidian group cause the most common and most significant clinical disease in domestic rabbits.

Coccidiosis

Numerous species of *Eimeria* are capable of infecting rabbits. Only a few of these are of clinical significance. These include *Eimeria stiedae, E. magna, E. irresidua,* and *E. intestinalis.* The organisms are transmitted by the fecal-oral route and require some time to sporulate before they are infective. Proper husbandry standards have decreased the incidence of coccidial infestation in rabbit colonies. Diagnosis of coccidiosis is based on clinical signs and demonstration of the organisms in fecal samples.

Coccidiosis occurs in rabbits in two forms. The hepatic form is caused by *E. stiedae.* The intestinal form is caused by several species of *Eimeria* (Figure 7-20). Although neither form is usually fatal, infected rabbits can become severely debilitated. Infections with hepatic coccidiosis may exhibit clinical signs related to liver dysfunction and blockage of bile ducts, which become chronically inflamed. Severely affected rabbits often lose weight and may develop hepatomegaly and icterus. Infections with the intestinal form may be asymptomatic

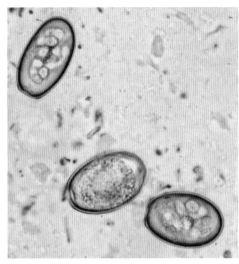

FIGURE 7-20. *Eimeria magna* oocysts, sporulated, from the feces of a domestic rabbit. (From Bowman D: *Georgis' parasitology for veterinarians,* ed 10, St. Louis, 2014, Saunders.)

or characterized by profuse, watery, or bloody diarrhea. Young rabbits seem to be most susceptible to developing clinical signs. Administration of sulfonamides in the drinking water may control outbreaks of infection, but addressing husbandry concerns provides greater benefits.

Encephalitozoonosis

Encephalitozoonosis, caused by the protozoal parasite *Encephalitozoon cuniculi,* is a latent, chronic disease. It is fairly common in domestic rabbits and may also infect rodents.

The organism is shed in the urine, and transmission is thought to occur by ingestion. Transplacental transmission also occurs. Clinical signs are usually not present, but neurologic signs such as depression, torticollis, and ataxia may occur. Lesions are consistently seen in the brain and kidney in the form of small, multiple, whitish foci, or subcapsular pitting of the kidneys from the scarring processes under the kidney capsule.

Lesions in the brain resemble those caused by *Toxoplasma gondii* infection and require microscopic evaluation to identify. Diagnosis is based on clinical signs and serologic testing. Treatment is lifelong and focused on minimizing the symptoms of the disease.

Miscellaneous Protozoal Parasites

Cryptosporidium cuniculus has been isolated from apparently healthy rabbits. The specific frequency of infection is not known. The organism is likely transmitted by fecal-oral route. No clinical signs are apparent in rabbits; however, rabbits may serve as reservoirs for infection of other animals. The rabbit is the intermediate host in the life cycle of *Sarcocystis cuniculi.* Transmission is by ingestion of infective oocysts. The organism does not usually cause clinical signs in rabbits, but encysted forms of the parasite are present in skeletal and cardiac muscle. These may initiate an inflammatory response and could result in eosinophilic myositis and myocarditis.

Nematodes

Many species of nematodes are known to infect wild rabbits. These include *Obeliscoides cuniculi, Nematodirus leporis, Trichuris leporis, Dirofilaria scapiceps, Protostrongylus boughtoni,* and *Passalurus ambiguus.* Of these, only *P. ambiguus* is found in domestic rabbits with any frequency. The organism is a species of pinworm and is generally considered nonpathogenic. Another nematode, *Baylisascaris procyonis,* infects raccoons. Migrating larvae can cause visceral larval migrans in rabbits.

Cestodes

Wild rabbits can be infected with tapeworms from the genera *Cittotaenia* and *Raillietina.* These are very rarely found in domestic rabbits. When husbandry conditions are poor, domestic rabbits can become infected with the larval stage of the tapeworms *Taenia pisiformis* and *T. serialis.* Infestation with other tapeworms or their larval stages is extremely rare.

ECTOPARASITES

Infestations with *Psoroptes cuniculi* are common in domestic rabbits. This species is a nonburrowing mite that feeds on the epidermis of the ear canal. The mite is transmitted by direct contact and completes its entire life cycle on the host. Clinically affected rabbits have painful inflammation of the ear. Intense pruritus is usually evidenced by shaking of the head and excessive scratching of the ears. The ear pinnae contain a dry, crusty, brown material with a foul odor (Figure 7-21). Skin beneath the dried exudate is raw. Mites are usually visible under this exudate with the unaided eye. Affected rabbits are usually treated with application of mineral oil or acaricides on the ears. Control of this parasite is difficult and requires careful attention to proper sanitation.

Cheyletiella parasitovorax is another nonburrowing mite that can infest rabbits. It is commonly referred to as the rabbit fur mite and usually causes a nonpruritic alopecia of the back and intrascapular area (Figure 7-22). This organism is transmitted by direct contact and is generally considered nonpathogenic. Care must be taken to control infestation because the organism has zoonotic potential.

Sarcoptic mange can occur in rabbits but is quite rare. Causative agents include *Sarcoptes scabiei* and *Notoedres cati.*

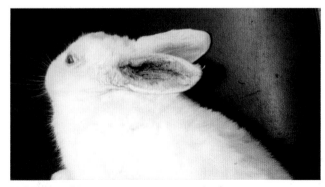

FIGURE 7-21. Ear mite (*Psoroptes cuniculi*) infestation. (From Jepson L: *Exotic animal medicine,* St. Louis, 2009, Saunders.)

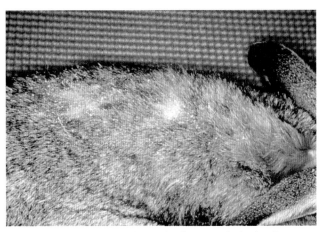

FIGURE 7-22. *Rabbit with infestation of Cheyletiella.*

Skin lesions are usually found initially on the muzzle and tend to be highly pruritic. *Haemaphysalis leporispalustris* is the only tick of any clinical significance in domestic rabbits. It is a three-host tick found primarily in North America. The larval stages parasitize birds. Ticks are of concern in rabbits primarily because they can serve as vectors of tularemia and possibly other infectious agents. Flea and lice infestations are also of concern as disease vectors. Lice and fleas are not usually seen unless husbandry conditions are poor.

Adult flies of the genus *Cuterebra* often lay eggs around outdoor rabbit hutches. When the larvae hatch, they penetrate the skin of the rabbit and encyst within the subcutaneous tissue. The cyst contains a fistulated opening to the skin. This condition is commonly referred to as warbles, and surgery is required to remove the larvae.

NONINFECTIOUS DISEASES

The primary noninfectious diseases of concern in rabbits are neoplasias. These are not frequently seen in laboratory rabbits but may develop in pet rabbits. Like mice and rats, certain rabbit strains seem to have a greater susceptibility to neoplastic diseases. Noninfectious diseases that are related to husbandry, age, and nutrition are also of concern.

NEOPLASIA

The most common neoplasia of domestic rabbits is uterine adenocarcinoma. This is a leading cause of death in intact pet female rabbits. Clinical signs include palpable uterine nodules, decreased fertility, and dystocia. Multiple tumors are usually present and grow rapidly. Metastasis, especially to pulmonary tissues, is common.

Lymphosarcoma, embryonal nephroma, and bile duct adenoma and carcinoma are also somewhat common in rabbits. They primarily affect juveniles and young adults, and a genetic factor may be involved. Lymphosarcoma usually presents with multiple, palpable abdominal masses and enlarged lymph nodes. Hepatomegaly and splenomegaly are also common. Biliary neoplasia rarely presents with clinical signs. Embryonal nephroma is slow growing and usually

benign. Other neoplasias that have been reported in rabbits include ovarian, testicular, stomach, urinary bladder, and skin cancers. All these are extremely rare.

AGE-ASSOCIATED DISEASES

The only significant age-associated diseases of rabbits are neoplastic in origin. Older females in particular may develop mammary carcinoma.

HUSBANDRY-RELATED DISEASES
Pododermatitis

Pododermatitis is commonly referred to as bumblefoot and is a common finding among rabbits, particularly if the animal is obese. Fecal contamination of the cage bottom is a predisposing condition. Wire-bottom cages and abrasive bedding are also implicated. Initially, round, ulcerated lesions occur on the plantar surfaces of the feet (Figure 7-23). Rapid bacterial invasion, most commonly with *Staphylococcus aureus,* usually follows. The condition is extremely painful, and affected animals are often reluctant to move. Treatment is directed to relieving the pain by placing the animal on a clean, solid surface. Local antiseptics and antibiotic ointments can be helpful.

Trauma

Vertebral fracture and luxation are the usual sequelae to improper handling. The condition manifests as posterior paresis or paralysis. Affected animals lose bladder and anal sphincter control and will have soiled fur on the hind quarters. If not recognized for several days, decubital ulcers and uremia occur. Rabbits that do not have severe spinal cord damage can recover various degrees of limb function. However, most rabbits with this condition are euthanized.

Moist Dermatitis

Moist dermatitis is commonly referred to as **slobbers**. The condition is the result of bacterial infection of skin that is chronically wet because of drooling (e.g., from malocclusion) or poor husbandry. A foul-smelling exudative

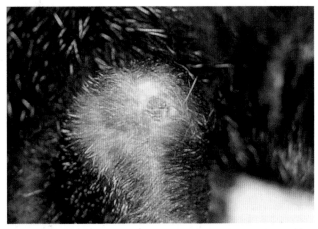

FIGURE 7-23. *Advanced pododermatitis (sorehocks) in the rabbit. (From Summers A: Common diseases of companion animals, ed 2, St. Louis, 2008, Mosby.)*

dermatitis is present around the folds of the dewlap. Treatment is aimed at correcting the cause. Topical or systemic antibiotics are usually helpful.

Buphthalmia

Buphthalmia (congenital glaucoma) is a hereditary condition with an autosomal recessive inheritance pattern with incomplete penetrance. It is common in New Zealand white rabbits. Affected animals have enlarged, protruding eyes, corneal opacity, and ulceration. One or both eyes can be infected, and rupture of the eye is possible. Diagnosis is based on clinical signs, and affected animals are usually euthanized.

Trichobezoars

Trichobezoars result from ingestion of hair during normal grooming, licking fur when animals are heat stressed, or maternal nest building (pseudopregnancy). Accumulations of hair tend to form into a large ball that can completely fill the stomach (Figure 7-24). Obstruction of the gastrointestinal tract results and affected animals will pass little or no feces. Anorexia and weight loss follow; the condition can be fatal if left untreated. Surgical removal of the hairballs may be needed. Prevention of the condition involves addition of proteolytic enzymes to the animal's diet.

Malocclusion

Mandibular prognathism, or malocclusion, is a genetic condition with an autosomal recessive inheritance pattern. It is common in domestic New Zealand white rabbits. The condition presents as an overgrowth of the mandibular incisors and prohibits the normal wearing of the incisors. Maxillary incisors tend to grow in a curve and may pierce the palate. Mandibular incisors tend to grow outwards

(Figure 7-25). Affected animals are usually unable to eat and may die of starvation. Treatment involves regular clipping of the incisors.

Other Diseases

Antibiotics that remove gram-positive flora (normal intestinal flora is disturbed) can result in gram-negative overgrowth with consequent septicemia.

Splay leg or hip dysplasia is observed in neonates. It is thoughts to be an inheritable condition or a teratologic (congenital) malformation. Environmental factors may also play a role, especially when animals are housed on slippery surfaces.

EUTHANASIA

Animals maintained in biomedical research facilities may be euthanized at the end of a research study to collect tissue samples for further analysis. Pet animals that are suffering are often humanely euthanized rather than allowed to live their final days in pain. Methods of euthanasia are listed in the *American Veterinary Medical Association Guidelines for the Euthanasia of Animals*. Acceptable methods of euthanasia for rabbits include administration of an overdose of inhalant or injectable anesthetic agents. Agents are usually administered by rapid intravenous or intraperitoneal injection. Rabbits involved in toxicology studies are sometimes anesthetized and then exsanguinated to allow for the collection of blood and tissue samples.

KEY POINTS

- Rabbits are classified as lagomorphs because of their unique dentition.
- The scientific name of the domestic rabbit used in biomedical research is *Oryctolagus cuniculus*.
- The breed of rabbit most commonly used in biomedical research is the New Zealand white.

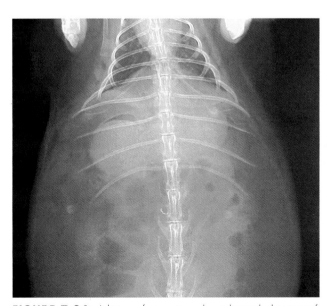

FIGURE 7-24. A history of anorexia and a radiograph showing soft tissue density in the stomach suggest the presence of trichobezoars in rabbits. (From Mitchell M, Thomas T: *Manual of exotic pet practice*, St. Louis, 2009, Saunders.)

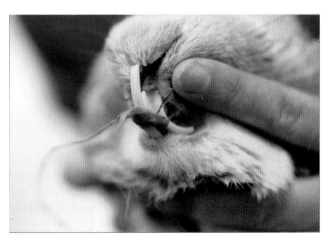

FIGURE 7-25. Overgrown maxillary and mandibular incisors, with hair matted around the lower teeth. (From Jepson L: *Exotic animal medicine*, St. Louis, 2009, Saunders.)

- The domestic rabbit was the first animal model of atherosclerosis; rabbits are also used in eye irritancy testing and for antibody production.
- Determination of gender in rabbits is accomplished by observing the shape of the external genitalia and appearance of secondary sex characteristics.
- Rabbits are usually housed in stainless steel or plastic cages with mesh floors that contain trays underneath to catch waste materials.
- Rabbits require high-fiber diets and are prone to development of hairballs when dietary fiber is inadequate.
- Restraint of rabbits can be accomplished manually and requires that their hindlimbs be well supported.
- Specialized rabbit restraint boxes are available.
- Ear tags, tattoos, and implanted microchips are used for permanent identification of individual rabbits.
- Injections can be given by subcutaneous, intravenous, intramuscular, or intradermal routes.
- Blood samples in rabbits can be easily collected from the marginal ear vein or central auricular artery.
- Rabbits are prone to a large number of infectious diseases, especially when husbandry conditions are poor.
- The most common bacterial infection of rabbits is Pasteurellosis.

REVIEW QUESTIONS

1. The scientific name of the domestic rabbit is
_____ _____.

2. The rabbit breed used most widely in biomedical research is the
_____ _____ _____.

3. The second pair of upper incisors are referred to as _____
_____ or _____ _____.

4. Rabbits have been used in studies of diet-induced
_____.

5. The round, expanded, muscular sac found at the terminal portion of the ileum in rabbits is referred to as
_____ _____.

6. Like rats and horses, rabbits are not able to _____.

7. Prevention of trichobezoars in rabbits involves the addition of
_____ _____ to the diet.

8. Improper handling of rabbits that causes injury to its spinal cord results in the condition referred to as _____
_____.

9. The most common sites for blood collection in the rabbit are
_____ _____ _____ or_____ _____ _____.

10. The most common bacterial infection of rabbits is
_____.

11. The causative agent of the disease characterized by sudden death or abortion and most often seen in does in the late stages of pregnancy is _____ _____.

12. Infection with the gram-negative organism *Francisella tularensis* is commonly referred to as _____ _____.

13. The causative agent for the highly zoonotic infection _____ is *Trichophyton mentagrophytes*.

14. Coccidiosis can occur in two forms in rabbits: _____ and _____ forms.

15. Infestations with the mite _____ _____ are common in laboratory rabbits.

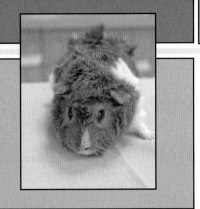

8 The Guinea Pig

KEY TERMS

Boar
Bumblefoot
Cavy
Coprophagia
Copulatory plug
Farrowing
Kurloff cells
Lordosis
Scurvy
Sow

LEARNING OBJECTIVES

After studying this chapter, you will be able to:

- Identify unique anatomic and physiologic characteristics of guinea pigs.
- Describe breeding systems used for guinea pigs.
- Identify unique aspects of guinea pig behavior.
- Explain routine procedures for husbandry, housing, and nutrition of guinea pigs.
- Describe various restraint and handling procedures used on guinea pigs.
- Describe methods of administering medication and collecting blood samples.
- List and describe common diseases of guinea pigs.
- Describe appropriate methods of euthanasia that may be used on guinea pigs.

TAXONOMY

The guinea pig is a small mammal native to South America. Although there is some disagreement in the scientific community regarding the taxonomy of guinea pigs, most scientists classify the animals in the order Rodentia, suborder Hystricognathi. Their scientific name is *Cavia porcellus*. Assessment of the amino acid sequence has some scientists considering whether guinea pigs might be more closely related to rodents in the gopher family. In the pet industry, the guinea pig is usually referred to as a **cavy**. The name guinea pig is somewhat of a misnomer because they are not pigs and not from Guinea. It is generally believed that the name originated from the method used to prepare the animals for cooking in South America, where they are considered a delicacy. In other literature, the characteristic squeals of guinea pigs are implicated as the source of the name. Guinea pigs were introduced to Europe in the sixteenth century by Dutch sailors. Although the name guinea pig is often used as a metaphor for "experimental subject," they are not as widely used for that purpose as mice and rats.

UNIQUE ANATOMIC AND PHYSIOLOGIC FEATURES

GENERAL CHARACTERISTICS

Guinea pigs have a number of unique characteristics that distinguish them from other rodents. Table 8-1 contains a summary of unique physiologic data. They have stocky bodies with relatively short, delicate limbs (Figure 8-1). There are four digits on each of the forelimbs and three on each of the hind limbs. Guinea pigs are more closely related to porcupines and chinchillas than mice and rats. The young are born precocious: fully haired, eyes open, and capable of eating solid food within a few hours after birth. True to their name, pig terms are used to describe the species. Male guinea pigs are known as **boars**, females as **sows**, and parturition is referred to as **farrowing.** Guinea pigs are docile animals and quite hardy when maintained properly.

An unusual feature seen in blood smears from guinea pigs is the presence of **Kurloff cells** (Figure 8-2). These cells are leukocytes that contain intracytoplasmic inclusions called Kurloff bodies. These cells are believed to be analagous to large granular lymphocytes or natural killer cells in other species. The number of Kurloff cells is greater in young guinea pigs and adult females than males and increases during estrus and pregnancy.

TABLE 8-1	Physiologic Values for Guinea Pigs
Usual life span as pet	5-6 years
Adult weight	Males, 900-1200 g; females, 700-900 g
Sexual maturity	Females, 2 mo; males, 3 mo
Type of estrous cycle	15-17 days
Length of estrous cycle	15-17 days
Ovulation	Spontaneous
Gestation period	59-72 days (average, 68 days)
Litter size	1-13 (2-4 is usual)
Normal birth weight	70-100 g
Weaning age	21 days (or at 180 g body weight)
Rectal temperature	37.2-39.5° C (99.0-103.1° F)
Average blood volume	70 ml/kg body weight
Heart rate	240-310 beats/min

(From Hillyer EV, Quesenberry KE: *Ferrets, rabbits, and rodents: clinical medicine and surgery*, St. Louis, 1997, Mosby.)

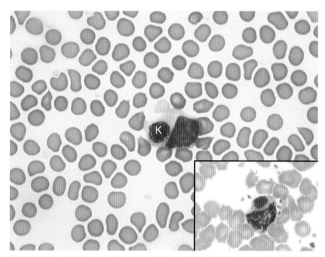

FIGURE 8-2. Lymphocytes with Kurloff's bodies. Peripheral blood smear—guinea pig. (From Quesenberry K, Carpenter JW: *Ferrets, rabbits, and rodents: clinical medicine and surgery*, ed 3, St. Louis, 2012, Saunders.)

TECHNICIAN NOTE Kurloff cells are unique to guinea pigs.

THE HEAD AND NECK

Like all hystricomorphs, guinea pigs have a large intraorbital foramen. Their ears have hairless pinna and large tympanic bullae, allowing easy examination of the microcirculation of the ear. The thymus is located subcutaneously on either side of the trachea. Although they have no laryngeal vesicle and very small vocal folds, guinea pigs are capable of a wide variety of characteristic vocalizations. Eleven distinct vocal patterns have been described.

Unlike other rodents, the dentition of guinea pigs includes a premolar in each quadrant of the oral cavity. The small gap between the premolars and molars is referred to as the diastema. Guinea pigs possess four pairs of salivary glands: parotid, mandibular, sublingual, and molar. These contain ducts that empty secretions directly into the oral cavity near the molars. The adrenal glands are bilobed and quite large. The soft palate is continuous with the rather large tongue. A hole in the soft palate, known as the palatal ostium, represents the opening between the oropharynx and the rest of the pharynx. This unique anatomic feature, and the fact that the oral cavity is narrow overall, makes endotracheal intubation extremely difficult to perform in this species.

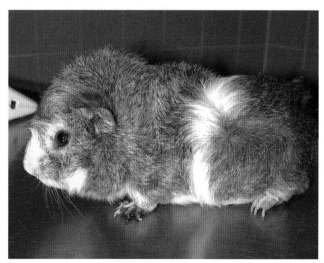

FIGURE 8-1. Normal guinea pig. (From Quesenberry K, Carpenter JW: *Ferrets, rabbits, and rodents: clinical medicine and surgery*, ed 3, St. Louis, 2012, Saunders.)

THORAX

Thoracic structures are similar to those of most other rodents, with a few exceptions. As mentioned previously, the thymus in immature animals is not located in the thoracic cavity as with other mammals. The right lung is composed of four lobes: cranial, middle, caudal, and accessory. The left lung is divided into three lobes: cranial, middle, and caudal.

ABDOMEN

The stomach of guinea pigs differs from that of most rodents in that there is no nonglandular portion. The cecum is a very large, thin-walled sac that occupies most of the central and left portion of the abdominal cavity. The liver is divided into six lobes: right, medial, left lateral, left medial, caudate, and quadrate. The spleen is relatively broad and the gallbladder is well developed. Ample sebaceous glands are present along the dorsum and around the anus. Secretions from the glands in the anal area are used for marking.

GENITOURINARY SYSTEM

The kidneys are characterized by a large renal pelvis. Urine is alkaline, highly crystalline, and usually appears creamy yellow or white. Females have a bicornuate uterus, and each uterine horn has a separate cervix. Although only a single pair of nipples is present, the female guinea pig is capable of raising rather large litters. Male guinea pigs also have a pair of inguinal nipples but mammary glands are not present. Accessory sex glands of the male include the prostate and vesicular, coagulating, and bulbourethral glands. The vesicular glands extend approximately 10 cm into the abdominal cavity. The testes are located in the inguinal canals, and these remain open throughout life. An os penis is present.

ANIMAL MODELS

The large tympanic bulla of the guinea pig allows easy visualization of internal ear structure and makes the guinea pig a good animal model for audiology studies. Their dietary need for vitamin C mimics primate physiology and makes them a good animal model for nutritional studies as well. Guinea pigs also exhibit unique antigen responses and are used extensively in immunologic studies, including hypersensitivity reactions and infectious diseases. The mature sow in particular is used as a source of serum complement for immunologic studies. Studies of hormonal effects of pregnancy also use guinea pigs because the sow can undergo ovariectomy before parturition and the young are born precocious and can be raised with minimal effort. Dermal studies are often performed with guinea pigs, and the animals are occasionally used as a source of intestinal epithelium cells.

REPRODUCTION

Determination of gender in guinea pigs can be accomplished in several ways. The genitalia in females contain a Y-shaped depression of tissue in the perineal area. The scrotal pouches and testes of adult males are usually quite obvious (Figure 8-3). In younger males, the application of digital pressure along the genitalia will extrude the penis from the prepuce.

Although not as prolific as other rodent species, guinea pigs can be easily bred. Guinea pigs reach sexual maturity at 2 to 3 months of age. The sow is nonseasonally polyestrous with an estrous cycle of 15 to 17 days. Ovulation is spontaneous with estrus lasting 6 to 11 hours. A postpartum estrus occurs approximately 2 to 10 hours after parturition. Vaginal cytology can be used to determine the stage of estrus; however, unique behavioral characteristics of the sow are also present during estrus. Sows will exhibit **lordosis**, which is a copulatory behavior characterized by arching of the back and swaying of the hindquarters.

It is recommended that sows intended for breeding be bred before the age of 6 months. The bony pelvic symphysis fuses between 6 and 9 months of age. If the sow is not bred before this age and subsequently becomes pregnant, the fused pelvic bones usually result in life-threatening dystocia. To avoid this problem, the female guinea pig is bred before the age of 6 months. Females bred before 6 months of age have cartilaginous fusion of the pelvic bones that is retained for life, allowing for parturition without dystocia.

> *TECHNICIAN NOTE* Sows intended for breeding should be bred before the age of 6 months.

Length of gestation is approximately 68 days. There is some variation with different strains of guinea pigs, and gestation periods can range from 57 to 72 days. In addition, larger litters tend to have shorter gestation periods and vice versa. Mating can be confirmed by the presence of a **copulatory plug** composed of coagulated material of secretions from the boar. Although sows do not build nests, pending

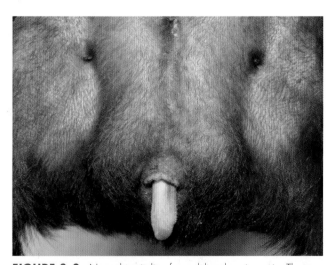

FIGURE 8-3. Normal genitalia of an adult male guinea pig. The scrotal sac is large and the penis is partially extruded. Males have a small os penis. Both male and female guinea pigs have one pair of inguinal nipples. The two nipples of the mammary glands are visible. (From Quesenberry K, Carpenter JW: *Ferrets, rabbits, and rodents: clinical medicine and surgery,* ed 3, St. Louis, 2012, Saunders.)

parturition is preceded by separation of the fused pelvic bones. This can occur as early as 2 days before parturition. Litter sizes can range from 1 to 13 pups, but 2 to 4 pups per litter is most common. The young are fully haired with open eyes. They generally stand within a few minutes after birth. Although capable of eating solid food within a few hours, the pups should remain with the sow until at least 5 days postpartum. Sows do not exhibit many maternal behaviors, but the sow will stimulate micturition and defecation in the pups for the first week. The sow lactates for approximately 3 weeks, at which time the pups should be fully weaned.

> **TECHNICIAN NOTE** Guinea pigs are born fully haired with eyes open and are able to eat solid food within a few hours after birth.

Guinea pig breeding programs may use intensive or nonintensive systems. As with rats and mice, the intensive systems use the postpartum estrus period. In most cases, a single boar is housed with 1 to 10 sows. The boar and sows remain together continuously with the young removed at weaning. Another variation of this system involves removal of the pregnant female just before parturition and then reintroducing her for a brief period just after parturition. This takes advantage of the postpartum estrus. The sow is then returned to a separate enclosure with the pups. This variation is often used when large harem groups are housed together to keep the pups from being trampled. In nonintensive systems, the sows are removed from the breeding group when pregnant and not rebred until after the young are weaned.

GENETICS AND NOMENCLATURE

There are three primary breeds of guinea pigs that are distinguished based on the direction of growth and length of their hair coat. The most common guinea pig in both pet and laboratory animal medicine is the English guinea pig (Figure 8-4). This variety has short, smooth, straight hair. The Peruvian guinea pig has a long, fine hair coat. The Abyssinian variety has a short, coarse hair coat that grows in whorls or rosettes (Figure 8-5). Within the guinea pig pet trade, several other breeds are described. These include the silkies, referred to as shelties in Great Britain. This long-haired breed is distinguished from the Peruvian breed in that the hair does not cover the face or part down the back. The teddy is a relatively new breed that is being shown in the United States; it has a coarse, short, and thick coat with kinked hair shafts without ridges or rosettes (Figure 8-6). The American crested cavy is a short-hair breed with a single whorl of a contrasting color on the forehead. Numerous color and hair coat combinations are possible because the three varieties can interbreed. Some of the more common varieties seen in pet guinea pigs include the selfs, agoutis, Himalayan, Dutch, roan, Dalmatian, and tortoiseshell. Selfs are smooth-coated guinea pigs whose coats are all one color. The agouti guinea pigs have short, silky hair

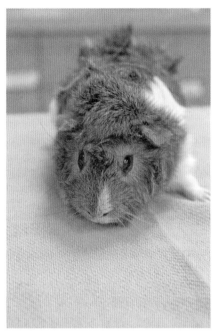

FIGURE 8-5. Abyssinian guinea pig.

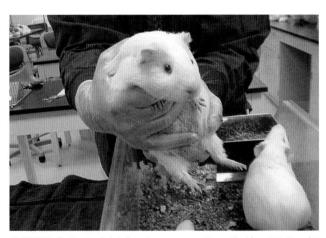

FIGURE 8-4. English (albino) guinea pig. (From Sheldon CC, Topel J, Sonsthagen T: *Animal restraint for veterinary professionals*, St. Louis, 2006, Mosby.)

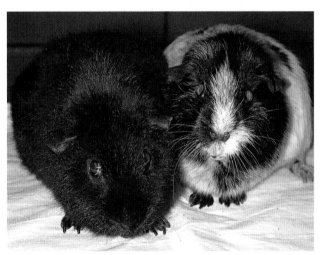

FIGURE 8-6. Two common guinea pig breeds: Teddy *(left)* and American *(right)*. (From Mitchell M, Thomas T: *Manual of exotic pet practice*, St. Louis, 2009, Saunders.)

that is interspersed with a second color throughout the coat. For example, the silver variety has a dark-colored coat interspersed with silver hairs. The Himalayan variety has a white, silky coat with black or chocolate ears, nose, and feet. Dutch guinea pigs have a self or agouti coloring on most of their bodies, a white "saddle" across the back, and a white "blaze" running from the forehead down to the nose. The Dalmatian variety is similar in coloring to the Dalmatian dog, with a white body interspersed with black spotting. The roan variety is similar to the agouti except that the body is black with interspersed white hairs and solid black hair on the head and feet. Tortoiseshell varieties are bicolored or tricolored and have markings similar to that of a tortoiseshell cat.

Guinea pigs used in biomedical research are usually the English variety. Several stocks are available. The most common outbred stocks used in biomedical facilities are the Duncan-Hartley and Hartley stocks. There are more than 14 inbred strains of guinea pigs available. The most common ones in use are strains 2 and 13.

BEHAVIOR

In their natural habitat—temperate forests, rainforests, and temperate grasslands—guinea pigs live in open, grassy areas. They do not dig their own burrows, but instead use burrows deserted by other animals or seek shelter in naturally protected areas. Guinea pigs are sociable animals and tend to live in groups. Pet guinea pigs are docile and rarely bite or scratch. Unlike other rodents that are nocturnal, guinea pigs are active most of the time during a 24-hour period.

Although not aggressive, they may make energetic attempts at escape when frightened. Explosive scattering of groups of frightened guinea pigs can present a challenge when moving animals from one cage to another. Some animals may become immobile for periods of up to 20 minutes when frightened. Guinea pigs also vocalize when in pain or distress and in response to other stimuli, such as the sound of a food bag being opened. A number of distinct vocalizations have been described, some of which cannot be heard with the human ear. They are creatures of habit and do not respond well to changes in their routine or care.

HUSBANDRY, HOUSING, AND NUTRITION

Guinea pigs are usually housed in solid-bottom stainless steel or plastic cages (Figure 8-7). If cages containing wire mesh bottoms or metal slatted bottoms are used, the animals should be introduced to these at a young age. Injuries to limbs are common when guinea pigs that are accustomed to solid-bottom cages are placed on wire mesh. Solid-bottom cages should be covered with a layer of bedding material. Bedding must be clean, nontoxic, absorbent, relatively dust free, and easy to replace. Corn cobs, shredded paper, or wood shavings are all suitable bedding materials. Sawdust and cedar shavings should be avoided because they can cause illness in the animals. Guinea pigs do not jump and are not likely to climb, so the cage does not require a covered top if the sides are at least 10 inches high. The cage should contain

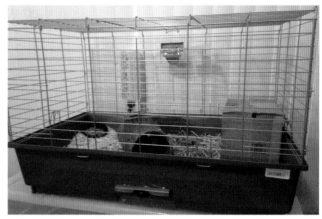

FIGURE 8-7. Pet guinea pig cage. (Courtesy of Pam Heeren, DVM.)

a small box or large piece of polyvinyl chloride tubing. This provides an enriched environment that allows the animals to exhibit normal burrowing behavior.

> **TECHNICIAN NOTE**   A cardboard box or piece of PVC pipe can be placed in the guinea pig cage to provide environmental enrichment.

Guinea pigs are highly susceptible to heat stress and do not tolerate temperatures greater than 90° F. An optimal environmental temperature range is 18° to 26° C (65° to 79° F) with 40% to 60% humidity. Guinea pigs are notorious for pushing partially chewed food up into the sipper tube of the water bottle. This often makes the water appear as if algal growth is present. This can also clog the tube and encourage bacterial growth. Guinea pigs must be given clean, fresh water in a clean water bottle with a clean sipper tube at least daily.

Guinea pigs also suck on their sipper tubes rather than lap from them as rats and mice do. For this reason, it is important that the sipper tube contain the appropriate size ball bearing to keep water from flowing freely out of the tube and getting the cage and bedding wet. It is not appropriate to place open feed or water containers on the cage floor because the animals will usually defecate in them.

Guinea pigs tend to develop meticulous dietary habits and do not respond well to changes in their diet or feeding methods. They should be fed a commercial high-quality feed designed specifically for guinea pigs. Rabbit feed is not an acceptable substitute because it generally contains too much fiber and not enough protein to satisfy the animal's nutritional needs. A major consideration with guinea pigs is their need for a dietary source of vitamin C. Guinea pigs are the only nonprimate mammal to have such a requirement; deprived of this vitamin, the animals will develop **scurvy**. Commercial guinea pig chow is supplemented with vitamin C. However, this vitamin is not highly stable and is easily destroyed by heat and ultraviolet light. Guinea pig chow that is retained for more than 90 days after its milling (manufacture) date will not contain adequate vitamin C. Ideally, vitamin C should be supplemented in the diet, either by adding a small amount to the water or by providing fresh vegetables that are high in vitamin C. If fresh vegetables are offered, care must be taken to choose those that are relatively low in fiber and water content. Cabbage and kale are acceptable sources of vitamin C. The vegetables must be thoroughly washed before being consumed by the animals. Vitamin C added to the drinking water lasts only a short time, so replenishing the water supply at least daily is essential. **Coprophagia** is an important component of guinea pig nutrition. Guinea pigs will lose weight if coprophagia is prevented.

> TECHNICIAN NOTE Vitamin C should be supplemented in the diet of guinea pigs.

RESTRAINT AND HANDLING

Specific handling and restraint techniques vary depending on the purpose of the manipulation. Pet guinea pigs are used to frequent handling and can be moved easily. Improper handling can result in thoracic compression, diaphragmatic hernia, and bruised lungs.

To remove a guinea pig from its cage, place one hand in front of the animal to stop its motion and place the other hand under the thorax. Gently scoop the animal up and move your hand from in front of the animal to support its hindquarters (Figure 8-8). Care must be taken to not grasp the animal tightly with a hand over the thorax or abdomen because damage to the lungs or liver can easily occur. For most technical procedures, guinea pigs can be placed on a towel on a flat surface and held in position. They rarely struggle or try to escape.

IDENTIFICATION

Cage cards or descriptions of a particular animal's color patterns can be used for identification purposes. Ear notching, ear tags, tattooing, and implantation of microchips are also used for permanent identification. Temporary identification can be accomplished with markers or dyes.

CLINICAL PROCEDURES

ADMINISTRATION OF MEDICATION

Guinea pigs are usually given medications orally or by subcutaneous (SC or SQ), intraperitoneal (IP), or intramuscular (IM) injection. The lack of readily accessible veins for injection or blood sampling is one reason why guinea pigs are not used extensively in biomedical research. They are quite docile and rarely require sedation or anesthesia for administration of medication, except for intravenous (IV) or intracardiac procedures.

INJECTION TECHNIQUES

Proper restraint is critical for correct administration of medications. In addition, the skin of the guinea pig is quite thick. In most cases, a fairly large-gauge needle (greater than 25 gauge) must be used for injections. The volume of fluid that can be injected at a specific site must also be considered. A maximum volume of 5 to 10 mL per site is acceptable for SC injections. IP injections should be limited to no more than 8 mL. No more than 0.5 ml should be administered by IM injection.

SC injections are quite easy to perform and can usually be completed by just one person. To administer an SC injection, remove the guinea pig from the cage and place it on a flat surface. Gently lift a generous amount of loose skin from over the back of the neck and insert the sterile needle into the SC space (Figure 8-9). IM injections are relatively simple with guinea pigs. The animal should be placed on a flat surface. One hand is used to hold the animal gently over the thorax. Care must be taken not to compress the thoracic cavity. The injection can then be administered in the gluteal or quadriceps muscles. Irritating substances should not be administered by IM injection.

> TECHNICIAN NOTE Guinea pigs have thick skin and large-gauge needles are needed for most injection techniques.

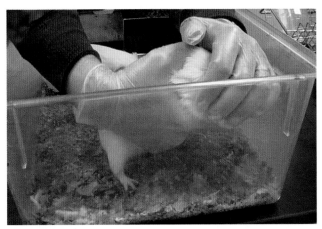

FIGURE 8-8. Removal of a guinea pig from its cage. (From Sheldon CC, Topel J, Sonsthagen T: *Animal restraint for veterinary professionals,* St. Louis, 2006, Mosby.)

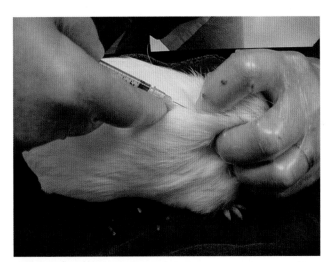

FIGURE 8-9. Subcutaneous administration in a guinea pig. (From Sheldon CC, Topel J, Sonsthagen T: *Animal restraint for veterinary professionals,* St. Louis, 2006, Mosby.)

Guinea pigs are sometimes used for toxicity studies and are routinely given intradermal injections for this purpose. To perform the procedure, the animal is restrained on a table as if for an SC injection. A small area on the back is shaved and cleaned (Figure 8-10). The injection is administered into the dermis with a 22- to 24-gauge needle. The presence of a wheal (bleb) verifies that the procedure was performed correctly.

IP injections are also commonly performed but usually require two persons: a handler/restrainer and the person giving the injection. The animal should be held with one hand supporting the hindquarters and the other hand placed gently around the shoulder area, under the front legs (Figure 8-11). The animal can then be turned on its back and tilted slightly so that its nose points toward the floor. Use a small-gauge needle (23 gauge or less) and administer the injection into the lower left quadrant of the abdomen. Aspirate before injection to ensure that no internal organs or blood vessels have been entered. If the urinary bladder, intestine, other organs, or blood vessels are punctured, fluid will enter the hub of the needle. The needle and syringe must then be discarded and the procedure started over. If no fluid is present, the material may be injected in a smooth motion and the needle withdrawn.

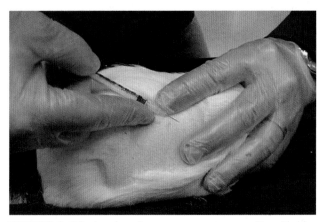

FIGURE 8-10. Intradermal injection in a guinea pig. (From Sheldon CC, Topel J, Sonsthagen T: *Animal restraint for veterinary professionals*, St. Louis, 2006, Mosby.)

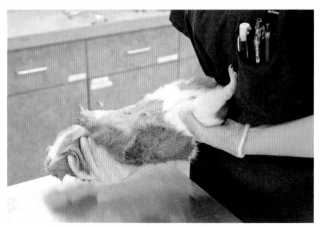

FIGURE 8-11. The guinea pig should be held with its head pointed downward when administering an IP injection.

> **TECHNICIAN NOTE** Tilting the guinea pig slightly so that its nose is toward the floor helps minimize the likelihood of penetrating an organ during IP injection.

IV injections are not commonly performed because they nearly always require that the animal be anesthetized. Vessels that may be used for IV injections include the lateral metatarsal, penile, lingual, cephalic, saphenous, and marginal ear veins.

ORAL ADMINISTRATION

Medications are usually administered orally by mixing the substance in the drinking water. Unpalatable medications may need the addition of 5 ml of sugar or syrup per liter of water so that the animals do not avoid drinking the water. Medications for oral administration may also be mixed in food if the animals are being fed a powdered or meal-type diet. A small syringe or dosing needle can be used to administer oral medications. The syringe can be introduced into the diastema of the mouth.

ANESTHESIA

Because laboratory animals tend to respond poorly to local or regional anesthesia, general anesthesia is usually administered when the guinea pig must undergo painful procedures. Like all species, many variables affect general anesthesia, including age of the animal, general health, species, strain or stock, and environment. Every animal must be individually dosed with enough medication to achieve the desired result. Guinea pigs, in particular, have highly variable responses to anesthetics, and a large range of anesthetic dosages have been reported for use in guinea pigs. The dose of anesthetics is always to effect. To determine whether anesthesia is adequate, the animal's vital signs and reflexes may be monitored. Monitoring of anesthetic depth in guinea pigs involves continuous assessment of the animal's respiratory rate. The heart rate and toe pinch response may also aid in evaluation of anesthetic depth.

General anesthetic agents are available in inhalant or injectable forms. Inhalant anesthetics used in guinea pigs include halothane, methoxyflurane, and isoflurane. The agent is usually administered by mask by a standard anesthesia machine. Methoxyflurane is safe for use in guinea pigs although it is not currently available in North America. Halothane has been linked to the development of hepatitis in guinea pigs.

Injectable agents for general anesthesia in guinea pigs include barbiturates, such as pentobarbital, and dissociative agents, such as ketamine. A variety of other pharmaceutical agents are also used. Table 8-2 lists some common anesthetics used in guinea pigs. The animal should be fasted for 3 hours before administration of anesthesia to allow emptying of the contents of their large cecum. To calculate the appropriate anesthetic dosage, an accurate weight must be determined, keeping in mind that the intestinal and cecal contents can contribute a significant amount to the weight of the animal.

TABLE 8-2	Common Injectable Anesthetic Agents Used in Guinea Pigs		
AGENT	**DOSAGE**	**ROUTE**	**COMMENTS**
Acepromazine	0.5-1.0 mg/kg	IM	Often used in conjunction with ketamine
Diazepam	0.5-3.0 mg/kg	IM	Sedation
Fentanyl/ droperidol	0.22-0.88 ml/kg	IM	Sedation
Ketamine	22-64 mg/kg	IM	Significant individual variation
Ketamine/ diazepam	20-30mg/ kg ketamine +1-2 mg/kg diazepam	IM	Anesthesia
Ketamine/ xylazine	50-75 mg/kg ketamine + 10 mg/kg xylazine	IP	Light anesthesia

BLOOD COLLECTION

The lack of readily accessible veins makes blood collection in guinea pigs quite challenging. The lateral saphenous and cephalic veins can be used to collect blood. However, these vessels are quite small and yield only a small volume of sample. In addition, the restraint required for these procedures is quite stressful to the animals unless they are first sedated.

Up to 8 mL of blood can be collected by the jugular vein (Figure 8-12), cranial vena cava (Figure 8-13), femoral artery,

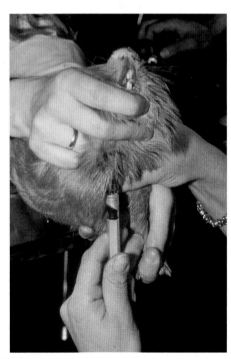

FIGURE 8-12. Restraint for jugular venipuncture in a guinea pig. Venipuncture of the jugular vein can be difficult because of the short, thick neck of guinea pigs and the stress caused by restraint. Tranquilization may be necessary. (From Quesenberry K, Carpenter JW: *Ferrets, rabbits, and rodents: clinical medicine and surgery*, ed 3, St. Louis, 2012, Saunders.)

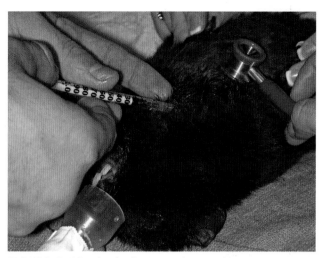

FIGURE 8-13. Blood collection via the cranial vena cava in an anesthetized guinea pig. (From Mitchell M, Thomas T: *Manual of exotic pet practice*, St. Louis, 2009, Saunders.)

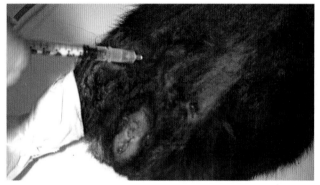

FIGURE 8-14. Blood collection via the femoral vein in an anesthetized guinea pig. (From Mitchell M, Thomas T: *Manual of exotic pet practice*, St. Louis, 2009, Saunders.)

or femoral vein (Figure 8-14). Cardiocentesis can also yield a significant volume of blood; however, this procedure is normally followed by euthanasia because of the high probability of complications. Samples collected from any of the above sites require that the animal be sedated or anesthetized.

> **TECHNICIAN NOTE** Most guinea pigs need sedation or anesthesia prior to undergoing blood collection.

DIAGNOSTIC IMAGING

Radiographs are often useful in diagnosing specific disease conditions. Guinea pigs require anesthesia or heavy sedation in order to obtain diagnostic-quality radiographs. Whole body radiographs are usually obtained and include both a lateral and a dorsoventral (or ventrodorsal) view (Figure 8-15). Skull radiographs may aid in the evaluation of malocclusion and usually require the lateral, dorsoventral, and lateral oblique projections. To enhance visibility of small structures, the animal can be placed on an elevated platform on the x-ray table to reduce the distance from the x-ray beam to the patient and thus magnify the image on the film.

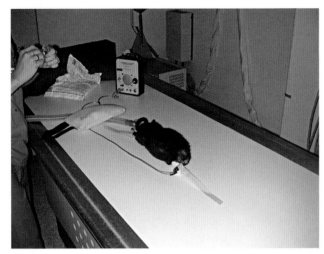

FIGURE 8-15. Positioning of an anesthetized guinea pig patient for a right lateral radiograph. (From Mitchell M, Thomas T: *Manual of exotic pet practice*, St. Louis, 2009, Saunders.)

COMMON DISEASES

Guinea pigs are prone to a number of bacterial and viral diseases. In addition, they are highly susceptible to illnesses related to nutritional and environmental parameters. Pet guinea pigs, in particular, are likely to become ill as a result of poor husbandry practices. Careful attention to proper caging, housing, and feeding techniques minimizes the likelihood of disease in this species.

INFECTIOUS DISEASES

Because guinea pigs are particularly susceptible to antibiotic toxicity, prevention of infectious disease is a primary consideration in this species. Stress can predispose the animals to infection. Excessive noise, temperature extremes, and changes to their environment are all stress factors that will increase the likelihood that the animals will develop disease.

Bacterial Disease

Pneumonia. Pneumonia is the most common bacterial disease in guinea pigs. The normal flora of the respiratory tract of guinea pigs includes several bacterial species that are capable of causing this disease. Animals that are under stress become predisposed to developing respiratory infection. Stress factors can include poor husbandry, improper nutrition, and excessive noise. Guinea pigs that live in close association with rabbits and rats may also develop pneumonia because these species harbor *Bordetella bronchiseptica*, a common causative agent of pneumonia in guinea pigs. Other bacterial agents implicated in the development of respiratory disease in guinea pigs include *Streptococcus pneumoniae*, *Pseudomonas aeruginosa*, and *Pasteurella multocida*. *Streptobacillus moniliformis* is also known to cause respiratory disease in this species and is of particular concern due to its zoonotic potential as the causative agent for rat bite fever in humans. *Yersinia pseudotuberculosis* causes a septicemic pneumonia in guinea pigs and is usually fatal.

TECHNICIAN NOTE   Stress factors that increase the likelihood of disease development in guinea pigs include excessive noise, temperature extremes, and changes to their environment.

Clinical signs of pneumonia may include dyspnea, oculonasal discharge from the eyes and nares, lethargy, and anorexia. Acute death is possible. Infected animals may also develop neurologic signs such as head tilt from the middle and inner ear infections occasionally seen in conjunction with pneumonia in guinea pigs.

Cervical Lymphadenitis. Cervical lymphadenitis, commonly known as lumps, is caused by *Streptococcus zooepidemicus*, although *Streptobacillus moniliformis* and *Yersinia pseudotuberculosis* have also been implicated. The bacterium is normally present in the conjunctiva and nasal cavity of guinea pigs. If the lining of the mouth becomes injured (usually by feeding coarse hay) or superficial wounds (e.g., bite wounds) penetrate the skin over the lymph nodes beneath the lower jaw and upper neck, the bacteria travel to the cervical lymph nodes. A discharge containing thick, creamy, yellow-white pus is released if the abscess breaks open.

Clinical signs include enlargement and abscessation of head and neck lymph nodes, fibrinopurulent pleuritis, myocarditis, and otitis. Abscessed areas are usually lanced and the animal treated with appropriate antibiotics. Because guinea pigs are highly susceptible to antibiotic toxicity, a bacterial culture and sensitivity test are usually performed to determine the most appropriate antibiotic therapy. When the abscesses are very large, surgical removal may be indicated.

Intestinal Infections (Bacterial Enteritis). Guinea pigs maintained in a laboratory animal facility rarely develop bacterial enteritis. Pet guinea pigs sometimes develop bacterial infections of the gastrointestinal tract. This is most commonly associated with feeding of unwashed vegetables or fecally contaminated food or water. The most common bacterial agents of this disease are *Salmonella typhirium* and *S. enteritidis*. Other bacterial agents implicated in enteritis in guinea pigs include *Yersinia pseudotuberculosis*, *Clostridium perfringens*, *Listeria monocytogenes*, and *Pseudomonas aeruginosa*. Clinical signs may include lethargy, weakness, anorexia, and weight loss. Diarrhea may or may not be present. Acute death may occur without prior clinical signs. Pregnant sows and weanlings are particularly susceptible.

Tyzzer's Disease. This disease has been reported in nearly all species of laboratory animals and is found throughout the world. The causative agent is the gram-negative, spore-forming, flagellated bacterium *Clostridium piliforme*. Definitive diagnosis often requires histologic examination of tissues from suspected infected animals. Poor sanitation and overcrowding predispose animals to this disease. Animals that are stressed, immunocompromised, or very young are most severely infected. Clinical signs include lethargy, rough hair coat, watery diarrhea, dehydration, and anorexia. The disease is often fatal in guinea pigs. Careful attention to proper sanitation and reduction of stress aid in prevention of this disease. The organism is difficult to eradicate from an animal facility because of the ongoing presence of resistant spores.

Mastitis. Lactating sows are prone to bacterial mastitis, especially as the pups approach weaning age. The agents most commonly implicated include *Pasteurella*, *Pseudomonas*, *Klebsiella*, *Staphylococcus*, and *Streptococcus* species. The mammary glands become inflamed and enlarged. Milk may be tinged with blood. The infection can become systemic and result in the death of the sow and pups. The pups should be immediately weaned and antibiotic therapy initiated in the sow.

Conjunctivitis. A number of bacterial agents have been identified that can cause conjunctivitis in guinea pigs, including *Chlamydia psittaci*, *Staphylococcus aureus*, *Streptococcus zooepidemicus*, and *Pasteurella multocida*. The disease is most severe in guinea pigs between 1 and 3 weeks of age. The most common clinical signs are ocular discharge, photophobia, and a reddened conjunctiva. Infected adults are often asymptomatic. Transmission can occur by direct contact or by aerosol transmission.

Viral Disease

Although several viral diseases of mice are capable of infecting guinea pigs, the infections are usually asymptomatic and self-limiting. However, guinea pigs can serve as reservoir hosts for some viral diseases of other animals, such as the Sendai virus. Most viral infections of pet guinea pigs are either mild or inapparent.

Cytomegalovirus. Cytomegalovirus is a latent viral infection found in 70% to 80% of guinea pigs. Infection is associated with minimal pathologic signs unless the animals are under stress or immunocompromised. The virus is transmitted transplacentally and by saliva and urine. Swelling of the salivary glands is the most common clinical sign. Eosinophilic intranuclear and cytoplasmic inclusion bodies are observed in salivary glands.

Mycotic Disease
Ringworm. *Trichophyton mentagrophytes* is the most common agent of ringworm in guinea pigs, although *Microsporum canis* has also been isolated from infected animals. Young guinea pigs are usually more susceptible than adults. The disease is often inapparent unless the animals are stressed. Ringworm in guinea pigs is generally characterized by patchy alopecia on the face, nose, and ears (Figure 8-16). The lesions are highly pruritic. The organisms are easily transmitted by direct contact and fomites. Ringworm has a high zoonotic potential.

Parasitic Disease
Guinea pigs are susceptible to infection with a number of ectoparasites and several parasitic protozoans and nematodes.

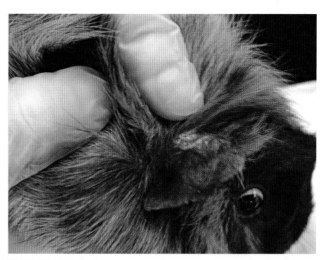

FIGURE 8-16. A guinea pig with a crusted area on the dorsal pinna consistent with dermatophytosis. A *Trichophyton* organism was cultured from the site. (From Mitchell M, Thomas T: *Manual of exotic pet practice*, St. Louis, 2009, Saunders.)

Clinical disease does not commonly occur unless the animals are immunocompromised or otherwise under stress.

Gastrointestinal Parasites. The protozoal parasites *Cryptosporidium wrairi* and *Eimeria caviae* can infect the gastrointestinal tract of guinea pigs. *C. wrairi* is usually the organism implicated in clinical infections. Young animals are most often infected. Infected animals exhibit weakness, lethargy, weight loss, and diarrhea. Transmission is by contact with contaminated food and water. Immune-competent animals usually recover in a few weeks. Intestinal parasites are usually not a significant problem in pet guinea pigs. Normal guinea pigs also harbor the coccidial organism *Eimeria caviae* and the protozoan *Balantidium coli* in the intestinal tract as well as the coccidian *Klebsiella cobayae* in the renal tubules. These organisms do not normally cause clinical disease. The nematode parasite *Paraspidodera uncinata* inhabits the cecum of guinea pigs and is not usually pathogenic. Overgrowth of the organism, however, may manifest as diarrhea and generalized unthriftiness.

> **TECHNICIAN NOTE** Parasitic infection rarely causes disease unless guinea pigs are stressed.

Ectoparasites. The most common ectoparasites of guinea pigs are lice and mites. Fleas, specifically *Ctenocephalides felis*, may also colonize guinea pigs, although these rarely cause clinical signs. The biting lice *Gliricola porcelli* (Figure 8-17) and *Gyropus ovalis* can cause alopecia and mild pruritis. Infestations of both burrowing and nonburrowing mites have been reported in guinea pigs. Infestation with the nonburrowing fur mite *Chirodiscoides caviae* is usually asymptomatic, although lesions are sometimes seen on the perineal or hip areas. The burrowing mite *Trixacarus caviae* can cause sarcoptic mange with significant pruritis and alopecia in

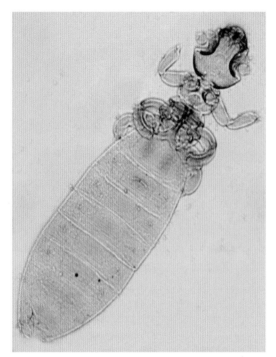

FIGURE 8-17. *Gliricola porcelli* (Mallophaga: Amblycera) of the guinea pig. (From Bowman D: *Georgis' parasitology for veterinarians,* ed 10, St. Louis, 2014, Saunders.)

affected animals (Figure 8-18). This is the most common problem seen in pet guinea pigs. Secondary infections are common, as is self-mutilation from the intense pruritus.

The organisms are transmitted by direct contact with either another host or contaminated bedding material. Infestations can be treated with pyrethrin powders or ivermectin. The environment must be thoroughly cleaned to prevent reinfestation.

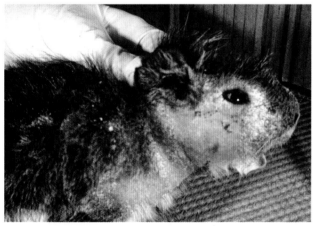

FIGURE 8-18. A guinea pig patient with severe *Trixacarus caviae* infestation. (Photograph courtesy Stephen D. White, DVM, DACVD.) (From Mitchell M, Thomas T: *Manual of exotic pet practice,* St. Louis, 2009, Saunders.)

NONINFECTIOUS DISEASES
Neoplasia
Cancer is a relatively rare problem of guinea pigs, even in older animals. Mammary tumors can occur in males and

females and are usually benign. Cavian leukemia/lymphosarcoma is a neoplasia with viral origin. There is some evidence that guinea pigs may develop pulmonary adenomas and basal cell epitheliomas. These conditions have not been well characterized in the guinea pig. Genetic factors appear to play a role in the development of neoplasias in guinea pigs.

AGE-ASSOCIATED DISEASES
Although there are a number of age-related diseases that can affect guinea pigs, most of these are not commonly seen. Chronic interstitial nephritis can occur in guinea pigs that are diabetic, but it is not a common problem. Nearly three fourths of adult female guinea pigs are likely to develop bilateral ovarian cysts (Figure 8-19). Alopecia is common in these animals. Affected animals can be treated by ovariohysterectomy. Guinea pigs older than 3 years are also susceptible to urolithiasis and cystitis. Treatment with antibiotics and relief of urinary obstruction are effective, but the condition is likely to recur.

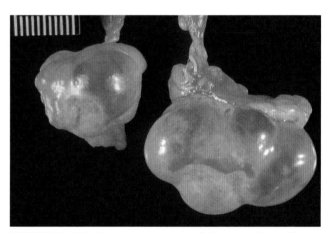

FIGURE 8-19. Ovarian cysts are identified in up to 75% of female guinea pigs and usually occur in both ovaries. (From Quesenberry K, Carpenter JW: *Ferrets, rabbits, and rodents: clinical medicine and surgery,* ed 3, St. Louis, 2012, Saunders.)

HUSBANDRY-RELATED DISEASES
Under normal circumstances, guinea pigs are hardy animals that rarely succumb to serious disease. They are, however, highly susceptible to illness when caging, housing, feed, or environmental conditions are inappropriate or unstable.

Pododermatitis
This condition is commonly referred to as **bumblefoot** and is a common finding among pet guinea pigs, particularly if the animal is obese. Fecal contamination of the cage bottom is a predisposing condition. Wire-bottom cages and abrasive bedding are also implicated. Hyperkeratosis of the foot pads is followed by ulceration of the surfaces of the feet (Figure 8-20). This allows for rapid bacterial invasion, most commonly with *Staphylococcus aureus*. Clinical signs include swelling of the feet, lameness, and inappetence. The condition is extremely painful, and affected animals are often reluctant to move. Infection can extend deep into the tissues

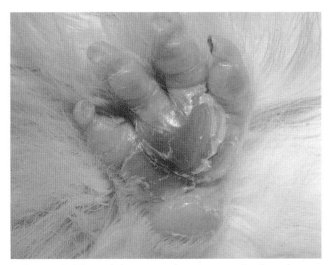

FIGURE 8-20. Pododermatitis in the guinea pig. Swollen soft tissues and ulceration, as seen here, should alert the clinician to potential underlying osteomyelitis; radiographs are warranted. (From Quesenberry K, Carpenter JW: *Ferrets, rabbits, and rodents: clinical medicine and surgery,* ed 3, St. Louis, 2012, Saunders.)

and lead to the development of osteomyelitis. Treatment involves debridement of the wounds and topical application of antibiotics. The feet are normally bandaged until healed, with regular bandage changes during the frequently long recovery period. Guinea pigs with severe infections may be treated with systemic antibiotics. To prevent recurrence, the flooring of the enclosure must be changed and overall sanitation must be improved.

> **TECHNICIAN NOTE** Untreated pododermatitis can lead to the development of osteomyelitis.

Trauma
One of the most common problems of pet guinea pigs is tibial fracture, usually from being dropped by children. Guinea pigs kept on wire mesh or metal slat cage floors may also fracture limbs if the animals catch their legs in them.

Alopecia
Hair loss or thinning of the hair is a common problem of sows in late pregnancy and during lactation. These sows tend to lose hair with each successive pregnancy, with the loss concentrated over the back. Juvenile guinea pigs also develop transient alopecia around the time of weaning. Alopecia is also seen when guinea pigs chew on their own hair or that of cagemates. The common name for this condition is barbering. Younger guinea pigs in particular can lose substantial amounts of hair when older, dominant cagemates chew their hair. Treatment is primarily aimed at removal of the offending animal.

NUTRITIONAL DISEASES
Scurvy
Like primates, guinea pigs cannot manufacture vitamin C and must therefore receive an adequate supply in the diet.

Vitamin C deficiency results in scurvy, which is characterized by inappetence, swollen, painful joints and ribs, reluctance to move, poor bone and teeth development, and spontaneous bleeding from the gums. Vitamin C content is quickly degraded in feed, especially if exposed to excessive heat, light, or moisture. All guinea pigs should receive supplemental vitamin C either added to the drinking water or by feeding a small amount of thoroughly washed, fresh kale or cabbage each day. Scurvy should be suspected in any guinea pigs that are anorectic, and aggressive vitamin C therapy should be administered.

> **TECHNICIAN NOTE** Vitamin C therapy is usually administered to all anorectic guinea pigs.

Metastatic Mineralization
Metastatic mineralization is thought to be the result of mineral imbalances in the diet of the guinea pig. Diets low in magnesium and potassium have been associated with development of calcium deposits in multiple locations throughout the body. Clinical disease is uncommon but has been reported in adult male guinea pigs. The most common clinical signs are stiff joints and generalized unthriftiness.

OTHER PROBLEMS
Antibiotic Toxicity
Administration of antibiotics is especially problematic in guinea pigs. They are particularly sensitive to antibiotics that target gram-positive organisms. Administration of these compounds causes imbalance in normal intestinal flora and subsequent overgrowth of clostridial and gram-negative organisms. Although most antibiotic toxicity occurs with oral administration, the condition has been identified when certain antibiotics are administered by injection or applied topically. The antibiotics most often implicated in this problem are the penicillins, erythromycin, lincomycin, and bacitracin. Streptomycin is directly toxic to guinea pigs and should never be administered in this species. When antibiotics are required, a culture and sensitivity test is used to identify the most appropriate agent. The therapeutic minimal dosage should always be used and the animal carefully monitored for signs of bacteremia. Antibiotics that seem to cause fewer problems include tetracycline, chloramphenicol, and the sulfonamides. It may be beneficial to feed guinea pigs a small amount (½ to 1 tsp) of plain yogurt daily during antibiotic therapy and for an additional 5 to 7 days after the medication is discontinued. Yogurt helps replace gram-positive enteric bacteria and may aid in restoring normal intestinal flora balance.

> **TECHNICIAN NOTE** Guinea pigs are particularly sensitive to antibiotics that target gram-positive organisms.

Malocclusion of Premolar Teeth
Malocclusion of the premolar teeth, commonly known as slobbers, results when the upper and lower premolar teeth

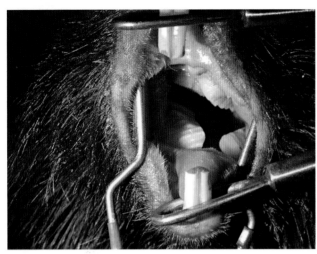

FIGURE 8-21. Guinea pig with malocclusion. Note the severe overgrowth of the mandibular premolars and molars, causing entrapment of the tongue. (Photograph courtesy Michelle G. Hawkins, VMD, DABVP [Avian].) (From Mitchell M, Thomas T: *Manual of exotic pet practice*, St. Louis, 2009, Saunders.)

do not properly meet (Figure 8-21). Dramatic weight loss is common and excessive drooling is a common sign. The condition is usually a direct result of overgrowth of the teeth. Guinea pigs have hypsodontic (open-rooted) teeth that grow continuously. The teeth are normally worn down by chewing. However, a genetic predisposition to overgrowth of the teeth is present, and animals with this condition should not be bred. The overgrown teeth cause abrasions of the cheeks and oropharynx. Treatment involves trimming or filing of the overgrown teeth, which must be performed under anesthesia. Force feeding may be needed to provide nutritional support during recovery. Guinea pigs with malocclusion require oral examination and trimming of the teeth.

Vaginitis and Preputial Infection

Accumulations of wet, soiled bedding can occur along the prepuce and in the vagina. Foreign body reactions result and secondary infection can occur, along with obstruction of urination and defecation. Accumulations of sebaceous material in the perineal area can also cause local inflammation and infection. Males occasionally develop scrotal plugs when bedding adheres to the moist prepuce. Treatment involves removal of the bedding and gentle cleansing of the area. The animals are usually placed on a different type of bedding until healed. Antibiotic therapy is sometimes indicated.

Heat Stress (Heat Stroke)

Guinea pigs are highly susceptible to heat stress when environmental temperatures rise above 85° F. High humidity (above 70%), inadequate shade and ventilation, crowding, and stress can also cause this condition, even when the ambient temperature is optimal. Animals that are overweight are especially susceptible. Clinical signs include hypersalivation, weakness, tachypnea, and pale mucous membranes. Treatment involves spraying or bathing the animal with cool water.

Diseases of Pregnancy

Dystocia. As mentioned earlier, sows must be bred before the age of 6 months to avoid potentially life-threatening dystocia. Obesity can also cause dystocia. Normally, a sow will deliver a litter in approximately 30 minutes, with one pup born approximately every 5 minutes. Clinical signs include depression, straining, and uterine bleeding. Cesarean section is usually indicated to deliver the young and save the sow's life.

Pregnancy Toxemia. Pregnancy toxemia is a serious condition that usually occurs in sows that are stressed or overweight sows in their first or second pregnancy. Fasting may also predispose guinea pigs to this disease. The condition appears to be related to reduced blood flow to the uterus, possibly as a result of the weight of the gravid uterus compressing the sow's blood vessels. Signs are usually acute and include inappetence, depression, weakness, reluctance to move, and incoordination. Dyspnea develops within 24 hours and death can occur in 2 to 5 days. Some afflicted sows may show no signs and suddenly die. Fasting and stress must be avoided, especially in the last several weeks of pregnancy.

EUTHANASIA

Animals maintained in biomedical research facilities may be euthanized at the end of a research study to collect tissue samples for further analysis. Pet animals that are suffering are often humanely euthanized rather than allowed to live their final days in pain. Methods of euthanasia are listed in the *American Veterinary Medical Association Guidelines for the Euthanasia of Animals*. Acceptable methods of euthanasia for guinea pigs include carbon dioxide chamber asphyxiation or administration of an overdose of inhalant or injectable anesthetic agents. Injectable agents are usually administered by rapid IV or IP injection. Carbon dioxide is administered by gradual displacement. The carbon dioxide is supplied as a humidified compressed gas or by a dry ice pack. The animals must not be permitted to come into contact with the dry ice container. Avoid placing large groups of animals in the carbon dioxide chamber simultaneously because this stresses the animals and reduces the effectiveness of the inhalation agent. Animals should be left in the carbon dioxide chamber for at least 5 minutes after obvious respiratory motions have ceased.

KEY POINTS

- The scientific name for the laboratory guinea pig is *Cavia porcellus*.
- Guinea pigs are commonly used in studies of audiology, nutrition, and immunology.
- Determination of sex in guinea pigs is accomplished by observing the shape of the external genitalia.
- Polygamous, intensive breeding systems are commonly used with guinea pigs.

- The English guinea pig is the most common breed used in biomedical research.
- Guinea pigs usually attempt to flee when frightened, although vocalization and immobilization may also occur.
- Guinea pigs are usually housed in solid-bottom cages covered with soft bedding material.
- Vitamin C must be provided in the diet of guinea pigs.
- Manual or chemical restraint is typically used for guinea pigs.
- Ear notching, ear tags, tattooing, and implantation of microchips are used for permanent identification.
- Injections are usually given by the subcutaneous or intramuscular routes.
- Guinea pigs do not have readily accessible veins.
- Larger volumes of blood can be collected from the jugular vein, cranial vena cava, femoral artery, or femoral vein.
- Guinea pigs are prone to a large number of bacterial and viral diseases, especially when husbandry conditions are poor.

REVIEW QUESTIONS

1. The scientific name of the laboratory guinea pig is
_____ _____.

2. Guinea pigs are unique in that babies are born
_____, eyes open and capable of eating solid food within a few hours of birth.

3. _____ is a variety of guinea pig with a short, coarse hair coat that grows in whorls or rosettes.

4. Like primates, guinea pigs have a dietary requirement for vitamin _____.

5. In an attempt to avoid dystocia, a sow must be bred before the age of _____ months.

6. Guinea pig food must be used within _____ days of milling.

7. The primary reason that guinea pigs are not used extensively in biomedical research is their lack of _____ _____ _____.

8. Leukocytes found in guinea pig blood smears that contain intracytoplasmic inclusions are referred to as _____ _____.

9. Guinea pigs are sometimes used for toxicity studies and routinely given _____ injections for this purpose.

10. Up to 8 mls of blood can be collected by using which vessels?

11. The most common outbred stocks of guinea pigs used in biomedical facilities are the _____ and _____ _____.

12. Pododermatitis in guinea pigs is associated with the bacterium _____ _____.

13. The common name for the disease known as cervical lymphadenitis is _____.

14. Lactating females may be prone to _____ _____, especially as the pups approach weaning age.

15. _____ should be suspected in guinea pigs that are anorectic and have not been on a diet with sufficient vitamin C.

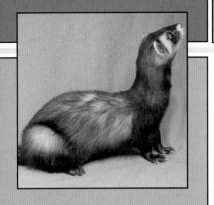

KEY TERMS

Aleutian disease
Hobs
Hyperestrogenism
Insulinoma
Jills

9 The Ferret

LEARNING OBJECTIVES

After studying this chapter, you will be able to:
- Identify unique anatomic and physiologic characteristics of ferrets.
- Identify unique aspects of ferret behavior.
- Explain routine procedures for husbandry, housing, and nutrition of ferrets.
- Describe various restraint and handling procedures used on ferrets.
- Describe methods of administering medication and collecting blood samples.
- List and describe common diseases of ferrets.

Ferrets are not widely used in biomedical research. Ferrets have been used in the past to hunt rats and rabbits and for their pelts. Pet ferrets are increasingly seen in companion animal veterinary practice.

TAXONOMY

The ferret is classified in the order Mustelidae, which includes minks, weasels, and skunks. The scientific name of the domestic ferret is *Mustela putorius furo.* Several color types are seen as pets. The domestic ferret is thought to have originated from the European ferret, *Mustela putorius.* The black-footed ferret, *Mustela nigripes,* is native to North America.

UNIQUE ANATOMIC AND PHYSIOLOGIC FEATURES

Anatomically, the ferret shares similarities with human beings, canines, and felines. Table 9-1 contains a summary of unique physiologic data for ferrets. Ferrets have a fine hair coat covered with denser, coarser guard hairs. A variety of color patterns exist (Figure 9-1).

The animals have a musky smell due to their active sebaceous glands. Secretions from the glands increase during breeding season. Neutering the animal may reduce the odor. Ferrets also possess paired anal glands that also secrete a serous yellow liquid with a strong odor. Surgical procedures are sometimes performed to remove the anal glands, which may lessen the odor in neutered males.

TECHNICIAN NOTE │ Neutering and removal of the anal glands are sometimes performed to minimize the odor of the ferret.

TABLE 9-1	Unique Physiologic Data for Ferrets
Average life span (years)	5-8
Average adult body weight (kg)	Male: 1000-2000; female: 600-900
Heart rate (beats/min)	180-250
Respiratory rate (breaths/min)	33-36
Rectal temperature (°C)	37.8-40
Daily feed consumption (g)	140-190
Daily water consumption (mL)	75-100
Recommended environmental temperature (°C)	39-64
Recommended environmental relative humidity (%)	40-65
Age at puberty (mo)	9-12
Estrus cycle length (days)	Continuous
Length of gestation (days)	41-42
Average litter size	8
Weaning age (weeks)	6-8

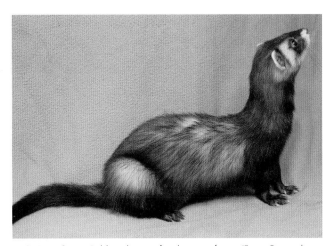

FIGURE 9-1. Sable coloring of a domestic ferret. (From Quesenberry K, Carpenter JW: *Ferrets, rabbits, and rodents: clinical medicine and surgery*, ed 3, St. Louis, 2012, Saunders.)

The intestinal tract appears as an undifferentiated tube with no obvious divisions between the ileum and colon. The intestine is relatively short, and no cecum or appendix is present.

The ferret's heart is cone-shaped and the cardiodiaphragmatic ligament that connects the heart to the sternum frequently contains large fat deposits. There is also a single brachiocephalic artery exiting the aorta rather than two carotid arteries. The single artery branches into the right and left carotid arteries.

ANIMAL MODELS

Ferrets were used in early studies of the influenza virus. Influenza infection in ferrets closely resembles infection in human beings regarding symptoms, viral distribution, and immunity. Ferrets have also been used in neuroendocrinology and toxicology research and to study canine distemper.

REPRODUCTION

Female ferrets are called **jills**. Male ferrets are **hobs**. Females tend to be larger than males. Males can be identified by the presence of the penis and testicles. The os penis is readily palpable. The vulva of female is ventral to the anus and appears as a small slit-like opening. During estrus, the vulva swells and appears fleshy (Figure 9-2). The ferret is seasonally polyestrus and an induced ovulator. Ferrets respond to changing photoperiods, with fertility increasing as the days lengthen. Female ferrets that are not induced to ovulate remain in estrus for a prolonged period. Persistent **hyperestrogenism** suppresses the bone marrow and increases the risk that the female will develop severe anemia.

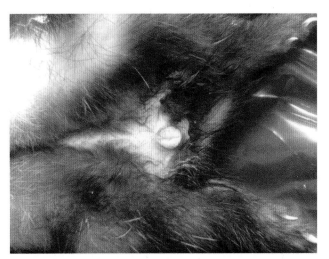

FIGURE 9-2. Swollen vulva of a ferret in estrus. (From Jepson L: *Exotic animal medicine*, St. Louis, 2009, Saunders.)

BEHAVIOR

The ferret is relatively easy to house and handle. This accounts in part for their increasing popularity both as pets and as research subjects. They are friendly, inquisitive animals and can be housed singly or in groups. They rarely bite unless frightened or in pain. However, females with litters often become aggressive, and males housed together usually fight during the breeding season.

Ferrets are burrowers and like to dig. Because vision is not well developed, they often bump into objects when let out of their cage. They are easily litter trained.

TECHNICIAN NOTE │ Ferrets rarely bite unless frightened or in pain.

HUSBANDRY, HOUSING, AND NUTRITION

Ferrets can be housed in cages used for cats, dogs, or rabbits that have been modified to prevent the animals from escaping. The bar spacing of some cages may be too large, so a Plexiglas panel can be placed over the cage front. The ferret's small feet can become injured in wire cage floors, so they are usually kept in solid-bottom cages. Nest boxes and soft towels may be provided to allow the animals to burrow and hide. Ferrets require somewhat cooler temperatures than most other small mammal species and are prone to heat stroke when kept at temperatures greater than 80° F. Ventilation must also be considered both to remove fumes from excreted wastes and to keep the temperature from rising excessively in the cage.

Ferrets are carnivorous and require a suitable diet. Commercial ferret chow is available, or high-quality kitten chow may be fed if it contains a protein content of at least 30%. Feed is often given in large, heavy bowls placed on the cage floor. The bowls must be made of an indestructible material and be heavy enough to not be easily tipped over. Water can also be provided in heavy bowls, or water bottles can be hung inside the cage. Sick ferrets can be syringe fed several times a day. A commercial product marketed for dogs and cats can be used. Esophagostomy tubes can be placed when long-term nutritional support is needed.

> **TECHNICIAN NOTE** Ferrets are carnivores and have a high dietary protein requirement.

HANDLING AND RESTRAINT

Most ferrets can be easily restrained by simply picking them up and cradling them in the crook of the arm. Some ferrets will wiggle and twist when attempts are made at restraint. If firmer restraint is needed, the loose skin over the back of the neck is grasped and the animal held suspended (Figure 9-3). This technique tends to calm many ferrets, and simple procedures such as nail clipping can be performed when the animal is held this way. For more invasive procedures, the animal can be held with a hand across the shoulders, the thumb under the chin, and fingers placed around the neck and behind the forelimbs. The other hand is used to restrain the hindquarters by placing a hand across the pelvis just cranial to the forelimbs. Injections and blood collection procedures can be performed with this restraint method (Figure 9-4). Ferrets can also be wrapped in a towel as a method of restraint (Figure 9-5).

IDENTIFICATION METHODS

Permanent identification of ferrets is usually accomplished with implantation of a microchip. However, tattoos, ear tags, and ear punches can also be used. Identification using photographs or description of markings is less accurate as the intensity of a ferret's color may change during the breeding season.

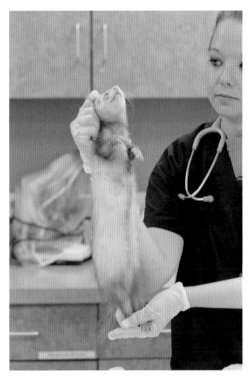

FIGURE 9-3. The ferret can be held by grasping the loose skin over the back of the neck and the animal held suspended.

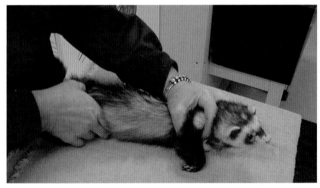

FIGURE 9-4. Restraint for invasive procedures. (From Sheldon CC, Topel J, Sonsthagen T: *Animal restraint for veterinary professionals*, St. Louis, Mosby, 2006.)

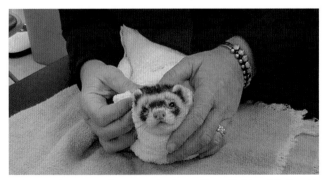

FIGURE 9-5. Towel restraint of a ferret. (From Sheldon CC, Topel J, Sonsthagen T: *Animal restraint for veterinary professionals*, St. Louis, 2006, Mosby.)

CLINICAL PROCEDURES

ADMINISTRATION OF MEDICATION
Injection Techniques

Injections can be given subcutaneously, intramuscularly, intraperitoneally, or intravenously. Subcutaneous injections are usually given by grasping the loose skin on the back over the shoulder area (Figure 9-6). In fall and winter months, ferrets usually develop a thick layer of fat in the subcutaneous space and a longer needle is required to penetrate this layer. Intramuscular injections are usually given in the quadriceps or semimembranous muscles, as in the domestic cat. Intramuscular injections usually require two people, one to restrain the animal and one to administer the injection. The ferret should be held by the scruff and the positioner should have his or her arm along the spine of the ferret. The restrainer grasps the hindlimbs (Figure 9-7). The person administering the injection then grasps the muscle of the thigh and enters the muscle at a 45-degree angle. It is important to aspirate prior to administering the injection to verify that a blood vessel has not been entered. Intraperitoneal injections into the lower abdomen are also relatively simple to perform. Intravenous injections are usually given into the cephalic, saphenous, or jugular veins. Sedation or anesthesia may be required if the animal is very fractious.

> **TECHNICIAN NOTE** Two people are needed when administering intramuscular injections to ferrets.

Blood Collection. The anterior vena cava and jugular vein are suitable locations for blood collection. The lateral saphenous or cephalic veins can be used but are difficult to visualize. For jugular collection, the ferret can be restrained in a manner similar to a cat with the legs extended over the table edge (Figure 9-8). Take care not to overextend the neck. The vein is somewhat more lateral in the neck than it is in cats. The head can be moved slowly up and down to enhance blood flow once the vessel has been penetrated. If the ferret resists the restraint, the animal can be wrapped in a towel and maintained in dorsal recumbency while the restrainer grasps the scruff.

Samples can also be collected from the anterior vena cava. The ferret should be restrained on its back with the neck extended. The forelimbs are pulled caudally. A second restrainer may be needed to immobilize the hind end and ensure the animal does not attempt to twist or wiggle out of the restraint position. The needle is inserted into the thoracic cavity between the first rib and the manubrium at an angle of 30 to 45 degrees (Figure 9-9).

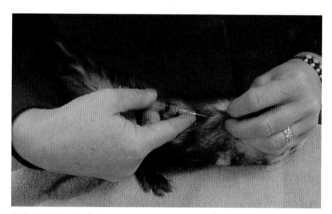

FIGURE 9-6. Subcutaneous injection in the ferret. (From Sheldon CC, Topel J, Sonsthagen T: *Animal restraint for veterinary professionals*, St. Louis, 2006, Mosby.)

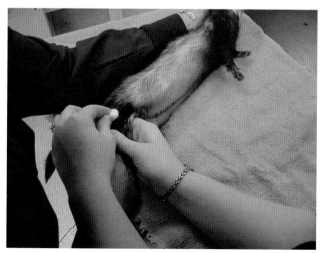

FIGURE 9-7. Intramuscular injection technique. (From Sheldon CC, Topel J, Sonsthagen T: *Animal restraint for veterinary professionals*, St. Louis, 2006, Mosby.)

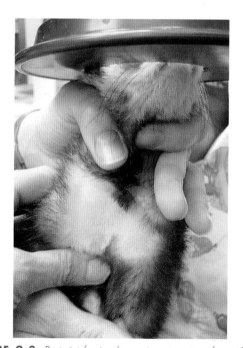

FIGURE 9-8. Restraint for jugular venipuncture in a ferret. Restrain the ferret in a manner similar to that used with a cat, with the legs pulled down and the head back. Shave the neck to improve visibility of the jugular vein in the lateral neck. After the vein is punctured, the head can be "pumped" up and down slowly to facilitate blood flow. (From Quesenberry K, Carpenter JW: *Ferrets, rabbits, and rodents: clinical medicine and surgery*, ed 3, St. Louis, 2012, Saunders.)

TECHNICIAN NOTE Blood samples can be collected from the jugular vein or anterior vena cava.

If very small amounts of blood are needed, the lateral saphenous or cephalic vein can be used. Small volumes of blood samples can be collected from the retroorbital sinus in the anesthetized animal, although for aesthetic reasons this procedure should not be performed in front of clients. Anesthesia is also required for blood collection from the tail artery since it is a painful procedure.

Bone Marrow Collection. Collection of bone marrow may be needed to evaluate anemic ferrets. The proximal femur is the most common site for collection of marrow samples. The iliac crest, tibial crest, and humerus can also be used. Aseptic technique is vital and the ferret must be anesthetized. For collection of bone marrow aspirates from the proximal femur, place the anesthetized ferret in lateral recumbency and aseptically prepare the site. A small incision is made over the site and a 20-gauge spinal needle introduced into the marrow cavity (Figure 9-10). Steady forward pressure while rotating the needle is needed. Core samples are collected with a similar technique using an 18-gauge needle.

Intravenous Catheters

Hospitalized ferrets and ferrets undergoing surgical procedures should have an intravenous catheter placed for administration of fluids. Intravenous catheters can be placed in the lateral saphenous or cephalic vein. The animal should be sedated or anesthetized for catheter placement. When the ferret cannot be anesthetized, a small amount of topical anesthetic should be placed over the venipuncture site. In very young or small ferrets, an intraosseous catheter can be placed in the proximal tibia or femur. Anesthesia is required and strict attention to aseptic technique is essential. Fluid therapy volumes are calculated in the same manner as for a feline patient. Fluids can also be administered subcutaneously.

TECHNICIAN NOTE Anesthesia is usually required to place an intravenous catheter in a ferret.

Oral Medications

Medications available in pill form are usually placed in suspension to administer as a liquid. Oral medications can be administered by a syringe or feeding tube (Figure 9-11). Ferrets do not have a cough reflex, so proper placement of the feeding tube in the stomach must be verified by aspiration of a small amount of stomach contents. Placement of a mouth gag is also needed to ensure that the animal does not chew on the tube.

Anesthesia

Agents used for anesthesia in ferrets are similar to those used for the domestic cat. Inhalation agents include sevoflurane and isoflurane. For procedures of short duration, inhalant anesthesia can be accomplished with an anesthetic mask or in an induction chamber. Short procedures can also be carried out with injectable anesthetics. An endotracheal tube should be placed for procedures of longer duration and anesthetic agents delivered by a precision vaporizer. Anesthetic depth can be evaluated by the same parameters as used for dogs and cats (e.g., palpebral reflex, heart and respiratory rate, muscle tension).

Ferrets should be fasted for no more than 8 hours prior to anesthesia. The ferret should receive a preanesthetic agent

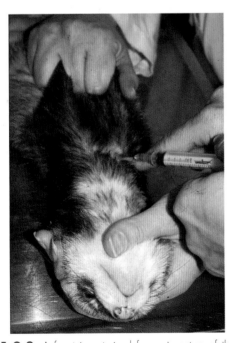

FIGURE 9-9. A ferret is restrained for venipuncture of the anterior vena cava. Both forelegs are pulled back, hindlegs are restrained, and the neck is extended. (From Quesenberry K, Carpenter JW: *Ferrets, rabbits, and rodents: clinical medicine and surgery*, ed 3, St. Louis, 2012, Saunders.)

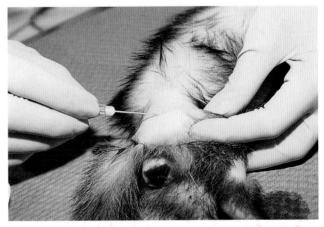

FIGURE 9-10. Collection of a bone marrow sample from the femur of a ferret with an enlarged vulva. The femur is stabilized while inserting a 20-gauge, 1.5-inch spinal needle medial to the greater trochanter. (From Quesenberry K, Carpenter JW: *Ferrets, rabbits, and rodents: clinical medicine and surgery*, ed 3, St. Louis, 2012, Saunders.)

or initial anesthesia via face mask or induction chamber. Endotracheal intubation is not difficult. A small amount of lidocaine can be used to minimize the possibility of laryngospasm.

Body temperature must be closely monitored in the anesthetized ferret and warmed fluids administered during surgical procedures.

Pain management is important in the postoperative period. Signs of pain in ferrets include tachypnea, a stiff gait, teeth grinding, shivering, half-closed eyelids, aggression, general malaise, and bristling of tail fur.

Diagnostic Imaging

Sedation or anesthesia is required to obtain diagnostic quality images of the ferret. Whole-body radiographs are commonly obtained. A stockinette may be used to aid in positioning of the ferret (Figure 9-12). Contrast radiography is also performed in ferrets. The ferret has a more rapid

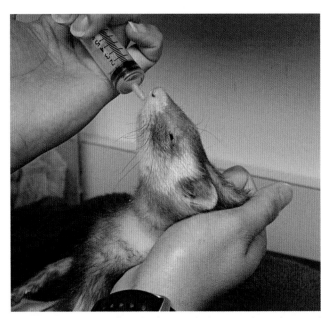

FIGURE 9-11. Scruffing the ferret with the nose directed upward facilitates the administration of oral medication. (From Mitchell M, Thomas T: *Manual of exotic pet practice*, St. Louis, 2009, Saunders.)

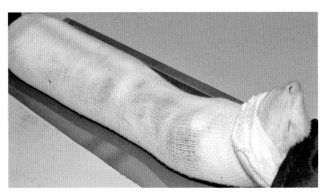

FIGURE 9-12. Utilizing stockinet for a ventrodorsal (VD) view of an unanesthetized ferret. Sandbags can be placed at either end. (From Brown M, Brown L: *Lavin's radiography for veterinary technicians*, ed 5, St. Louis, 2014, Saunders.)

gastrointestinal transit time, so contrast radiographs must be taken more frequently than they would be in dogs and cats. Techniques used for radiology are similar to those used on feline patients.

Other Procedures

A variety of clinical diagnostic and therapeutic techniques are performed on pet ferrets. These include urinary catheterization, tracheal wash, and fine needle aspiration. The procedures for most of the techniques performed on ferrets are done in a manner similar to that used for feline patients. Blood transfusions are also administered to anemic ferrets. Detectable blood groups have not been identified in ferrets, so cross-matching of donor samples is not needed.

COMMON DISEASES

Ferrets are susceptible to many of the same viral and bacterial diseases as dogs and cats as well as infection with the human influenza virus. A complete review of all ferret diseases is beyond the scope of this text. Information on the most commonly encountered diseases of pet ferrets is presented below.

VACCINATION

Routine vaccination of pet ferrets against canine distemper is recommended. Ferrets used in biomedical research also receive immunizations against canine distemper and diseases caused by *Bordetella* and *Pseudomonas* species.

Infection with canine distemper has a near 100% mortality rate in unvaccinated ferrets. The vaccines are administered subcutaneously although some localities may require intramuscular administration of rabies vaccine. Canine distemper vaccine is usually administered at the age of 6 to 8 weeks with additional boosters approximately every 2 weeks for a total of three doses. Annual re-vaccination is required. The rabies vaccine is usually administered at 3 months of age and an annual booster vaccine administered.

> **TECHNICIAN NOTE** Ferrets are vaccinated against canine distemper virus and rabies virus.

INFECTIOUS DISEASES
Bacterial Diseases

Ferrets may develop bacterial infections with a variety of agents, including *Helicobacter mustelae*, *Clostridium botulinum*, *Staphylococcus aureus*, *S. zooepidemicus*, *Escherichia coli*, and *Desulfovibrio* species.

Helicobacter mustelae is a gram-negative bacillus and most ferrets are exposed by weaning age. Severe *Helicobacter* infections can occur in ferrets under stress and are usually characterized by gastrointestinal dysfunction and result in anorexia and weight loss. Gastric ulcers can result from infection.

The most serious bacterial infection of ferrets is infection with the campylobacter-like organism *Desulfovibrio*. This bacterium is the causative agent of proliferative bowel disease. Clinical signs include tenesmus and production of small, frequent bowel movements that often contain frank blood and mucus. Rectal prolapse can occur. The disease can be fatal if untreated.

A large number of bacterial agents have been implicated in development of bacterial pneumonia in ferrets. These include *Streptococcus zooepidemicus,* other streptococcal species, numerous mycobacterial species, *Escherichia coli, Klebsiella pneumoniae, Pseudomonas aeruginosa, Bordetella bronchiseptica, Pneumocystis carinii,* and *Listeria monocytogenes.* Infection is rare but evidence suggests hospitalization in areas where dogs and other carriers of the organisms are present may result in clinical disease in ferrets.

Viral Diseases

Canine Distemper.
Canine distemper is a serious disease in unvaccinated ferrets and is nearly always fatal. Clinical signs of infection are seen 7 to 10 days after exposure and are similar to those seen in dogs. Photophobia, mucopuru-

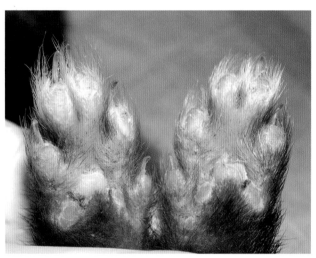

FIGURE 9-13. Hyperkeratotic footpads in a ferret diagnosed with canine distemper virus (CDV). (From Quesenberry K, Carpenter JW: *Ferrets, rabbits, and rodents: clinical medicine and surgery,* ed 3, St. Louis, 2012, Saunders.)

lent oculonasal discharge, hyperkeratosis of the footpads, a papular rash on the chin and inguinal area, and bronchopneumonia may be seen (Figure 9-13). Infected ferrets usually die within a week of developing symptoms. Those that initially survive may die of a neurotropic form of the disease weeks to months later.

Rabies.
Although ferrets are susceptible to rabies, the disease is rarely seen in this species. Routine vaccination against rabies has further reduced the incidence of this disease. When present, the typical signs are nervous system abnormalities similar to those seen in other mammals. Depending on state and local laws, unvaccinated ferrets that bite a human being may be euthanized and screened for rabies.

Influenza.
Ferrets are susceptible to infection from both influenza type A and B viruses. Transmission is usually the result of contact with aerosol droplets from infected humans in the household. Clinical signs are similar to that seen in humans and include pyrexia, sneezing, nasal discharge, and lethargy and must be differentiated from the symptoms of canine distemper (Table 9-2). Conjunctivitis may also occur as well as secondary bacterial infections. Treatment is aimed at reducing the severity of symptoms and maintaining hydration.

Coronavirus and Rotavirus.
Coronavirus is the causative agent of epizootic catarrhal enteritis (ECE). This disease is a highly transmissible diarrheal disease of ferrets characterized by anorexia, lethargy, and green mucoid diarrhea that may progress to a loose, grainy stool resembling birdseed (Figure 9-14). Young ferrets are often asymptomatic carriers that are capable of infecting adult ferrets. Rotavirus infection causes diarrhea in young ferrets. Mortality is high in neonatal ferrets. Adult ferrets may exhibit a green, mucoid diarrhea. Treatment involves fluids and antimicrobial therapy.

Another coronavirus has been implicated in the development of a progressive systemic disease in ferrets that resembles feline infectious peritonitis. Clinical signs include

TABLE 9-2	Clinical Distinctions between Canine Distemper Virus and Influenza Virus Infections	
CLINICAL FINDINGS	**CANINE DISTEMPER VIRUS**	**INFLUENZA**
Nasal and ocular discharge	+++ (Mucopurulent)	++ (Mucoserous)
Sneezing	+	+++
Coughing	+	+++
Pyrexia	+++ (>40°C)	++[b]
Dermatitis (chin, lips, inguinal)	+++	—
Footpad hyperkeratosis	++	—
Central signs	+[a]	—
Outcome	Almost 100% fatal	Self-limiting[c]

Frequency of clinical signs: +, may be present; ++, common; +++, usual presentation; —, absent.
[a]Central nervous system signs seen in advanced stages of disease (rarely the only signs).
[b]Pyrexia occurs early in the course of disease and may be resolved by the time of presentation.
[c]Influenza virus infection can be fatal in neonates.
(From Quesenberry K, Carpenter JW: *Ferrets, rabbits, and rodents: clinical medicine and surgery,* ed 3, St. Louis, 2012, Saunders.)

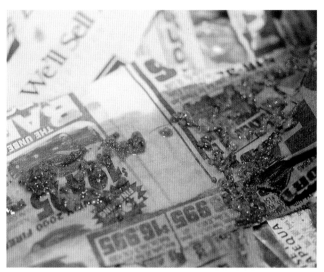

FIGURE 9-14. Grainy, loose feces in a ferret with chronic diarrhea, consistent with infection ferret enteric coronavirus (epizootic catarrhal enteritis). (From Quesenberry K, Carpenter JW: *Ferrets, rabbits, and rodents: clinical medicine and surgery*, ed 3, St. Louis, 2012, Saunders.)

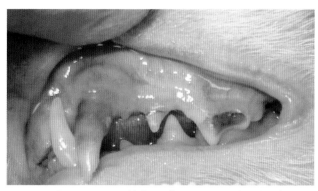

FIGURE 9-15. Fractured left maxillary canine tooth with pulp exposure in a ferret. Note the discoloration of the tooth and discoloration of the mucosa overlying the root. (From Holstrom, SE: *Veterinary dentistry: a team approach*, ed 2, St. Louis, 2013, Saunders.)

weight loss, diarrhea, and anemia. There is no effective treatment and mortality is high.

Aleutian Disease. Hobs is a chronic progressive disorder caused by a parvovirus, the **Aleutian disease** virus (ADV). The virus causes hypergammaglobulinemia. Clinical signs include glomerulonephritis, bile duct proliferation, weight loss, ataxia, and progressive wasting. CNS signs can also occur. Secondary infections are common due to immune suppression. Different strains of ADV vary in their virulence. Infection can remain latent for years before clinical signs develop. Transmission is by direct contact with infected body fluids or contaminated fomites. There is no definitive treatment for infected ferrets.

Parasite Infections

With the exception of coccidia, intestinal parasites are uncommon in ferrets. *Toxocara cati, Toxascaris leonina, Ancylostoma* species, *Dipylidium caninum, Filaroides* species, *Mesocestoides* species, and *Giardia* species have all been reported in ferrets. Three species of coccidia have been seen in ferrets: *Eimeria furo, Eimeria ictidea,* and *Isospora laidlawii.* Most coccidial infections are subclinical.

Ectoparasites of ferrets include *Sarcoptes scabei, Ctenocephalides* species (fleas), and *Otodectes cyanotis* (ear mites). Diagnosis and treatment of parasite infections is much the same as for dogs and cats.

Infections with the canine heartworm *Dirofilaria immitis* have been reported in ferrets and can cause coughing, lethargy, weakness, and dyspnea when even a single adult worm is present. Right-sided heart failure and sudden cardiac death can occur. Diagnosis includes radiographs to evaluate the ferret for right-sided heart enlargement. Microfilaria are seen in only about 50% of infected ferrets. Diagnostic tests used with canine and feline blood samples may not detect the presence of heartworms when worm burden is very low.

Heartworm-preventative medications should be administered to ferrets in heartworm-endemic areas.

> **TECHNICIAN NOTE** Ferrets in heartworm-endemic areas should be given heartworm-preventative medications.

NONINFECTIOUS DISEASES
Dental Disease

Ferrets have a relatively high incidence of dental disease. This may result from dietary factors, such as feeding of hard, dry kibble, or as a result of inappropriate chewing on objects. Ferrets often develop periodontal disease that progresses with age, and the disease is similar to that seen in feline patients. Fractures of the teeth are also common (Figure 9-15). Treatment is similar to procedures performed on feline patients and can include dental scaling, extractions, and endodontic therapy.

> **TECHNICIAN NOTE** Dental disease is common in pet ferrets.

Urolithiasis

Urolithiasis is relatively rare in ferrets that are fed high-quality ferret or kitten food. When present, the most common urinary calculi is struvite. Calcium oxalate and cystine calculi can also occur. Uroliths occur more often in male than female ferrets.

Neoplasia

Neoplasia is a common presentation in pet ferrets. Several types of neoplastic diseases have been reported in ferrets. Adrenocortical neoplasia, **insulinoma**, mast cell tumors, and malignant lymphoma are particularly common.

Insulinoma is a tumor of the beta cells of the pancreatic islets and is the most common neoplasm of the ferret. Unlike the insulinoma of dogs and cats, the disease in ferrets does not metastasize readily. Diagnosis is based on clinical signs, including ataxia, as well as a persistent hypoglycemia. Treatment involves surgical excision but recurrence is likely.

Adrenocortical neoplasms are the second most common neoplasm in the pet ferret and are associated with hypersecretion of estrogen in females and testosterone in males. Typical signs include alopecia that is progressive and bilaterally symmetrical (Figure 9-16). Vulvar swelling in neutered jills may also occur. Behavioral changes in neutered hobs are also possible. The disease may be treated with surgical excision or the symptoms managed medically.

Malignant lymphoma is the third most common neoplasia in the domestic ferret. It can occur at any age and has no gender predilection. Lymphoma denotes solid-tissue tumors composed of neoplastic lymphocytes in visceral organs or lymph nodes throughout the body. Cutaneous and gastric lymphomas also occur (Figure 9-17). A variety of grading systems are used to classify lymphoma. Anemia is the most common clinical sign. Histologic or cytologic examination is needed to diagnose the disease. Treatment protocols include chemotherapy, radiation, or palliative care.

> **TECHNICIAN NOTE** Adrenocortical tumors, insulinoma, and malignant lymphoma the most common neoplasms of ferrets.

Benign basal cell tumors are the most common skin neoplasm in the ferret. Benign mast cell tumors are the second most common skin tumors and are treated effectively with surgical excision. Neoplasia of the scent glands also occurs and is commonly malignant.

A number of tumors of the liver are also seen in pet ferrets, with malignant biliary cystadenoma seen most often. Tumors of the oral cavity are also seen occasionally in ferrets and are usually associated with a poor prognosis. Squamous cell carcinoma is the most common tumor of the oral cavity.

Hyperestrogenism

Aplastic anemia is a common problem in intact female ferrets. Female ferrets undergo a persistent estrus if not bred, and the resultant prolonged estrogen exposure leads to anemia. Clinical signs include lethargy, anorexia, pale mucous membranes, and petechial hemorrhage. Affected females must be immediately treated and an ovariohysterectomy performed. Pet ferrets not intended to be bred should be spayed.

Miscellaneous Diseases

Ferrets are susceptible to dermatophytosis caused by *Microsporum canis*. Clinical signs are similar to those in cats. Megaesophagus is an uncommon but usually fatal disease in ferrets. Clinical presentation is similar to that seen in dogs and cats. Gastrointestinal foreign bodies are common in young or bored ferrets. Ferrets are curious animals and will chew and may ingest nearly any object they come into contact with, including towels or other forms of bedding. Anorexia and passage of abnormal stools are common presenting signs. Prolonged anorexia predisposes ferrets to hepatic lipidosis.

EUTHANASIA

Ferrets are usually euthanized by administering an overdose of barbiturate by intravenous injection. A carbon dioxide chamber may also be used, but sedation before placement in the chamber may be needed to avoid undue stress on the animals.

KEY POINTS

- The scientific name of the domestic ferret is *Mustela putorius furo*.
- Ferrets have been used in neuroendocrinology and toxicology research and the study of human influenza infection and canine distemper.
- Domestic ferrets are highly susceptible to heat stroke.

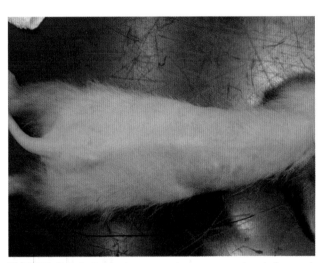

FIGURE 9-16. Bilateral symmetrical alopecia in a female ferret with hyperadrenocortism. (From Jepson L: *Exotic animal medicine*, St. Louis, 2009, Saunders.)

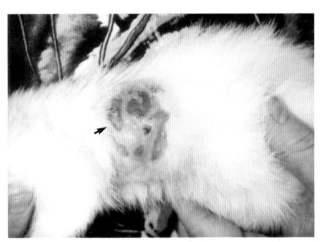

FIGURE 9-17. Cutaneous lymphoma in a ferret. Surgical excision of this ulcerated neoplasm *(arrow)* was accomplished and, despite several recurrences, the ferret was still alive 3 years later. (From Quesenberry K, Carpenter JW: *Ferrets, rabbits, and rodents: clinical medicine and surgery*, ed 3, St. Louis, 2012, Saunders.)

- Ferrets can be given injections by subcutaneous, intramuscular, intraperitoneal, or intravenous routes.
- Blood samples are usually collected from the jugular vein or anterior vena cava in the anesthetized animal.
- Ferrets are susceptible to many of the same infectious diseases as dogs and cats.

REVIEW QUESTIONS

1. The scientific name of the domestic ferret is _____ _____ _____.

2. Anatomically, ferrets are similar to _____, _____, and _____.

3. The active _____ gland gives ferrets the musky smell.

4. Ferrets have been used to study _____ _____ because the infection closely resembles the infection in humans.

5. Ferrets rarely bite unless _____ or ___ _____.

6. Ferrets are prone to _____ _____ if exposed to temperatures over 80° F.

7. Ferrets can be fed kitten chow as long as it is over _____% protein.

8. The _____, _____, _____, or _____ _____ are the best sites for blood collection in ferrets.

9. Coronavirus is a causative agent of _____ _____ _____, a highly transmissible diarrheal disease in ferrets.

10. Infections with the _____ _____ virus are often fatal in unvaccinated ferrets.

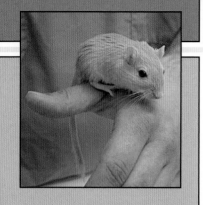

10 Gerbils and Hamsters

LEARNING OBJECTIVES

After studying this chapter, you will be able to:

- Identify unique anatomic and physiologic characteristics of hamsters and gerbils.
- Describe breeding systems used for hamsters.
- Identify unique aspects of hamster and gerbil behavior.
- Explain routine procedures for husbandry, housing, and nutrition of hamsters and gerbils.
- Describe various restraint and handling procedures used on hamsters and gerbils.
- Describe methods of administering medication and collecting blood samples.
- List and describe common diseases of hamsters and gerbils.

TAXONOMY

HAMSTER

The hamster is classified in the order Rodentia, suborder Sciurognathi, family Cricetidae. There are several species of hamsters kept as pets and used in biomedical research. The most common species are the Syrian or golden hamster, *Mesocricetus auratus*, and the Chinese hamster, *Cricetus griseus*. Other species seen occasionally as pets include the Armenian or gray hamster, *Cricetulus migratorius,* and the European hamster, *Cricetus cricetus*. Another species, the Djungarian hamster, *Phodopus songorus*, is seen in the pet industry and is usually referred to as the dwarf hamster (Figure 10-1). Chinese hamsters are sometimes included in the dwarf varieties as well. The various species differ in chromosome number and physical characteristics. This chapter will focus primarily on the Syrian hamster.

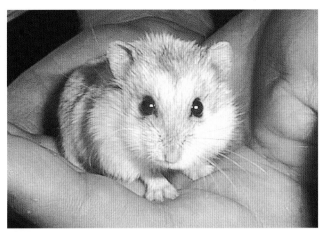

FIGURE 10-1. Siberian dwarf hamsters are popular pets. (From Bassert JM, McCurnin DM: *McCurnin's clinical textbook for veterinary technicians*, ed 7, St. Louis, 2007, Saunders.)

TABLE 10-1	Normal Physiologic Reference Values for Hamsters
Average life span (mo)	18-36
Average adult body weight (kg)	Male: 87-130; female: 95-130
Heart rate (beats/min)	310-470
Respiratory rate (breaths/min)	38-110
Rectal temperature (°C)	37.6
Daily feed consumption (g)	10-15
Daily water consumption (mL)	9-12
Recommended environmental temperature (°C)	21-24
Recommended environmental relative humidity (%)	40-60
Age at puberty (weeks)	Male: 8; female: 6
Estrus cycle length (days)	4-5
Length of gestation (days)	15-18
Average litter size	5-10
Weaning age (days)	19-21

TABLE 10-2	Normal Physiologic Reference Values for Gerbils
Average life span (mo)	24-39
Average adult body weight (kg)	Male: 46-131; female: 50-55
Heart rate (beats/min)	260-600
Respiratory rate (breaths/min)	85-160
Rectal temperature (°C)	38.2
Daily feed consumption (g)	5-7
Daily water consumption (mL)	4
Recommended environmental temperature (°C)	18-22
Recommended environmental relative humidity (%)	45-55
Age at puberty (weeks)	Male: 9-18; female: 9-12
Estrus cycle length (days)	4-7
Length of gestation (days)	23-26
Average litter size	3-8
Weaning age (days)	21-28

Hamsters live in the semiarid regions of southeast Europe and Asia Minor. The origin of the Syrian hamster in the United States has been traced to a zoologic expedition to Syria in 1930. A female hamster and 11 neonates were found in a burrow in a wheat field. The female cannibalized all but three of the young. The remaining neonates, one female and two males, were taken and bred. In 1931 hamster colonies were established in England and France. In 1938 the hamster was introduced to the United States, and by 1971 the hamster was already the third most commonly used laboratory animal.

GERBIL

Gerbils are small, friendly rodents that are native to harsh desert environments. The scientific name of the species most often seen in biomedical research is *Meriones unguiculatus* and is in the same taxonomic family as mice and hamsters. This species originates in Mongolia, southern Siberia, and northern China and is commonly referred to as the Mongolian gerbil. There are nearly 90 other species of gerbils. Very few of these are kept as pets.

UNIQUE ANATOMIC AND PHYSIOLOGIC FEATURES

GENERAL CHARACTERISTICS

Hamsters are stout-bodied, short-tailed rodents with short legs and prominent dark ears. Table 10-1 contains a summary of unique physiologic data. Unlike mice and rats, the tail is well haired. The Syrian hamster is slightly larger than a mouse and has a smooth hair coat. The female is usually larger and more aggressive than the male. Hamsters have the shortest gestation of all the laboratory species and are virtually free from spontaneous disease. They are the only commonly used laboratory animal that hibernates. They are inquisitive animals that are relatively easy to handle and seldom bite.

Table 10-2 contains a summary of unique physiologic data for gerbils. Their overall body shape is long and slim when compared with that of hamsters. The hindlimbs are particularly long, allowing the animal to stand nearly upright and jump relatively high.

> TECHNICIAN NOTE   Hamsters are the only commonly used laboratory animal that hibernates.

Gerbils consume very little water. In their natural habitat they acquire their water solely from food sources during periods of drought. Like hamsters, the tail is covered with hair. Both sexes have a prominent sebaceous gland located on the abdomen that is covered with darker hair than found on the rest of the body. The gland is more noticeable in males than females. Secretions from this gland are used in marking territory.

THE HEAD AND NECK

Like mice and rats, hamsters possess harderian glands, which are located behind the eyeball. Their eyes are small, black, and somewhat bulging. Hamsters are born with a full set of teeth. There are no deciduous teeth. Their incisors are open rooted and grow continuously throughout life. Molars are rooted. There are no canine or premolar teeth. Teeth crowns morphologically resemble human crowns. This feature allows retention of fine particles, making the hamster susceptible to dental caries comparable to human beings.

> **TECHNICIAN NOTE**   Hamsters are susceptible to dental caries.

Cheek Pouches

Hamsters have large **cheek pouches** that represent evaginations of the lateral buccal wall. Each is 35 to 40 mm long, extending back to the shoulder region, and 4 to 8 mm wide when empty. The cheek pouches are considered an immunologically privileged site because of an absence of an intact lymphatic drainage pathway. The absence of lymphoid tissue in this area prevents the immune system from normal responses. Hamsters often carry large amounts of food in their cheek pouches (Figure 10-2). This trait has earned the hamster its name, taken from the German word *hamstern*, which means "to hoard." Females will hide their offspring in the cheek pouches when they feel threatened.

> **TECHNICIAN NOTE**   The cheek pouches of hamsters are considered an immunologically privileged site.

THORAX AND ABDOMEN

The left lung of hamsters is composed of a single lobe. The right lung is divided into five small lobes.

Typical of most rodents, the hamster and gerbil stomach is compartmentalized. The forestomach is a nonglandular compartment that functions in pregastric fermentation of ingesta. The forestomach is separated from the glandular

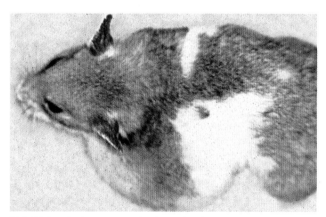

FIGURE 10-2. Hamster cheek pouch. This Syrian (golden) hamster has a peanut in the cheek pouch, which can extend halfway down the length of the body. (From Hnilica, KA: *Small animal dermatology: a color atlas and therapeutic guide*, ed 3, St. Louis, 2011, Elsevier.)

portion by a sphincterlike muscular structure that regulates movement of ingesta between the sections.

Costovertebral (flank) glands are present on the flank of hamsters. They are better developed in males than in females. These are bilateral sebaceous glands seen as coarse, dark pigmented hair areas. Secretions from the glands are used in territorial marking and play a role in mating behavior. The hamster possesses a large amount of brown adipose tissue. The primary function of this tissue is temperature regulation. Vascularity of brown fat tissue is four to six times greater than that of white adipose tissue; blood is warmed as it passes through this tissue.

Gerbils of both sexes have a ventral sebaceous gland that appears as a distinct orange-tan oval area of alopecia on the midventral region. The secretions are used for territorial marking. In males entering puberty, the gland enlarges and secretes a musky substance.

> **TECHNICIAN NOTE**   Gerbils have ventral sebaceous glands used for territory marking.

GENITOURINARY SYSTEM

The renal papilla extends well into the ureters in hamsters. This makes urine collection fairly simple in this species. Female hamsters have paired vaginal pouches. Female hamsters have six to seven pairs of mammary glands. Gerbils have four pairs of mammary glands. Gerbils produce only very small quantities of highly concentrated urine.

ANIMAL MODELS

Hamsters are popular as research subjects because of their rapid reproductive rate and ease of reproduction. They are relatively free of spontaneous diseases but are susceptible to many introduced pathogenic agents. The physiologic characteristics of the cheek pouch tissues make it an excellent site for evaluation of the carcinogenic potential of many agents. They are susceptible to diabetes mellitus, human leprosy, and brucellosis. Dental caries and gallstones can be induced in the species with dietary modifications. Studies of hypothermia take advantage of changes in hamster physiology when they are hibernating.

Radiobiology research is aided by the fact the Syrian and Chinese hamsters are highly resistant to the deleterious effects of radiation. In addition, their short life span and rapid reproductive rate make them an excellent model for studies of reproductive physiology.

Among the unique features that make the gerbil a good animal model are its very low water requirement and highly concentrated urine. Gerbils are therefore used in some endocrine function studies. The Mongolian gerbil is also prone to develop high serum and hepatic cholesterol levels, even when on low-fat diets. They are used extensively in the study of lipid metabolism. Strains have been developed with a condition that is similar to idiopathic epilepsy in humans. Gerbils also have anatomic variations that make them susceptible to stroke. Their unique resistance to radiation makes them useful models for radiobiologic studies.

REPRODUCTION

Determination of gender in hamsters is relatively simple and can be accomplished without handling the animals. Males have large fat pads along the inguinal canal that make the rear end of the animal appear rounded when viewed from above. The **flank gland** is also more prominent and darker in color in males. Females have a more pointed appearance to their rear end. Adult females are also larger than males and have a smaller anogenital distance than males.

Determination of gender in gerbils can be accomplished by evaluating anogenital distance, as with mice (Figure 10-3). Females are polyestrous and monogamous pairs can be left together for life. The male assists in caring for the young and so should be left in the cage with the female. Female gerbils are polyestrous, spontaneous ovulators. The gestation period is fairly short (approximately 25 days), but females bred during the postpartum period often have delayed implantation and gestation periods in excess of 3 weeks. The development of the young is similar to that seen in mice, but neonatal gerbils develop somewhat more slowly.

> **TECHNICIAN NOTE** Gerbils bred as monogamous pairs can be left together for life.

Puberty in both male and female hamsters occurs between 6 and 8 weeks. Female hamsters are continuously polyestrous, with an estrus cycle of about 4 days. Shortly after ovulation the female will produce a creamy white vaginal discharge. This usually occurs around the second day of the estrous cycle. The female is usually bred in the evening of the third day after the appearance of the vaginal discharge. The female is typically placed in the male's cage on that evening. If mating does not occur within 5 minutes or the female becomes aggressive, she is removed from the cage. If mating does occur, the female and male may be left together until the next morning. A vaginal plug is present for several hours after mating.

Hamsters have a 15- to 18-day gestation period, the shortest of all small rodents. The female is usually caged singly approximately 2 days before parturition and until the pups are weaned. Pups are born hairless, eyes and ears closed, weigh 2 to 3 g, and have teeth. Average litter size is 4 to 12 pups. It is important that the new litter is not disturbed for at least 1 week after birth. When a new litter is disturbed, the female may cannibalize the pups. The pups can eat solid food after 1 week and are usually weaned at approximately 21 days; the female will resume estrous cycling a few days after weaning.

GENETICS AND NOMENCLATURE

The various species of hamsters differ significantly in phenotype as well as genotype, with each species having a different diploid chromosome number. Some of the species can interbreed, and a variety of hybrids are possible.

Inbred Strains

The common stock of Syrian hamster is the golden Syrian, designated as the Lak:LVG(SYR). Approximately 36 inbred strains are available. The most common strains are the MHA/SsLak and PD4/Lak, white strains with pink eyes that are susceptible to dental caries; the LSH/SsLak and CB/SsLak, brown and white hamsters; and the LHC/Lak, a cream-colored variety.

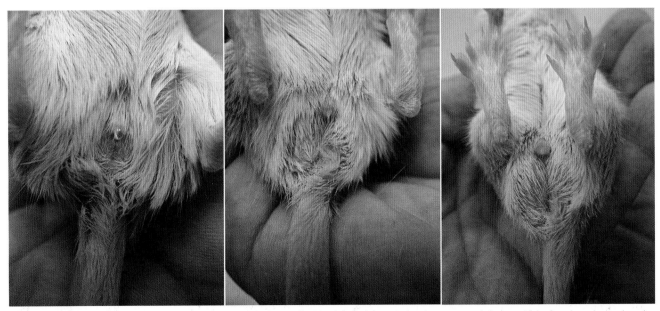

FIGURE 10-3. External genitalia of the male *(right, middle)* and female *(left)* gerbil. Note that the anogenital distance of the female is shorter than that of the male. The adult male can also be determined by the presence of testicles in the scrotum *(right)*, but the frightened gerbil may retract the testicles from the scrotum *(middle)*. (From Mitchell M, Thomas T: *Manual of exotic pet practice*, St. Louis, 2009, Saunders.)

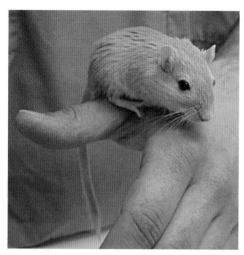

FIGURE 10-4. Most gerbils are relatively docile and easily handled for physical examination. (From Mitchell M, Thomas T: *Manual of exotic pet practice,* St. Louis, 2009, Saunders.)

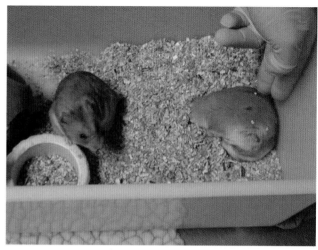

FIGURE 10-5. Hamsters are usually maintained in shoebox cages. (From Sheldon CC, Topel J, Sonsthagen T: *Animal restraint for veterinary professionals,* St. Louis, 2006, Mosby.)

BEHAVIOR

Like other rodents, hamsters are nocturnal animals. This should be considered when keeping pet hamsters because they are quite active in the evening. Hamsters are unique among rodents in that they are capable of hibernating under certain conditions. **Hibernation** can be stimulated by exposure to cold temperatures (less than 5° C), restriction of the food supply, or a shortening of their light cycles. Hamsters do wake up and feed during hibernation. Hibernation occurs in cycles of approximately 3 days. Physiologic changes during hibernation include reduced heart and respiratory rates and decreased body temperature. They remain sensitive to both tactile and thermal stimulation. Adult female hamsters are particularly aggressive to other adults, both male and female. Fights between hamsters can be vicious and often fatal.

Gerbils are highly social and inquisitive animals that are quite easy to handle (Figure 10-4). They rarely bite and do not tend to become aggressive toward cagemates unless overcrowded. They tend to do well when housed in pairs or groups. Ideally, pairs to be housed together should be introduced before puberty. Unlike most other rodents, gerbils are not nocturnal. When gerbils are fearful, startled, or excited, they often thump their hindlimbs on the cage floor. Gerbils are intensely curious and rarely run or hide. They dig and burrow in bedding material; in their native habitat they are known to construct elaborate tunnels.

HUSBANDRY, HOUSING, AND NUTRITION

Hamsters are solitary animals. Pet hamsters are usually housed individually in shoebox cages with bedding of corn cobs, soft paper, or hardwood shavings. Colony housing of hamsters can be successful when the young are reared together (Figure 10-5). Group-housed animals should have readily available hiding places within the enclosure. Hamsters are notorious escape artists, and their enclosure must be secure. They easily climb the sides of most cages.

> **TECHNICIAN NOTE**   Hamsters and gerbils are usually housed in solid-bottom shoebox cages.

Solid-bottom shoebox cages with ample soft bedding material are preferred for housing of gerbils. Gerbils do not tend to climb but are capable of jumping rather large heights. Cages should have secure-fitting lids to prevent escape. Gerbils tend to eliminate very small amounts of wastes, so cage cleaning is usually only performed weekly. Ambient temperature should be 65° to 70° F, with a relative humidity of 50% to 60%. Temperature extremes must be avoided because this may induce seizures in gerbils.

Hamsters and gerbils can be fed commercial rat chow. The gerbil diet may be supplemented with small amounts of sunflower seeds and clean, fresh vegetables. However, excessive supplementation must be avoided because gerbils tend to develop obesity.

Because of their broad muzzle, hamsters are unable to eat through wire hopper feeders. Hamster feed is usually placed directly on the floor of the cage. Hamsters are rather orderly and will carry their food in their cheek pouches to their preferred location. They tend to set aside an area of the cage for urination and defecation.

> **TECHNICIAN NOTE**   Hamster food should be placed directly on the cage floor.

RESTRAINT AND HANDLING

Before attempting to restrain a hamster, always make sure the animal is fully awake and aware of your presence. If startled or suddenly awoken, hamsters often bite. To move a hamster to a new cage, simply scoop it up in your hand. Alternatively, place a small can in the cage for the animal to enter, then carry the animal in the can. Hamsters can also be picked up by grasping the loose skin over the neck (Figure 10-6).

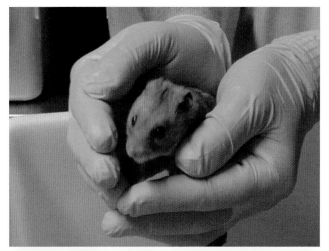

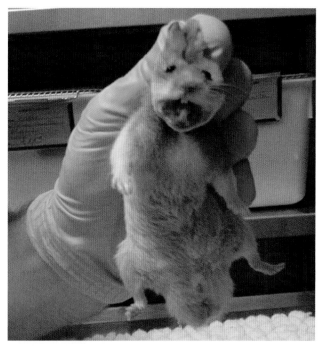

FIGURE 10-8. Hold the hamster in the palm of your hand. (From Sheldon CC, Topel J, Sonsthagen T: *Animal restraint for veterinary professionals*, St. Louis, 2006, Mosby.)

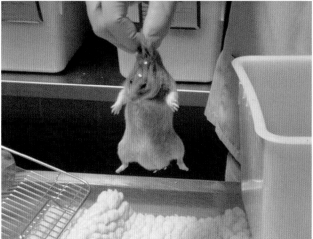

FIGURE 10-6. Transferring a hamster. (From Sheldon CC, Topel J, Sonsthagen T: *Animal restraint for veterinary professionals*, St. Louis, 2006, Mosby.)

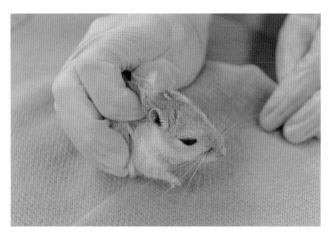

FIGURE 10-7. Grasp the loose skin over the shoulders.

If firmer restraint is needed for technical procedures, a whole-handed grip is needed. The loose skin of the neck must be fully gathered. Hamsters have a large amount of loose skin in this area and can easily turn and bite if the handler does not gather the skin fully (Figure 10-7). The animal is then placed

in the palm of the hand (Figure 10-8). Gerbils should not be picked up by the tail because the skin can slip off. The subsequently exposed tissue eventually becomes necrotic.

IDENTIFICATION

Cage cards can be used when animals are individually housed. For group-housed animals, ear notching, ear tags, tattooing, and implantation of microchips are used for permanent identification. Temporary identification can be accomplished with markers or dyes.

CLINICAL PROCEDURES

ADMINISTRATION OF MEDICATION

Because of their small size, administration of parenteral and oral medications can be quite challenging in hamsters. As with mice, some procedures require that the animal be anesthetized. Depending on which techniques are used, two people may be required to complete a procedure.

INJECTION TECHNIQUES

Hamsters and gerbils are usually given injections by the subcutaneous (SC) or intraperitoneal (IP) routes. Intramuscular (IM) injections are not usually practical because of the relatively small muscle mass present. The volume of fluid that can be injected at a specific site must also be considered. An accurate weight is critical to ensure correct dosages. Medications used in hamsters and gerbils must usually be diluted to deliver the correct dose accurately. Dilutions cannot be so great as to require excessive volumes for injection.

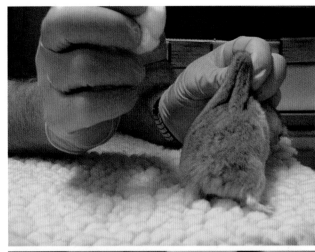

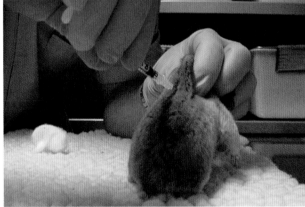

FIGURE 10-9. Subcutaneous injection in the hamster. (From Sheldon CC, Topel J, Sonsthagen T: *Animal restraint for veterinary professionals,* St. Louis, 2006, Mosby.)

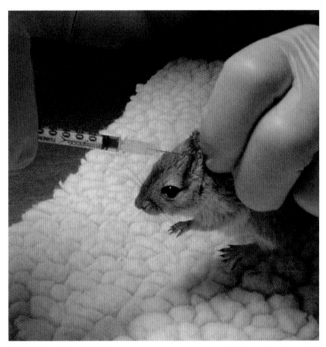

FIGURE 10-10. Subcutaneous injection in gerbil. (From Sheldon CC, Topel J, Sonsthagen T: *Animal restraint for veterinary professionals,* St. Louis, 2006, Mosby.)

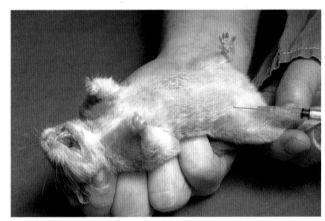

FIGURE 10-11. Intraperitoneal injection in the hamster. (From Thomas JA, Lerche P: *Anesthesia and analgesia for veterinary technicians,* ed 4, St. Louis, 2011, Mosby.)

SC injections are usually given under the loose skin over the shoulder area. A maximum volume of 3 to 4 ml can be administered at this site with a 21-gauge needle. To perform the injection in hamsters, hold the hamster's scruff with the animal facing away from you and form a tent of skin. Clean the injection site, insert the needle from the caudal aspect of the skin tent, and complete the injection (Figure 10-9).

For gerbils, grasp the loose skin over the shoulders to make a skin tent. Lift the animal slightly so that its front feet are suspended. Introduce the needle into the skin tent and complete the injection (Figure 10-10). Similar volumes and needle sizes are used for IP injections. IP injections should be administered with the animal restrained in the palm of the hand and the animal's nose tilted downward. The injection can be given in the lower abdomen in either the right or left quadrant.

Firm restraint is required for IP injections. Administer the injection in the lower right or left quadrant of the abdomen (Figure 10-11). Always aspirate before injection to verify that no internal organs have been entered.

> **TECHNICIAN NOTE** Hamsters and gerbils are usually given injections by the subcutaneous (SC) or intraperitoneal (IP) routes.

When IM injections must be given, the quadriceps or gluteal muscles are usually used. Injection volumes should be very small (less than 0.5 mL) and given with a 22-gauge or smaller needle. The animal should be monitored closely because self-mutilation of the limb is a common problem after IM injection in hamsters. Intravenous injections can be administered by the cephalic, lateral metatarsal, or jugular veins.

ORAL ADMINISTRATION

Medications can be administered orally by mixing the substance in the drinking water. Unpalatable medications may need the addition of a small amount of sugar or syrup so that the animals do not avoid drinking the water. Medications for oral administration may also be mixed in food if the animals are being fed a powdered or meal-type diet.

A ball-tip feeding needle can also be used to administer oral medications. An 18-gauge, 4-in needle is appropriate. The hamster must be firmly restrained in the palm of the hand. Care must be taken to extend the neck of the animal during the procedure and ensure that the animal does not move. The needle is lubricated, usually with the material to be administered, and then placed in the diastema of the mouth. The needle is passed along the roof of the mouth and into the esophagus. Once proper placement is verified, the material can be administered by a syringe attached to the end of the needle. It is important that the needle not be rotated once placed because the tip could rupture the esophagus. Flexible rubber catheters (8 Fr) may also be used to administer oral medications to hamsters. However, the animal is likely to bite the tube, so an oral speculum must first be placed.

ANESTHESIA

Routine anesthesia is rarely performed on pet hamsters or gerbils. Surgical procedures performed on hamsters or gerbils in biomedical research may include ovariectomy, thymectomy, and adrenalectomy. Anesthetic techniques for hamsters and gerbils include injectable and inhalant anesthesia. Short-term procedures typically use single-dose injectable anesthetics. Inhalant anesthetics are usually administered by face mask. Isoflurane is an acceptable anesthetic agent. A commonly used injectable anesthetic is a combination of ketamine and xylazine administered by IP injection. Hamsters and gerbils should not be fasted before anesthesia. Their small size and high metabolism predispose them to hypoglycemia and hypothermia if food is withheld.

BLOOD COLLECTION TECHNIQUES

Most blood collection techniques require that the hamster be anesthetized. For pet hamsters, blood may be collected from the jugular, saphenous, cephalic, or tail vein or cranial vena cava venipuncture. For the cephalic, saphenous, and tail veins, puncture the vessel with a small-gauge needle and collect the sample into a hematocrit tube. The volume of blood collected should not exceed 10% of the blood volume, or approximately 8.0 mL/kg of body weight. Small Microtainer tubes with a variety of anticoagulant additives are useful for these small blood volumes (Figure 10-12).

If very small volumes of blood are needed, a toenail clip can be used. Blood can also be collected from the retroorbital sinus or by cardiocentesis. Both techniques require that the animal be anesthetized. If using the retroorbital sinus technique, the capillary tube can be introduced at either the medial or lateral canthus of the eye. The tube should be directed medially when using the lateral canthus. The technique for retroorbital sinus blood collection by the medial canthus is similar to that described for mice. Cardiac blood sampling and retroorbital sinus collection are not usually performed on pet hamsters because of the high probability of cardiac tamponade. The anesthetized animal is placed in dorsal recumbency, and a small-gauge

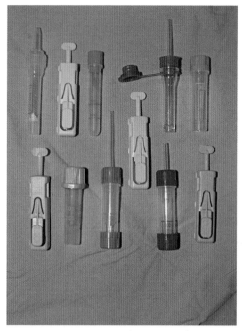

FIGURE 10-12. Microtainers with a variety of anticoagulant additives and lancets in a variety of styles are available for blood sampling of hamsters and gerbils. (From Mitchell M, Thomas T: *Manual of exotic pet practice*, St. Louis, 2009, Saunders.)

needle is introduced underneath and slightly left of the manubrium.

DIAGNOSTIC IMAGING

Anesthesia is required to facilitate proper positioning of hamsters and gerbils for radiographic studies. Whole-body radiographs are usually obtained and both lateral and ventrodorsal or dorsoventral images are taken. The animal can be taped to the x-ray cassette on the tabletop. If greater detail is needed, mammography film or a dental x-ray unit can be used. The cassette with the animal taped on top can be placed on a platform to decrease the distance to the x-ray beam and thus magnify the image on the film.

> *TECHNICIAN NOTE* Anesthesia is required to facilitate proper positioning of hamsters and gerbils for radiographic studies.

COMMON DISEASES

Although hamsters and gerbils are susceptible to many bacterial and viral diseases, spontaneous diseases are very rare. Some genetic varieties tend to be more susceptible to disease than others. The "teddy bear" hamsters tend to be more predisposed to disease and sensitive to antibodies and other drugs than golden hamsters. Because of their unique behavioral characteristics (e.g., nocturnal state, hibernation), early signs of illness are frequently overlooked in hamsters. One early sign of illness is irritability in a usually even-tempered animal. Sick hamsters are usually reluctant to move about, and their eyes often look dull and sunken. Hamsters and gerbils often become anorectic when ill, and subsequent weight loss can worsen the condition.

INFECTIOUS DISEASES
Bacterial Disease
Proliferative Ileitis. **Proliferative ileitis**, also called wet tail, regional enteritis, or transmissible ileal hyperplasia, is the most common infectious disease of hamsters. The causative agent is the intracellular bacteria *Lawsonia intracellularis.* A synergistic effect from several bacterial agents may also be involved. Clinical signs of disease are usually present only in weanling animals. Signs include watery diarrhea, dehydration, anorexia, and depression. The presence of moist, matted fur on the tail and ventral abdomen is also indicative of this disease. Gross lesions include the thickening and congestion of the ileum, enlarged mesenteric lymph nodes, and peritonitis. The intestinal epithelium becomes hyperplastic and ileal obstruction, intussusception, or impaction may occur, even after apparent recovery from infection. Affected animals often die within 48 hours. Animals that are under stress, particularly when husbandry practices are poor and animals are overcrowded, are most susceptible. The disease can reach epidemic proportions very quickly. If administered early in the course of the disease, antimicrobial therapy can help reduce the mortality rate in epidemic outbreaks. Care must be taken to monitor the animals for signs of **antibiotic-associated enterocolitis**. Sick hamsters should be isolated. Mechanisms to minimize stress factors are critical to control this disease.

Antibiotic-Associated Enterocolitis. Hamsters treated for bacterial infections are highly susceptible to enterocolitis. The mechanism for this disease is similar to that described for guinea pigs. Some antibiotics may have toxic effects even in very small, single doses. A large number of antibiotics have been implicated, including penicillin, erythromycin, gentamicin, ampicillin, and cephalosporins. Administration of antibiotics is thought to allow for overgrowth of *Clostridium difficile,* and subsequent release of toxins from this organism causes the clinical signs. Signs include anorexia, dehydration, rough hair coat, and copious diarrhea.

Tyzzer's Disease. **Tyzzer's disease** has been reported in nearly all species of rodents and is found throughout the world. The causative agent is the gram-negative, spore-forming, flagellated bacterium *Clostridium piliforme.* Definitive diagnosis often requires histologic examination of tissues from suspected infected animals. Poor sanitation and overcrowding predispose animals to this disease. Weanling and immunocompromised animals are most severely infected. Clinical signs include diarrhea, dehydration, and anorexia. Careful attention to proper sanitation and reduction of stress aids in prevention of this disease. The organism is difficult to eradicate from an animal facility because of the ongoing presence of resistant bacterial spores.

Other Bacterial Infections. A variety of bacteria are capable of causing pneumonia in hamsters. These include *Pasteurella pneumotropica* and *Streptococcus pneumoniae.* Clinical signs are nonspecific. Depression, anorexia, nasal and ocular discharges, respiratory distress, and chattering have all been reported in infected animals. The primary control mechanism is to eliminate environmental stress. Treatment with antibiotics can be helpful although care must be taken to avoid antibiotic-associated enterocolitis.

Several types of infectious agents can cause diarrhea in the hamster. Hamsters are carriers of *Campylobacter jejuni.* Although they are usually asymptomatic, they represent a potential source of human infection and may cause disease in hamsters under stress. *Salmonella* species have also been isolated from both hamsters and gerbils with signs of enteritis.

Viral Disease
Lymphocytic Choriomeningitis. Although primarily a disease of mice, the lymphocytic choriomeningitis virus can infect most rodents, including gerbils and hamsters. Clinical signs vary depending on the specific strain of the virus. Lymphocytic infiltration of a variety of organs can occur, and immune complexes associated with the virus can cause glomerulonephritis. The cerebral form, a result of lymphocytic infiltration of the meninges, is characterized by convulsions, photophobia, and weakness. Hamsters rarely have clinical signs of disease and can serve as reservoirs for infection in a research facility. The virus is transmissible to human beings and can cause flulike symptoms. Prevention of this viral disease requires exclusion of wild rodents from the population and assurances that animal feed is not contaminated from wild rodents or arthropod vectors. Because of the high zoonotic potential of this virus, treatment is usually not attempted and infected animals must be eliminated from the colony.

Other Viral Disease. Viral disease is not seen in gerbils. Hamsters can be infected with the **hamster parvovirus** and the hamster polyoma virus. The hamster parvovirus is associated with high mortality in weanlings. The disease is characterized by incisor abnormalities, testicular atrophy, and domed crania. The presence of epitheliomas on the face, neck, flanks, or abdomen is pathognomonic for hamster polyoma virus. In the research setting, treatment is not usually undertaken.

Mycotic Disease
Although infections with dermatophytes are possible, these are almost unheard of in hamsters. A pet hamster may rarely be infected with dermatophytes. Diagnosis and treatment are similar to that used in small animal veterinary practice. Dermatophytosis is a significant zoonotic concern.

Parasitic Disease
Hamsters and gerbils can be infected with a number of internal and external parasites. Parasite infections are rarely

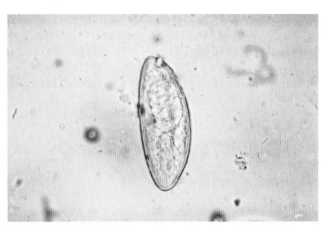

FIGURE 10-13. *Syphacia muris ova.* (From Mader DR: *Reptile medicine and surgery,* ed 2, St. Louis, 2006, Saunders.)

of concern in laboratory hamsters. Protozoal parasites that may be found in hamsters include *Trichomonas* and *Giardia*. However, these are of no clinical significance. Some parasites of hamsters, particularly cestode parasites, are of zoonotic concern.

Gastrointestinal Parasites. The cestode *Rodentolepis nana* may infect hamsters and gerbils and is of zoonotic concern. *Hymenolopsis diminuta* can also infect hamsters. Infections with either of these parasites can cause intestinal obstruction and enteritis. Several other parasites are capable of infecting hamsters and gerbils, including *Syphacia obvelata* (the mouse pinworm) and *Syphacia muris* (the rat pinworm) (Figure 10-13). Clinically significant infections are extremely rare. However, infected hamsters may serve as a reservoir for infection in other species.

Ectoparasites. Mite infestations with *Demodex criceti* or *Demodex aurati* have been reported in gerbils and hamsters, particularly those older than 18 months. Some researchers have suggested that infestation with *D. aurati* results in more severe clinical signs than seen with *D. criceti* infestation. Significant pathology can occur from other concurrent diseases. Clinical signs include alopecia over the rump, back, and neck. Diagnosis is by demonstration of the mites in a deep skin scraping. Infected hamsters usually respond well to treatment with topical acaricides. Hamsters may also become infested with the ear mite *Notoedres*. This mite can cause dermatitis of the ears, face, feet, and tail. Treatment with ivermectin is usually effective.

NONINFECTIOUS DISEASES
Neoplasia
Spontaneous tumors are rare in hamsters and gerbils. When they do occur, they are nearly always benign. The most common benign neoplasias are gastrointestinal polyps and adenomas of the adrenal cortex. Affected hamsters have signs similar to those seen with Cushing's disease. Malignant tumors that can occur include lymphosarcoma and gastrointestinal or adrenal carcinoma.

AGE-ASSOCIATED DISEASES
Amyloidosis
The most common cause of death in aged hamsters is **amyloidosis**. Evidence of this condition has been documented in as many as 85% of hamsters older than 18 months. The condition occurs as a result of amyloid deposits in the glomeruli of the kidney and is initially subclinical. As the animal ages, renal function becomes impaired and clinical signs consistent with azotemia are seen. Amyloid deposits can occur in other organs as well. Anorexia, rough hair coat, and depression are common signs. A genetic factor has been suggested. There is no effective treatment for this condition.

Polycystic Disease
The occurrence of cysts is high in hamsters older than 1 year. The most commonly affected site is the liver. Cysts may also be found in the pancreas and seminal vesicles. The lesions generally are of no clinical significance. Older gerbils may develop chronic interstitial nephritis, and cystic ovaries are often commonly seen in older females.

Cardiovascular Disease
Aged hamsters are prone to cardiomyopathy and atrial thrombosis. Cardiovascular disease occurs with relatively the same incidence in both sexes, but onset in females tends to occur at an earlier age.

HUSBANDRY-RELATED DISEASES
Trauma
Trauma from fighting is more common among females than males. Fighting can be vicious and bite wounds often become infected with *Staphylococcus aureus*. Pet hamsters and gerbils may also incur traumatic injury. This is a particular problem when owners (and their young children) are not accustomed to proper handling and drop the animal.

Barbering. As with other rodents, in the absence of pruritus, evidence of alopecia is most likely from barbering. This condition results from chewing of hair by cagemates. Alopecia is often restricted to the whiskers and the hair around the muzzle and eyes. Removal of the animal that has no evidence of hair chewing usually resolves the problem.

Nasal Dermatitis. **Nasal dermatitis** is also referred to by the common names red nose, sore nose, or stress-induced chromodacryorrhea, and is a common condition of juvenile gerbils. The disease is characterized by nasal dermatitis and alopecia around the upper lip and external nares. The disease has been associated with *Staphylococcus* infection but is related to stress factors such as loss of a cagemate, incompatible mating, and overcrowded conditions. The condition may be self-limiting or topical treatments may be needed. Mechanisms to reduce stress must also be addressed.

Nutritional Diseases. Hamsters are very sensitive to vitamin E deficiency. A deficiency of this vitamin can lead to skeletal muscular dystrophy. This may be a significant problem in pet hamsters that are fed seed-based diets. Balanced diets formulated specifically for hamsters are commercially available; however, hamsters also thrive on commercial rat and mouse diets.

EUTHANASIA

Hamsters and gerbils that are maintained in biomedical research facilities may be euthanized at the end of a research study to collect tissue samples for further analysis. Pet animals that are suffering are often humanely euthanized rather than allowed to live their final days in pain. Acceptable methods of euthanasia are listed in *American Veterinary Medical Association Guidelines for the Euthanasia of Animals.* Suitable methods of euthanasia for hamsters include overdose of inhalant anesthesia, IP overdose injection of barbiturates, and carbon dioxide chamber asphyxiation. The dose of pentobarbital to induce death is usually two to three times that required for anesthesia. Carbon dioxide is administered by gradual displacement. The carbon dioxide can be supplied as a humidified compressed gas or as a dry ice pack. The animals must not be permitted to come into contact with the dry ice container. Avoid placing large groups of animals in the chamber simultaneously because this stresses the animals and reduces the effectiveness of the inhalation agent. Animals should be left in the carbon dioxide chamber for at least 5 minutes after obvious respiratory motions have ceased.

KEY POINTS

- The most common species of hamster used in biomedical research is the Syrian or golden hamster, *Mesocricetus auratus.*
- The scientific name of the laboratory gerbil species most often seen in biomedical research is *Meriones unguiculatus.*
- Because of their very low water requirements and highly concentrated urine, gerbils are routinely used in endocrine function studies.
- The Mongolian gerbil is prone to development of high serum and hepatic cholesterol levels and is used extensively in the study of lipid metabolism.
- Hamsters have the shortest gestation of all the laboratory species, are virtually free from spontaneous disease, and are the only commonly used laboratory animal that hibernates.
- The anatomy of the hamster closely resembles that of human beings; hamsters are prone to dental caries.
- Prominent cheek pouches in hamsters represent an immunologically privileged site and are used as a site for studies of human carcinogens.
- Determination of sex in hamsters is accomplished by viewing the secondary sex characteristics.
- Hamsters and gerbils are usually housed individually in shoebox cages.

- Medications are usually given subcutaneously or intraperitoneally, and blood is collected from the retroorbital sinus or by cardiocentesis in the anesthetized hamster.
- The most common infectious disease of hamsters, commonly referred to as wet tail, is regional enteritis, also known as transmissible ileal hyperplasia.
- The most common cause of death in aged hamsters is amyloidosis.
- Determination of sex in gerbils is accomplished by observing anogenital distance.
- Breeding pairs of gerbils are usually housed together for life.
- Gerbils should never be picked up by the tail because the layer of skin over the tail may slough off.
- Nasal dermatitis, also referred to by the common names red nose, sore nose, or stress-induced chromodacryorrhea, is a common condition of juvenile gerbils.

REVIEW QUESTIONS

1. The scientific name for the Syrian or golden hamster is _____ _____.

2. The _____ _____ of the hamster are considered an immunologically privileged site because of an absence of an intact lymphatic drainage pathway.

3. Changes in hamster physiology when they are hibernating make them a good animal model for studies of _____.

4. Hamsters have been used to study _____ _____ because their teeth are comparable to human teeth.

5. The _____ are dark-pigmented glands in the hamster that secrete substances used to mark territory.

6. A common renal disease of geriatric hamsters is _____.

7. The most common infectious disease of hamsters is _____ _____, also called wet tail, regional enteritis, or transmissible ileal hyperplasia.

8. Radiobiology research is aided by the fact the Syrian and Chinese hamsters are highly resistant to the deleterious effects of _____.

9. The scientific name of the species of gerbil most often seen in biomedical research is _____ _____.

10. Gerbils are native to _____ environments.

11. Gerbils are prone to develop high serum and hepatic _____ levels, even when on low-fat diets.

12. Gerbils are very _____ and _____ animals that are easy to handle.

13. Gerbils should not be picked up by the _____ to avoid sloughing.

14. Due to the gerbil's high _____ rate, it should not be fasted prior to anesthesia.

15. A common condition of juvenile gerbils characterized by nasal dermatitis is also referred to by the common names _____ _____, _____ _____, or _____ _____.

11 Other Species

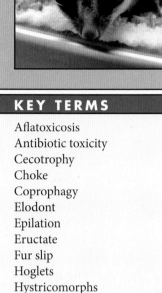

OUTLINE

KEY TERMS

Aflatoxicosis
Antibiotic toxicity
Cecotrophy
Choke
Coprophagy
Elodont
Epilation
Eructate
Fur slip
Hoglets
Hystricomorphs
Lumpy jaw
Marsupial
Metabolic bone disease
Ocular proptosis
Patagium
Pododermatitis
Ptyalism
Quills
Self-anointing behavior
Slobbers
Trichobezoars

LEARNING OBJECTIVES

After reviewing this chapter, the reader will be able to:

- Identify unique anatomic and physiologic characteristics of unique exotic pets and nontraditional laboratory animals.
- List and describe uses of unique exotic pets and nontraditional animals as models for animal diseases.
- Describe breeding systems used for unique exotic pets and nontraditional laboratory animals.
- Identify unique aspects of behavior of unique exotic pets and nontraditional laboratory animals.
- Explain routine procedures for husbandry, housing, and nutrition of unique exotic pets and nontraditional laboratory animals.
- Describe restraint and handling procedures used on unique exotic pets and nontraditional laboratory animals.
- Describe methods of administration of medication, collection of blood samples, and common diseases of unique exotic pets and nontraditional laboratory animals.

Because scientists are working toward reducing the numbers of higher species used in biomedical research and focusing on refining research techniques so that the most appropriate animal model species are used, a number of other animals are now being used in biomedical research. Many of these species are also kept as pets and may be seen in the veterinary clinic. Although specific data on the numbers of these species used in research is not available, numerous research institutions use nontraditional, specifically invertebrate, animals in basic research. Although a detailed discussion of all these species is beyond the scope of this chapter, an overview of the types of research in which these animals are involved and common concerns in their care follows. Greater detail is given for species that are commonly kept as pets.

HEDGEHOGS

Hedgehogs have become popular pets in spite of being illegal to own in some localities. Individuals who breed, transport, sell, exhibit, or use hedgehogs for research or teaching purposes must be licensed by the U.S. Department of Agriculture (USDA). Importation of hedgehogs from Africa into the United States is illegal. Hedgehogs are not routine subjects for biomedical research due in part to the difficulty in handling them and the lack of readily accessible veins.

There are 12 species of hedgehogs in the family Erinaceidae within the order Insectivora. The most commonly encountered species is the central African hedgehog *(Atelerix albiventris)* (Figure 11-1). The central African hedgehog—also known as the white-bellied, four-toed, or African pygmy hedgehog—is native to the savannah and steppe regions of central and eastern Africa. Because importation of this species is now banned, the pet hedgehogs in the United States are captive-bred.

> **TECHNICIAN NOTE** The scientific name of the hedgehog species commonly kept as pets is *Atelerix albiventris*.

Hedgehogs are nocturnal and will hide in burrows during daylight hours. At night they search out their preferred food of insects, earthworms, slugs, and snails. Males and females are territorial and have a preference to live individually. They are active diggers and swim and jog around their natural habitat.

UNIQUE ANATOMY AND PHYSIOLOGY

Physiologic data for hedgehogs is located in Table 11-1. The most unique anatomic feature is the spines or **quills**. The dorsal surface of the animal is covered in a dense coat of several thousand smooth spines. There is a thin epidermis and a thick dermal layer. The spines are composed of keratin and are periodically replaced. When the hedgehog feels threatened, it will raise the spines and pull into a rolling position.

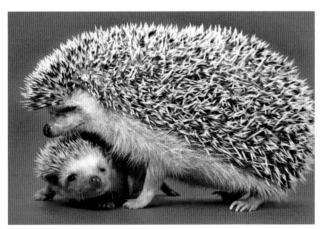

FIGURE   11-1. Captive African hedgehog with young. (From Quesenberry K, Carpenter J: *Ferrets, rabbits, and rodents*, ed 3, St. Louis, 2012, WB Saunders.)

Hedgehogs have **brachydont** (closed-rooted) teeth. Their first incisor in each quadrant is large and projects forward. The molar teeth are flattened and suited for crushing food items. The stomach is simple, there is no cecum, and the colon is smooth.

Gender is determined by visual observation. The male prepuce opens on the midabdomen while the female urogenital opening is just cranial to the anus. African hedgehogs are polyestrous and breed throughout the year. The estrus cycle for *A. albiventris* lasts 3 to 17 days, and ovulation is believed to be induced. The gestation period is 34 to 37 days, and pups are born hairless, with closed eyes and ears. The spines are visible shortly after birth. Hedgehogs are usually bred at 6 months of age. The pregnant female must be provided with a large cage and an additional hiding place and be given strict privacy just prior to and for at least a week after delivery. The environmental temperature should be maintained at around 90° F. Young are called **hoglets** and are usually weaned at around 6 weeks.

BEHAVIOR

Hedgehogs emit multiple vocalizations. Box 11-1 summarizes vocalization of African hedgehogs.

TABLE 11-1	Biologic and Physiologic Data for African Pygmy Hedgehogs
Average body weight	Captive: male 400-600 g, female 300-400 g
Life span	Average 4-6 years, may live to 8 years
Body temperature	95.7° F-98.6° F (35.4° C-37.0° C)
Adult dental formula	2 (I3/2:C1/1:P3/2:M3/3) = 36 (variations have been noted)
Gastrointestinal transit time	12-16 hours
Heart rate	180-280 beats per minute
Respiratory rate	25-50 breaths per minute
Age at sexual maturity	2-3 months
Reproductive life span	Female, 2-3 years; male, throughout life
Gestation	34-37 days
Milk composition	Protein, 16 g/100 g; carbohydrate, trace; fat, 25.5 g/100 g
Litter size	3-4 (range, 1-9)
Birth weight	10-18 g
Eyes open	14-18 days
Deciduous teeth eruption	Begins on day 18: all deciduous teeth erupted by 9 weeks
Permanent teeth eruption	Begins at 7-9 weeks
Age at weaning	5-6 weeks (start eating solids at 3 weeks)

(From Quesenberry KE, Carpenter JW: *Ferrets, rabbits, and rodents*, ed 3, St. Louis, 2012, WB Saunders.)

BOX 11-1 | African Pygmy Hedgehog (Atalerix albiventris) Vocalizations

SOUND	DESCRIPTION
Snorting/huffing Hissing/grunting	Aggressive or warning sounds produced by sharp vibrating exhalations through the nostrils. Generally made when the animal is disturbed, when it encounters another animal, or when it is in the process of rolling up.
Screaming	A severe distress call given when the animal is in distress or pain.
Twittering/whistling	High-pitched sound of neonates. Whistling stimulates contact by the dam.
Clucking	High-pitched contact call of the dam to neonates, also made by courting males.
Snuffling	Made as hedgehogs search for food.
Inaudible sounds	Hedgehogs can make and hear sounds in the 40- to 90-kHz range, above the range of human hearing.

(From Mitchell M, Tully T: *Manual of exotic pet practice*, St. Louis, 2008, WB Saunders.)

Both males and females demonstrate a unique behavior called **self-anointing,** whereby the animal takes an item such as fish, wool, and various plants into its mouth, mixes it with saliva, and applies the mixture to its spines with its tongue. Hedgehogs that are handled regularly from a young age are usually quite tame and rarely bite.

HUSBANDRY, HOUSING, AND NUTRITION

Hedgehogs are usually maintained in individual cages. Because they are very active, the primary enclosure should be at least 2 × 3 feet with a secure lid. The cage should be taller than the animal when it is stretched out. Hedgehogs are able to climb and escape through small holes. Enrichment devices are needed, especially a hiding spot or nest box. A cardboard box or a piece of large-diameter polyvinyl chloride pipe is suitable. The bedding material must be soft and absorbent and about 3 inches deep to allow for normal digging behavior. Avoid cedar bedding and similar aromatic shavings as they can cause dermatitis. Unless the animal is frequently let out of the cage into a larger area, an exercise wheel or ball is also needed. The exercise wheel must be made of solid material and not wire grid. Preferred environmental temperature is between 75° F and 80° F with a relative humidity of less than 40%. When hedgehogs are hospitalized, it is recommended that the environmental temperature be between 80° F and 84° F and the animal be maintained in a quiet area with low

lighting. Oxygen cages or incubators are often used for hospitalized hedgehogs.

> **TECHNICIAN NOTE** Environmental enrichment for hedgehogs should include a nest box and several inches of bedding material.

Identification

Hedgehogs are solitary animals in the wild and are usually housed individually. An individual animal can be identified with a cage card. A microchip can also be implanted in the subcutaneous dorsal fat pad between the shoulders (between the spines). Nontoxic marker or fabric paint applied to the dorsal spines can be used for temporary identification.

Nutrition

Wild African hedgehogs primarily feed on insects but also consume a variety of other items, such as frogs, eggs, fruit, and fungi. Commercially available hedgehog food is suitable but is usually supplemented with small amounts of mixed vegetables, fruit, and insects because it is not known whether the hedgehog food is nutritionally complete. Food must be rationed to prevent obesity, which is common in captive hedgehogs.

RESTRAINT AND HANDLING

A double layer of latex gloves or light cotton gloves should be worn when handling hedgehogs. The spines can be painful and allergenic. Even very tame hedgehogs will roll up or become difficult to handle. Examine the animal in a quiet room with low light. Grasp the scruff before the hedgehog rolls into a ball. If the animal is already rolled up, it may be coaxed to unroll by holding it facedown over a table (Figure 11-2). In many cases, chemical restraint will be required to perform a complete physical examination or for other procedures.

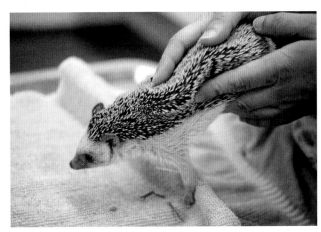

FIGURE 11-2. Holding a rolled-up hedgehog face-downward over a table may induce extension of the legs as the animal seeks to reach the surface to avoid falling. (From Quesenberry K, Carpenter J: *Ferrets, rabbits, and rodents*, ed 3, St. Louis, 2012, WB Saunders.)

CLINICAL PROCEDURES

Administration of Medication

The ideal site for subcutaneous injection is the haired skin of the ventrum or legs. Injections can also be given in the spiny areas, but the skin is less vascular so medications are absorbed slowly. Intramuscular injections can be given in the triceps, quadriceps, or gluteal muscles. The cephalic, femoral, or lateral saphenous veins can be used for intravenous injections using a small-gauge needle.

> *TECHNICIAN NOTE* Subcutaneous injections given in the less vascular, spiny areas of the hedgehog's skin are absorbed slowly.

Fluids can be administered subcutaneously or intravenously. Intravenous catheter placement is not advised because the animal is likely to dislodge the catheter when it balls up. A femoral or tibial intraosseous catheter can also be placed using a 22- or 25-gauge needle or 1-in spinal needle. A 5-Fr polyvinylchloride feeding tube may be placed in the dorsal cervical area for use if long-term fluid therapy is needed.

Oral medication may be administered by mixing it with a fruit-flavored liquid. If the animal does not accept the medication, it may be inserted into a mealworm or other dietary items that the animal prefers. Topical medications are not advisable due to the presence of the spines as well as the animal's fastidious grooming habits.

Blood Collection

Sedation is usually required for blood collection. The jugular vein or cranial vena cava can be used to collect samples. The jugular vein is not readily visualized but is in the same general location as in other mammals. The femoral, lateral saphenous, or cephalic veins may also be used to collect small-volume samples.

Diagnostic Imaging

Anesthesia is usually required for proper patient positioning. The presence of the spines reduces radiographic detail. A lateral and a ventrodorsal whole body view are usually obtained.

> *TECHNICIAN NOTE* Sedation or anesthesia is required for blood collection and diagnostic imaging procedures in hedgehogs.

Anesthesia

Anesthesia is required to complete a thorough physical examination, for diagnostic testing, and for treatment of wounds. Routine neutering surgery is not commonly performed because the animals are usually housed singly. Hedgehogs should be fasted for 4 to 6 hours and fluids administered.

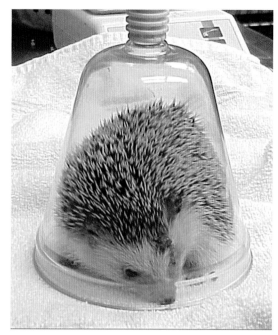

FIGURE 11-3. Anesthetic induction of the African pygmy hedgehog (*Atalerix albiventris*) is readily accomplished with a standard dog face mask. (From Mitchell M, Tully T: *Manual of exotic pet practice*, St. Louis 2008, WB Saunders.)

Monitoring for hypothermia and administering analgesic agents is vital. Anesthesia is usually induced by delivering isoflurane via face mask or induction chamber or by placing the entire animal in a large dog face mask (Figure 11-3). Injectable agents such as ketamine, alone or in combination with other medications, can also be used. For prolonged procedures, the animal may be intubated with a 1.0- to 1.5-mm endotracheal tube or feeding tube. When indicated, spines can be removed by clipping at the skin surface or applying steady traction near the base of the spine. Alcohol should not be used to prepare the surgical site due to the increased likelihood of hypothermia.

COMMON DISEASES

Pet hedgehogs are susceptible to a number of bacterial, mycotic, neoplastic, and husbandry-related diseases. The following section summarizes some of the more common presentations.

Infectious Disease

Bacterial. Respiratory infections with *Bordetella bronchiseptica*, *Pasteurella multocida*, and *Corynebacterium* spp. have been reported in pet hedgehogs. Clinical signs include rhinitis, pneumonia dyspnea, and lethargy. Sudden death can occur.

Dental disease with a bacterial component is also common and is characterized by the presence of calculus, gingivitis, and periodontitis. Dental cleaning and antibiotic administration should be performed. The addition of abrasive items to the diet may help prevent recurrence.

Salmonella spp. can cause enteritis in hedgehogs. Hedgehogs may be asymptomatic carriers of *Salmonella*. Owners must be advised of the zoonotic potential of the bacteria.

Viral. Few viruses have been reported in pet hedgehogs. They are susceptible to foot-and-mouth disease, herpes simplex virus type 1, and rabies. These viral diseases have mostly been reported in European hedgehogs and hedgehogs imported from Africa. With the ban on importation, the African hedgehogs kept as pets in the United States are not likely to be infected with viral disease.

Mycotic. African hedgehogs are susceptible to *Trichophyton mentagrophytes*, *Arthroderma benhamiae*, and *Microsporum* spp. Affected animals will show classic signs of dermatophytosis, including pruritic dermatitis of the face as well as quill loss. Treatment is usually with systemic antifungal agents. Owners must be advised of the zoonotic potential of this disease.

Parasitic. Hedgehogs are likely to harbor a number of ectoparasites. Most notable are the mites *Chorioptes* spp., *Caparinia*, and *Notoedres* spp. Infection may be subclinical or show evidence of pruritis. Clinical signs of infestation with *Caparinia* include hyperkeratosis, seborrhea, quill loss, and white or brownish crusts at the base of the quills and around the eyes (Figure 11-4). Crusting lesions around the head and ears are characteristic of *Notoedres* infestation. The ear mite *Otodectes cynotis* may also infest pet hedgehogs. Although a variety of endoparasites have been demonstrated in wild hedgehogs, infection in pet hedgehogs is extremely rare.

> **TECHNICIAN NOTE** Hedgehogs are susceptible to infestation with a number of species of mites.

Noninfectious Disease
Nutritional. Hedgehogs in captivity have a tendency to become obese. An obese hedgehog may be unable to roll

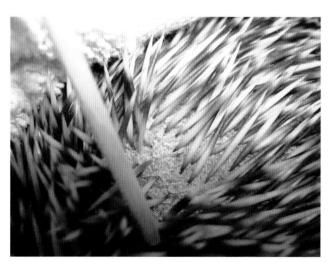

FIGURE 11-4. Hyperkeratosis of skin in a hedgehog secondary to *Caparinia tripolis* infestation. (From Miller W, Griffin C, Campbell K: *Muller and Kirk's small animal dermatology*, ed 7, St. Louis, 2013, WB Saunders.)

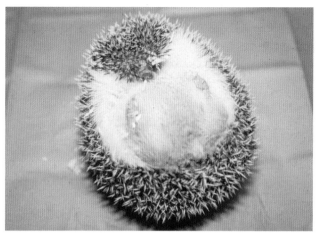

FIGURE 11-5. Obesity in a hedgehog. This hedgehog is so obese that it cannot roll up completely. (From Quesenberry K, Carpenter J: *Ferrets, rabbits, and rodents*, ed 3, St. Louis, 2012, WB Saunders.)

up (Figure 11-5). Weight reduction requires gradual calorie reduction. Rapid weight loss may lead to hepatic lipidosis. Hedgehogs raised primarily on an insect diet are also prone to calcium deficiency. A varied diet is recommended to avoid this and other potential vitamin deficiencies.

> **TECHNICIAN NOTE** Obesity is a common problem in captive hedgehogs.

Neoplasia. Neoplastic diseases are quite common in hedgehogs and can affect a variety of organs (Table 11-2). Semiannual examinations are recommended to evaluate for the presence of masses or other signs of neoplasia, including weight loss, anorexia, lethargy, diarrhea, dyspnea, ascites, and neurologic signs.

Miscellaneous Conditions. Pet hedgehogs have a high incidence of dilated cardiomyopathy. The disease can occur in hedgehogs as young as 1 year. Clinical signs include dyspnea, weight loss, lethargy, and ascites. High incidence of cystitis and urolithiasis is also seen in pet hedgehogs, possibly due to genetics or dietary factors. **Ocular proptosis**, corneal ulcers, and other ocular injuries can occur in hedgehogs. The shallow orbit of the hedgehog may be a predisposing factor for ocular disease. Lameness caused by ingrown toenails, arthritis, nutritional deficiencies, **pododermatitis**, or constriction of a foot or digit by fibrous foreign material also occurs in pet hedgehogs.

SUGAR GLIDERS

Sugar gliders (*Petaurus breviceps*) are small, nocturnal **marsupials** native to Australia, Tasmania, and Indonesia. There are several subspecies that differ slightly in appearance, specifically size and color patterns. They are highly social and are best housed in pairs or small groups. Like

TABLE 11-2 Neoplasms of the African Pygmy Hedgehog by Organ System

ORGAN SYSTEM	NEOPLASM	ORGAN AFFECTED	METASTASES
Integument	Mast cell tumor	Skin	Rare, usually locally invasive
	Mammary tumors	Mammary gland	Y
	Squamous cell carcinoma	Junction of quilled and unquilled skin	Rare, usually locally invasive
	Neurofibroma	Skin	Likely based on clinical signs
	Fibrous histiocytoma	Skin	N
Vascular/ hemolymphatic	Lymphosarcoma	Multicentric or gastrointestinal	Y
	Myeloproliferative disease/ myelogenous leukemia	Lymphatic and hemopoietic organs	Y
	Hemangioma	Eye	N
		Ventricle wall	N
Neuroendocrine	C-cell carcinoma	Thyroid	N
	Follicular adenoma	Pituitary	N
	Adenocarcinoma	Parathyroid	N
	Adenoma	Pancreas	N
	Adenoma	Adrenal	N
	Islet cell tumor	Upper GI tract	Locally invasive
	Cortical carcinoma	Nerve sheath	Y
	Pheochromocytoma		N
	Neuroendocrine		Y
	Schwannoma		N
Musculoskeletal	Osteosarcoma	Multicentric	Y
		Bone	N
		Subcutaneous	N
Gastrointestinal	Squamous cell carcinoma	Oral	Rare, usually
	Fibrosarcoma plasmacytoma	Oral	Locally invasive
	Acinic cell carcinoma	Intestinal	Locally invasive
	Hepatocellular carcinoma	Eye, retrobulbar	Locally invasive
	Adenocarcinoma	Liver	Locally invasive
		Stomach	Y
		Colon	Y
Reproductive	Granulosa cell tumor	Uterus	N
	Adenoma/adenosarcoma	Uterus	Locally invasive
	Leiomyosarcoma	Uterus	N
	Adenosarcoma	Uterus	N
	Adenoleiomyosarcoma	Uterus	N
	Spindle cell tumor	Vagina	N
	Neurofibrosarcoma	Testicular tunic	Unknown
Respiratory	Bronchoalveolar carcinoma	Lung	Y
	Squamous cell carcinoma	Lung	N

(Data from Greencar CB: Spontaneous tumors of small animals, *Vet Clin North Am Exot Anim Pract* 7:627-651; Heatley J, Maulden G, Cho D: Neoplasia in the captive African hedgehog (*Atalerix albiventris*), *Semin Av Exot Pet Med* 14(3):182-192, 2005; Mitchell M, Tully T: *Manual of exotic pet practice*, St. Louis, 2008, WB Saunders.)

all marsupials, the female sugar glider has a pouch in which the young are raised. Sugar gliders are not routine subjects for biomedical research, and there are a few U.S. states that prohibit ownership of sugar gliders by private individuals.

TECHNICIAN NOTE Sugar gliders are highly social and are best housed in pairs or small groups.

UNIQUE ANATOMIC AND PHYSIOLOGIC CHARACTERISTICS

Sugar gliders have a gliding membrane, the **patagium**, between the front and hindlimbs (Figure 11-6). This structure is responsible for the ability of the animal to glide through the air for distances up to 50 m. A variety of coat colors are available, including white face, leucistic (pure white with black eyes), albino, mosaic, piebald, platinum, and white-tipped tail. Eyes are large, widely spaced, and somewhat protruding. The second and third digits are fused to assist with gliding. The tail serves as

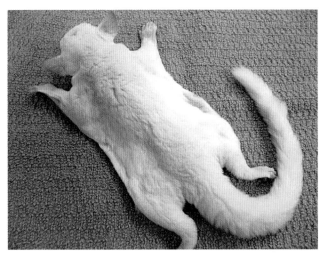

FIGURE 11-6. The patagium, or gliding membrane, of sugar gliders stretches between the front and hind legs. (From Quesenberry K, Carpenter J: *Ferrets, rabbits, and rodents*, ed 3, St. Louis, 2012, WB Saunders.)

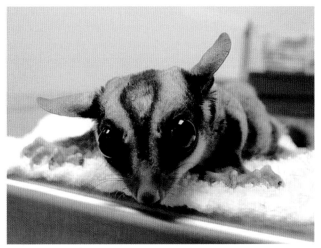

FIGURE 11-7. The male sugar glider has a frontal scent gland on its head. (From Quesenberry K, Carpenter J: *Ferrets, rabbits, and rodents*, ed 3, St. Louis, 2012, WB Saunders.)

a stabilization aid during gliding and is somewhat prehensile. In contrast to small mammals of similar size, the life span is quite long, with 10 to 12 years not unusual in captive sugar gliders.

> **TECHNICIAN NOTE** The gliding membrane, or patagium, is the structure that allows the sugar glider to glide through the air.

Females are seasonally polyestrous with a 29-day estrous cycle. Gestation is 15 to 17 days after which the young (joeys) migrate to the pouch. The young nurse in the pouch for 70 to 74 days then remain in the nest until weaning at around 120 days. Females become sexually mature at 12 months and males at 12 to 15 months.

BEHAVIOR

Sugar gliders are highly social, playful, and inquisitive. They require regular handling and exercise for at least several hours every day. Those not receiving sufficient socialization or lacking environmental enrichment are likely to become aggressive or depressed. They are highly vocal and respond best to handling in the evening hours due to their nocturnal nature. Sugar gliders handled during the day may exhibit aggression and irritability. Self-mutilation is common in solitary housed sugar gliders. Ideal housing for sugar gliders is to house one male with several females.

Both genders have scent glands, and secretions from the glands are used to mark territory. The scent glands are located in the pouch of the female and on the forehead and ventral aspect of the throat of the male (Figure 11-7).

HUSBANDRY, HOUSING, AND NUTRITION

Sugar gliders require a much larger cage than similarly sized small mammals. They are very active and require space to climb and jump. Wire caging is ideal, but the spacing must be small enough to prevent escape. Commercially available bird cages can be used, but those with only vertical bars are not

suitable because they do not allow for normal climbing activity. Ideal temperatures are between 75° F and 80° F. Food and water dishes should be placed in several locations in the cage, and a nest box must be provided. A pouch can be hung from an upper area of the cage to serve as a nest box. Other cage furniture—such as branches, shelves, solid exercise wheels, swings, and chew toys—should also be provided (Figure 11-8). Be sure that the branches are free of pesticides or other harmful chemicals. The cage should be located in an area that is not subject to significant daytime disturbances, when the animals are generally sleeping in the nest box. Additionally, because they are very active in the evening, the cage should probably not be placed near human sleeping areas.

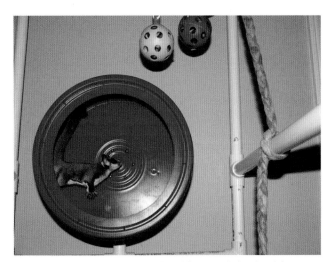

FIGURE 11-8. Sugar gliders should be provided with solid exercise wheels. (From Quesenberry K, Carpenter J: *Ferrets, rabbits, and rodents*, ed 3, St. Louis, 2012, WB Saunders.)

Nutrition

Sugar gliders are omnivores and consume a variety of plant-based material and insects. The ideal diet contains approximately 50% fruit sugars, such as fresh nectar, maple syrup, honey, and artificial nectar products. The remainder of the diet should consist of protein sources such as insects (mealworms and crickets) or commercially available feed (pelleted insectivore diets or monkey chow).

RESTRAINT AND HANDLING

Sugar gliders are best examined early in the day when they are less active. Thorough examinations require that the animal be sedated or anesthetized. Docile animals can be restrained in a small towel or placed in a pouch. The head should be grasped at the jawline from behind and the body cupped in one hand. The towel or pouch can then be folded back to expose one area at a time. The sugar glider can also be picked up by the base of the tail and lifted while allowing the animal to grasp a surface with its front feet to allow for palpation of the abdomen.

CLINICAL PROCEDURES

Administration of Medication

Injections can be administered intramuscularly in the epaxial muscles or the biceps femoris. Subcutaneous injections are usually administered over the shoulder region. Intravenous injections can be administered into the cephalic or lateral saphenous veins, but sedation or anesthesia is usually required.

Fluid therapy can be administered by oral, subcutaneous, or intraosseous routes. Administer subcutaneous fluids along the shoulder. Avoid the patagium area because fluids are poorly absorbed in this location and edema can cause discomfort. Intraosseous fluids can be administered in the proximal femur or tibia.

> **TECHNICIAN NOTE** Sugar gliders require sedation or anesthesia when intravenous injections are administered, blood samples are collected, or diagnostic imaging procedures are performed.

Blood Collection

Sedation or anesthesia is required to collect blood samples from sugar gliders. Only small volumes of no more than 1% of body weight can safely be taken. A 25- to 27-gauge needle and tuberculin syringe can be used. The jugular vein and cranial vena cava are preferred sites in adult sugar gliders. Smaller samples of 0.25 to 0.5 ml can be collected from the medial tibial artery or the cephalic, lateral saphenous, femoral, or ventral coccygeal veins.

Diagnostic Imaging

Proper positioning of sugar gliders for imaging studies requires general anesthesia. Young that are not attached to a teat should be removed from the pouch prior to imaging. The patagium must be reflected away from the body.

Anesthesia

Analgesics and sedatives followed by inhalant anesthesia decreases the risk of wide fluctuations in heart rate during surgical procedures. Isoflurane or sevoflurane delivered by face mask provides rapid anesthesia. The respiratory rate and body temperature should be constantly monitored. Transient apnea is also likely to occur during induction. Endotracheal intubation is difficult and not generally performed. An intraosseous catheter can be placed and fluid administered during surgery.

A brief period of fasting (approximately 4 hours) is recommended prior to surgery. Alcohol should not be used to perform the surgical preparation due to its cooling effects. Commonly performed surgical procedures include castration, ovariohysterectomy, removal of the paracloacal glands, and repairs to the patagium. Skin is often closed with tissue glue. Elizabethan collars are not effective in this species.

COMMON DISEASES

Infectious Disease

Clinically relevant viral diseases have not been documented in sugar gliders. Bacterial, fungal, and parasitic agents have been implicated in disease of sugar gliders.

> **TECHNICIAN NOTE** Clinical disease is not common in well-managed captive sugar gliders.

Bacterial. Infectious disease can infect the gastrointestinal system, pouch, respiratory tract, urinary tract, and reproductive organs. Culture and sensitivity is needed to identify the most appropriate antimicrobials.

Bacterial enteritis is common in captive sugar gliders, especially when husbandry practices are poor. *Escherichia coli* and *Clostridium* spp. have been implicated in infection. Sugar gliders may also become infected with *Pasteurella multocida*, usually transmitted from rabbits housed in the same area. Sudden death is a common result. It is presumed that sugar gliders are also prone to many of the same bacterial diseases as other marsupials, although this has not been well documented. Other potential infectious agents include *Yersinia pseudotuberculosis, Salmonella* spp., *Mycobacterium* spp., and *Cryptococcus neoformans*. Sugar gliders may also become infected with *Leptospira* spp. This disease has significant zoonotic potential, and careful attention to proper handling procedures is vital to prevent transmission to humans or other pets.

Actinomyces israelii causes a condition commonly referred to as "**lumpy jaw**." The bacterium infects the face and neck, and the condition is characterized by the presence of a slowly enlarging hard lump. Ocular discharge and weight loss also occur, and infection can spread to the lungs and intestinal tract. The disease is fatal if left untreated.

Parasitic. Parasitic infections are not common in well-managed sugar gliders. Infections with *Trichomonas, Giardia,* and *Toxoplasma* have been reported. Fleas and lice are extremely rare in captive sugar gliders. Neurologic disorders, including seizures and sudden death, have been associated with aberrant migration of the raccoon ascarid *(Baylisascaris procyonis)* in sugar gliders housed outdoors. Gastrointestinal infections with the nematodes *Parastrongyloides, Paraustrostrongylus,* and *Paraustroxyuris* spp. and liver infection with the trematode *Athesmia* spp. are also possible.

Noninfectious Disease

Nutritional. Wild sugar gliders feed on a variety of food sources that vary by season and include tree sap, nectar, and insects. Captive sugar gliders also require a varied diet. Fresh fruits and vegetables and a daily source of protein are needed. Protein can be provided using commercially available protein pellets, mealworms, crickets, or small amounts of cooked skinless chicken. A multivitamin supplement including balanced calcium/phosphorus with vitamin D_3 is also recommended. Fresh water must be available at all times.

Sugar gliders fed a high-protein or high-fat diet or not given sufficient exercise are prone to obesity. Other common diet-related conditions in captive sugar gliders include anemia and hypoproteinemia (due to lack of dietary protein), hypocalcemia (due to calcium/phosphorus imbalance and lack of vitamin D_3), and hypoglycemia. Clinical signs of general malnutrition include dehydration, weakness, and lethargy. **Metabolic bone disease**, also known as nutritional osteodystrophy or nutritional secondary hyperparathyroidism, occurs when vitamin D is insufficient or with low calcium or an improper calcium:phosphorus ratio. Affected animals present with pain and hind-limb paresis and are usually hypocalcemic and hypoproteinemic. Severe cases may present with pathologic fractures and seizures. Other conditions thought to be related to poor nutrition include foreign body intestinal impaction, rectal prolapse, cataracts, cystitis, crystalluria, and urolithiasis.

Neoplasia. Lymphoid neoplasia is relatively common in captive sugar gliders. Tumors have also been described in the oral cavity, spleen, liver, kidney, pouch, jaw, and lymph nodes. The ingestion of aflatoxins can also lead to cancer.

Miscellaneous Conditions

Aflatoxicosis. Aflatoxicosis can occur when sugar gliders consume toxins produced by certain fungi that are in or on food sources. Common sources of aflatoxins include contaminated peanuts and crickets that have been fed contaminated corn. Therefore, it is important not to feed peanuts o sugar gliders and to know what kind of feed the insect supplier feeds its insects.

Dental Disease. Periodontal disease can occur in captive sugar gliders fed soft diets. A diet that includes insects that have hard exoskeletons may help minimize this potential disease. Advanced tooth decay or fractures resulting in exposed pulp usually require extraction.

Ophthalmic Disorder. Trauma to the eyes may result due to the slightly bulging eyes of sugar gliders. Corneal scratches are common in animals that rub against cage toys

or from bite wounds when fighting occurs among cagemates. Ulceration, conjunctivitis, or retrobulbar abscess can result.

Stress-Related Disorders. Lack of proper socialization, poor nutrition, lack of environmental enrichment, exposure to predatory species, and failure to provide for the nocturnal nature of sugar gliders can lead to a number of stress-related conditions. Self-mutilation is common, especially of the penis, scrotum, tail, and limbs (Figure 11-9). Treatment includes wound care as well as management of the underlying cause.

> *TECHNICIAN NOTE* Self-mutilation is a common stress-related condition in sugar gliders.

In males with severe injuries of the penis, amputation may be necessary. Males urinate from the base of the penis rather than the tip, so amputation does not interfere with urination. Other manifestations of stress include **coprophagy**, hyperphagia, polydipsia, and pacing. Alopecia may also result due to the increased adrenal activity caused by stress.

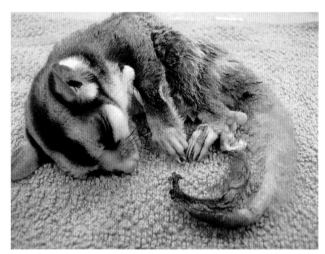

FIGURE 11-9. Self-mutilation of the tail is common in solitary, stressed sugar gliders. (From Quesenberry K, Carpenter J: *Ferrets, rabbits, and rodents,* ed 3, St. Louis, 2012, WB Saunders.)

CHINCHILLA

The scientific name for the chinchilla is *Chinchilla laniger.* Chinchillas are rodents that originated in the mountainous regions of Peru, Argentina, Bolivia, and Chile. At one time, they were hunted for their fur and nearing extinction in the wild. They live in large social groups in burrows. They are popular as pets and used in biomedical research in limited numbers. In the 1940s and 1950s, chinchillas were used to develop a vaccine for cholera. They have also been used by the U.S. National Aeronautics and Space Administration (NASA) for sleep research studies; much of the knowledge gained from those studies has been applied to assisting astronauts on their missions.

UNIQUE ANATOMIC AND PHYSIOLOGIC CHARACTERISTICS

Chinchillas are **hystricomorphs** and more closely related to guinea pigs than to rats and mice. The teeth are all open rooted (**elodont**) and grow continuously. Physiologic data for the chinchilla are located in Table 11-3. They have more hairs per square inch of skin than any other animal. As many as 60 hairs may be present in each hair follicle. The palmar and plantar surfaces of the feet are hairless, and there are four toes on the front and rear feet. Chinchillas have very large tympanic bullae. This makes them an excellent animal model for auditory research, specifically relating to noise-induced hearing loss and childhood middle ear infections. Unlike most rodents, the chinchilla has a fairly long life span, often in excess of 10 years. They have a rounded body, large ears, short forelegs, long hind limbs, and a long tail. The limbs are adapted for leaping, with the tail acting as an organ of balance. A variety of coat colors are available as a result of selective breeding.

> **TECHNICIAN NOTE** Chinchillas may have as many as 60 hairs per hair follicle.

Female chinchillas have two uterine horns and two cervices, one pair of inguinal mammary glands, and two lateral thoracic pairs of mammary glands. Males have testes contained within the inguinal canal or abdomen, rather than a scrotum. Males have accessory glands that produce secretions that form a vaginal plug in the female reproductive tract after mating.

Determination of gender can be accomplished by evaluating the anogenital distance. The distance is greater in males than females. The penis can also be everted from the urethral orifice to confirm gender.

The average age at puberty is approximately 8 months. Female chinchillas are seasonally polyestrous and estrus lasts

TABLE 11-3	Physiologic Values for Chinchillas
Usual life span as pet	10 years (up to 20 years reported)
Adult weight	Males, 400-500 g; females 400-600 g
Sexual maturity	8 months
Type of estrous cycle	Seasonally polyestrous (November to May)
Length of estrous cycle	30-50 days
Ovulation	Spontaneous
Gestation period	105-118 days (average, 111 days)
Litter size	1-6 (2 is usual)
Normal birth weight	30-50 g
Weaning age	6-8 weeks
Rectal temperature	98.6-100.4° F (37-38° C)
Heart rate	100-150 beats per minute

(Quesenberry K, Carpenter J: *Ferrets, rabbits, and rodents,* ed 3, St. Louis, 2012, WB Saunders.)

3 to 4 days. Breeding females are often housed in groups with a single male. The male is usually removed from the cage during parturition and until the young are weaned. If kept as monogamous pairs, the male can usually remain in the cage. Length of gestation is approximately 111 days and the young are precocious, born fully haired and able to walk within an hour. Litter size is usually two, and the young usually begin to eat solid food by about 1 week of age and are weaned at about 6 to 8 weeks.

BEHAVIOR

Chinchillas are highly intelligent but somewhat shy. They are also very agile and tend to be most active at dusk, early morning, and nighttime. If handled regularly when they are young, chinchillas become quite tame and rarely bite.

Like guinea pigs, chinchillas have distinct vocalizations, and at least 10 different sounds have been identified. These may be specific to certain behaviors, such as predator avoidance, sexual behavior, and offensive behavior. They may raise and lower the tone of their vocalizations.

HUSBANDRY, HOUSING, AND NUTRITION

Chinchillas can be housed in pairs or small groups. They are very active and require a large and interesting environment. The cage should allow sufficient space for climbing and jumping. Large, multilevel cages with ramps and platforms are ideal. Wire mesh cages are most appropriate provided that the openings in the mesh floor are no wider than ½ by ½ inches. A solid floor in at least a portion of the cage bottom is recommended. A small box with soft bedding such as plain pine shavings or shredded newspaper provides a hiding place. Polyvinyl chloride pipes of about 4 to 5 inches in diameter can also be used as hiding places. A 15-inch exercise wheel and parrot toys can be used for additional environmental enrichment.

Acceptable temperature range is 65° to 80° F; however, chinchillas do best in relatively cooler temperatures with humidity 50% or lower. Dampness and high temperatures predispose the animals to disease. Heat stroke is likely with temperatures above 86°F. Chinchillas usually develop matted fur when in humid environments. It is also important that the cage be located in an area away from other pets, especially predatory species.

> **TECHNICIAN NOTE** High humidity and high temperatures predispose chinchillas to disease.

Dust Baths

Chinchillas require daily access to a "dust bath," which is a normal component of the animal's grooming behavior. The animal rolls in a small box containing about a 1-in depth mixture of sand and earth to clean itself (Figure 11-10). Commercially available sanitized dust bath products can be used or a 9:1 mixture of silver sand and kaolin with aluminum magnesium silicate (Fuller's earth) provided. Dust bath access should be limited because the animals tend to

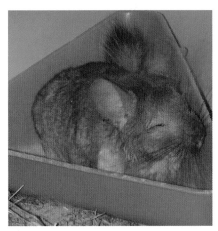

FIGURE 11-10. A chinchilla enjoying a dust bath. Dust baths are essential for chinchillas' skin maintenance and coat health. (Photo courtesy of Michelle G. Hawkins, VMD, DABVP [Avian].) (From Mitchell M, Tully T: *Manual of exotic pet practice*, St. Louis 2008, WB Saunders.)

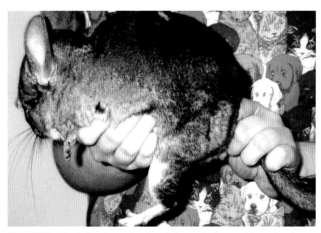

FIGURE 11-11. Grasp the chinchillas at the base of the tail with one hand and support the chest with the other when carrying or examining the animal. (From Quesenberry K, Carpenter J: *Ferrets, rabbits, and rodents*, ed 3, St. Louis, 2012, WB Saunders.)

overuse it; subsequent clouds of dust that remain in the cage can predispose the animals to conjunctivitis.

Nutrition

Commercial chinchilla feed is available and should be supplemented with fresh alfalfa or timothy hay. High-calcium diets may predispose the animals to urinary calculi. Chinchillas eat and defecate mainly at night. Like rabbits and guinea pigs, they pass both a dry, pelleted feces and a soft feces intended for **cecotrophy**. Fresh water must be available at all times and should be delivered with a water bottle instead of a bowl to decrease the chance of contamination.

RESTRAINT AND HANDLING

Chinchillas are very docile and rarely bite if accustomed to regular handling from a young age. Minimal manual restraint is ideal for routine examination. They can be removed from the cage by grasping and lifting the base of the tail and using the opposite hand to support the rest of the body. They may be restrained cupped in the hand or wrapped in a towel (Figure 11-11). Chinchillas are easily stressed by aggressive restraint. "**Fur slip**" can result from improper handling or anything that overexcites the chinchilla. The condition is characterized by loss of a small patch of fur (**epilation**) that exposes the smooth underlying skin. The fur can take several months to regrow and frequently regrows in a different shade. It is essential that the chinchilla be handled gently and calmly to avoid this. Should any procedure require more than minimal restraint, chemical restraint should be used. Isoflurane or sevoflurane delivered by mask is an appropriate agent for chemical restraint (Figure 11-12). Ketamine alone or in combination with diazepam can also be administered by IM injection for chemical restraint.

CLINICAL PROCEDURES
Administration of Medication

Medications and fluids can be administered by the oral, subcutaneous, or intraperitoneal routes. Care must be

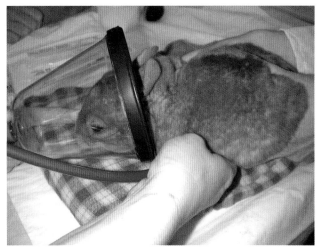

FIGURE 11-12. Inducing a chinchilla using a gas anesthetic agent. (From Mitchell M, Tully T: *Manual of exotic pet practice*, St. Louis 2008, WB Saunders.)

taken when grasping the skin to introduce the needle into the subcutaneous space to avoid causing fur slip. Butterfly catheters can be used to deliver fluids or other medications subcutaneously.

Intraperitoneal administration can also be used to administer medications and fluids. The animal should be placed in dorsal recumbency so that gravity displaces the organs away from the injection site. The injection site should be disinfected and the needle inserted at a 20- to 30-degree angle off the abdominal wall.

Intravenous catheters can be used for administration of fluids. It is recommended that the animal be anesthetized prior to catheter placement. A 24- to 26-gauge intravenous catheter is used, and a small incision made in the skin prior to placement to minimize the likelihood of the small-gauge catheter becoming kinked as it penetrates the skin.

In animals that are severely dehydrated, an intraosseous catheter is preferred. The proximal femur and tibia are the preferred sites for catheter placement. The patient should be anesthetized if possible. A small amount of lidocaine infiltrated into the insertion site can be used to minimize pain, especially when the animal is too debilitated to safely anesthetize. A spinal needle with a stylet is used, and careful attention to aseptic technique is vital.

Medications and fluids can also be administered per os unless the animal has gastrointestinal system dysfunction. A syringe can be used or the medication mixed with food or a fruit-flavored electrolyte solution.

Blood Collection

Venipuncture in the chinchilla generally involves fairly aggressive restraint and requires that the animal be anesthetized. The preferred blood vessels are the jugular vein, cranial vena cava, or femoral veins. Very small quantities of blood can be collected from the cephalic or lateral saphenous veins. A 25- or 27-gauge needle with a 1- or 3-ml syringe or an insulin syringe can be used to collect blood samples from chinchillas.

Diagnostic Imaging

Sedation or anesthesia is needed to properly restrain chinchillas for imaging studies. A minimum of two whole body views are usually obtained. Preferred views are lateral and ventrodorsal or dorsoventral.

> **TECHNICIAN NOTE** Chinchillas require sedation or anesthesia when intravenous injections are administered, blood samples are collected, or diagnostic imaging procedures are performed.

Anesthesia

Anesthesia may be needed when performing a comprehensive physical examination or for surgical and therapeutic procedures. Common surgical procedures performed on chinchillas include ovariohysterectomy, castration, fracture repair, and foreign body removal. The procedures are similar to those performed in other small mammals except that the body tissues of the chinchillas are somewhat more fragile and require gentle handling. The long, narrow oral cavity of the chinchilla makes endotracheal intubation difficult. Using a laryngoscope may help visualize the glottis, but care must be taken to avoid damage to the soft tissues or mandible. A rigid endoscope may be helpful in placing an endotracheal tube. A small amount of lidocaine should be applied to the glottis to decrease the likelihood of laryngospasm.

Chinchillas should be fasted only about 2 hours prior to anesthesia. A face mask or induction chamber can be used to deliver isoflurane or sevoflurane to induce and maintain anesthesia. Regular monitoring of the heart rate, respiratory rate, and body temperature is needed for anesthetized chinchillas. A Doppler unit can be used to monitor the heart rate (Figure 11-13). Supplemental heat should also be provided (e.g., circulating water blanket, forced air blankets).

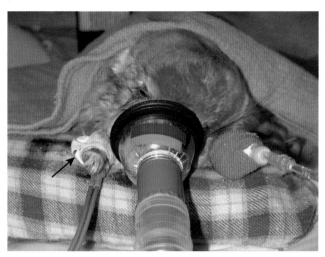

FIGURE 11-13. An anesthetized chinchilla. Oxygen and anesthetic gas are being provided via a face mask. An intravenous catheter is being used to deliver fluids via the cephalic vein. The heart rate is being monitored via a Doppler unit. (From Mitchell M, Tully T: *Manual of exotic pet practice*, St. Louis 2008, WB Saunders.)

COMMON DISEASES

Chinchillas are prone to many of the same diseases as other rodents. Sick chinchillas often show signs of weight loss and labored breathing and a general unkempt appearance to the hair coat. Sick chinchillas should be handled as little as possible.

Infectious Disease

Infectious diseases are rare in pet chinchillas or those used in biomedical research. Like guinea pigs, chinchillas are particularly susceptible to **antibiotic toxicity**. Prevention of infectious disease is a primary consideration in this species. Chinchillas are particularly sensitive to antibiotics that target gram-positive organisms. Administration of these compounds causes imbalance in normal intestinal flora and subsequent overgrowth of gram-negative organisms. Although most antibiotic toxicity occurs with oral administration, the condition has been identified when certain antibiotics are administered by injection or applied topically. The antibiotics most often implicated in this problem are the penicillins, erythromycin, and lincomycin. When antibiotics are required, a culture and sensitivity test is used to identify the most appropriate agent. The therapeutic minimal dosage should always be used and the animal carefully monitored for signs of bacteremia. Antibiotics that seem to cause fewer problems include chloramphenicol, ciprofloxacin, metronidazole, and the sulfonamides. Oral medications may be administered with a small syringe or eye dropper or mixed in the food or water.

Although there have been reports of ranch-raised chinchillas with disease thought to have a viral cause, no species-specific viral diseases have been identified in chinchillas. Chinchillas are susceptible to human herpesvirus 1, but infections are extremely rare.

Chinchillas are particularly susceptible to antibiotic toxicity.

Bacterial. Many of the bacterial infections seen in pet chinchillas are opportunistic pathogens that cause disease in animals that are stressed or immunocompromised. *Pseudomonas aeruginosa* and *Escherichia coli* are the most commonly implicated agents and cause a variety of clinical signs depending on the affected organ. *Yersinia pseudotuberculosis* and *Y. enterocolitica* are also fairly common and cause enteritis in chinchillas. Clostridial enterotoxemia, salmonellosis, and *Klebsiella* infections have also been reported in pet chinchillas. Other infectious diseases have been reported primarily in fur-ranched chinchillas, such as infections with *Listeria monocytogenes.*

Mycotic. Chinchillas can be infected with the dermatophytes *Trichophyton mentagrophytes, Microsporum canis,* and *M. gypseum.* Infection is characterized by small, scaly patches of alopecia. These occur most commonly on the face, behind the ears, or on the forelimbs (Figure 11-14). Infection with *Histoplasma capsulatum* has also been reported in chinchillas. *H. capsulatum* may be a contaminant present in timothy hay used for food.

Parasitic. Most normal chinchillas harbor the protozoal parasite *Giardia.* When the animals are stressed or when husbandry conditions are poor, the number of *Giardia* organisms may increase and result in gastroenteritis. Gastroenteritis is also associated with *Cryptosporidium, Eimeria chinchilla,* and *Sarcocystis.*

Neurologic disorders have been associated with aberrant migration of the raccoon ascarid *Baylisascaris procyonis* in chinchillas housed outdoors. Neurologic signs may also result from infection with *Toxoplasma gondii,* although this is not common.

Noninfectious Disease

Most noninfectious diseases of chinchillas are due to poor husbandry practices. Their dense hair coat makes chinchillas particularly sensitive to warm, humid climate conditions, and heatstroke is not uncommon. A variety of nutritional disorders and traumatic injuries are also seen in captive chinchillas.

Nutritional. Chinchillas with anorexia may develop hepatic lipidosis. Affected animals may also be dehydrated and prone to develop hyperglycemia with resulting ketonuria.

Dental Disorders. Dental problems, especially malocclusion, also occur and are similar to those seen in rabbits. The teeth grow continuously and must be clipped or the animal provided with appropriate materials to gnaw. Malocclusion, commonly referred to as "**slobbers**," is characterized by excessive salivation (**ptyalism**) and alopecia of the chin and skin (Figure 11-15). If left untreated, the animal eventually develops anorexia and weight loss. Periodontitis and abscess of the cheek teeth also occur. Malnutrition results and signs of hypoglycemia leading to seizures, coma, and death can follow.

The teeth of chinchillas grow continuously and may need to be clipped to avoid malocclusion.

Gastrointestinal Disorders. Noninfectious gastrointestinal disorders usually result from husbandry practices that are not appropriate for the species. **Choke** is the common name for the condition that results from the presence of a foreign body in the oropharynx or esophagus. Common foreign bodies that may occlude the esophagus are small

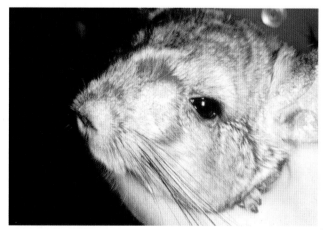

FIGURE 11-14. Fungal Dermatitis. Chinchilla with dermatophytosis on the face. (From Hnilica KA: *Small animal dermatology,* ed 3, St. Louis, 2011, WB Saunders.)

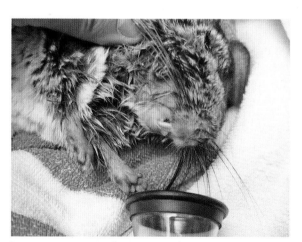

FIGURE 11-15. Dental Disease. Wet fur around the mouth and chin (slobbers) in a chinchilla is caused by increased salivation secondary to dental disease. (From Mayer J, Donnelly T: *Clinical veterinary advisor: Birds and exotic pets,* St. Louis, 2012, WB Saunders.)

treats, such as raisins, or items that the animal swallows without thoroughly chewing (often due to malocclusion). Like other rodents, chinchillas are unable to vomit. The trapped material results in irritation, which causes the animal to retch and cough. Small pieces of the material can become dislodged and aspirated into the respiratory system, leading to pneumonia. Obstruction of the esophagus that results in the inability of the animal to release gas from the stomach (**eructate**) can result in gastric tympany (bloat). Once the obstruction is removed, the bloat usually resolves.

Constipation and diarrhea are also common presentations in pet chinchillas. Sudden changes in the diet, lack of adequate fiber in the diet, stress, **trichobezoars**, and obesity are common causes of constipation. Diarrhea can also result from sudden dietary changes or stress.

Trauma. Bite wounds to the pinna and tibial fractures are common traumatic injuries in chinchillas. Group-housed chinchillas are prone to bite wounds from females during breeding season. The wounds often become abscessed and may require surgical removal of that portion of the pinna. Tibial fractures can occur when the cage bars are improperly spaced and the chinchilla catches its hind limb in the bars. Repair of such fractures is difficult, and amputation is sometimes needed.

Miscellaneous Conditions. Even in aged chinchillas, neoplasia is extremely rare. Cataracts may develop with age. Cardiac diseases such as heart murmurs, dilated cardiomyopathy, congenital septal defects, and valvular disease have been reported in chinchillas and are generally diagnosed in young chinchillas.

Some chinchillas will barber their own fur or that of cage mates. Affected animals have areas of alopecia, usually along the shoulders, flanks, sides, and paws. A variety of factors have been implicated as causes of barbering, including boredom, stress, and malnutrition. Barbering must be differentiated from fur slip, mentioned previously (Figure 11-16).

Fur rings can be present around the penis and under the prepuce that prevent the penis from going back into the prepuce. Affected males may groom excessively, urinate frequently or strain to urinate, and repeatedly clean their penis. Sedation or anesthesia may be needed to remove the fur ring.

Exposure to high environmental temperatures, particularly when humidity is also high and ventilation is inadequate, may result in heat stroke. Affected animals are usually ataxic with tachypnea and infected mucous membranes.

> **TECHNICIAN NOTE** Heat stroke is likely when chinchillas are exposed to high environmental temperatures.

WOODCHUCK

The scientific name for the woodchuck is *Marmota monax.* Laboratory woodchucks can be housed in rabbit-type cages and fed commercial rodent chow. Woodchucks have been

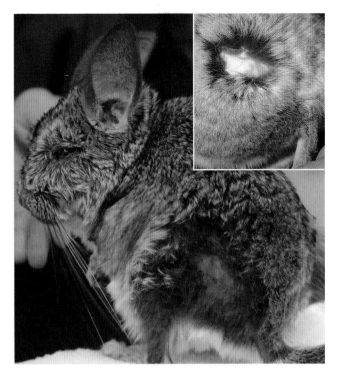

FIGURE 11-16. A chinchilla with fur biting, a behavioral problem, on its flank. The inset shows fur slip, a protective reaction that results in the release of a large patch of fur revealing smooth, clean skin underneath. (From Quesenberry K, Carpenter J: *Ferrets, rabbits, and rodents,* ed 3, St. Louis, 2012, WB Saunders.)

used as a model for hibernation and obesity. This species is also prone to develop spontaneous malignant hepatoma and hepatocellular adenocarcinoma. The latter is usually caused by chronic hepatitis from the woodchuck hepatitis virus, which is closely related to the hepatitis B virus. Woodchuck hepatitis virus occurs naturally in a majority of woodchucks in the mid-Atlantic states. Therefore, the woodchuck is a valuable animal model for human hepatocellular adenocarcinoma. Specific research is aimed at developing improved therapies to treat chronic hepatitis and subsequent liver cancer in human beings.

ARMADILLO

The scientific name for the armadillo is *Dasypus novemcinctus.* Armadillo means "little armored thing" in Spanish. The primary use for armadillos in biomedical research is in the study of human leprosy. Their normally low body temperature (27° to 36° C) enables *Mycobacterium leprae* to grow in the living organism. Armadillos are also susceptible to trypanosomiasis and schistosomiasis. They give birth to monozygous quadruplets, making them useful for genetic studies. Armadillos are usually kept in solid-bottom cages with thick bedding, which prevents them from developing sore feet. They are capable of burrowing or digging out of earthen-bottom cages.

> **TECHNICIAN NOTE** Armadillos are animal models for the study of human leprosy.

FARM ANIMALS

The United States Department of Agriculture (USDA) regulates the use of farm animals that are not used for agricultural production. The specific requirements for care and housing of these animals are addressed in the Guide for the Care and Use of Agricultural Animals in Research and Teaching (see Chapter 1). Farm animals used in biomedical research can be housed in a manner similar to that used for agricultural production or in specially designed laboratory facilities. The agricultural species most commonly seen in biomedical research are swine, sheep, and goats. Cattle and horses are used less often in biomedical research but have made significant contributions to scientific knowledge.

Farm animals used in biomedical research may be laboratory reared or farm raised. If reared in a stressful environment, immune response, health, and growth may suffer. The animal may often respond with unusual behavior. Farm animals for use in biomedical research can be obtained with conventional microbial status or be specific pathogen free (SPF). In sheep the most common SPF animal produced is one free of Q fever. Q fever is a rickettsial disease caused by *Coxiella burnetii* that does not often manifest with clinical signs in sheep. However, the disease is zoonotic and has occasionally been fatal in human beings. Human beings can develop clinical signs, including fever, chills, profuse sweating, malaise, anorexia, myalgia, severe headaches with retrobulbar pain, and nausea and vomiting. The fever lasts 9 to 14 days and is recurrent. Chronic infections can cause endocarditis, pneumonitis, pericarditis, and hepatitis. Cattle, sheep, goats, and ticks are natural reservoirs for the organism. Infected animals can shed massive numbers of organisms at parturition, and caretakers are advised to don gloves when working with parturient animals.

There are a number of respiratory, enteric, and central nervous system diseases that are excluded from SPF swine. Regardless of their source, the combination of shipping stress, high body temperatures after activity, and change in diet make them susceptible to respiratory and gastrointestinal diseases that are caused by normal flora bacteria. Livestock are usually fed commercial feeds, but care must be taken to avoid feeds designed for production of meat or milk because they tend to contain excessive amounts of protein. Environmental enrichment strategies for farm animals include group housing, addition of toys, and regular interaction with caretakers. Toys can include empty plastic jugs or food treats.

SWINE

Swine, specifically *Sus scrofa*, are friendly and docile animals but will react poorly to improper handling or stressful environmental conditions. They are extremely social and do well in group housing and when provided with regular human interaction. Swine breeds used in research include farm breeds and minipigs. Farm swine breeds are large species that achieve adult weights in excess of 500 pounds. Minipigs tend to reach adult weights of 200 to 250 pounds.

Swine share many physiologic and anatomic features with human beings, particularly characteristics of the cardiovascular and integumentary systems. Pigs have been used to evaluate mechanisms to prevent restenosis, the renarrowing of an artery after balloon angioplasty. Cardiac stents—small, expandable mesh tubes used to prop open clogged arteries—have been implanted in swine. Pigs have been used as models for studies of stress and its relation to hypertension and atherosclerosis.

The pig is also one of the best models for studying the healing process of skin wounds because the repair process is similar to that found in human beings. In the areas of immunology and transplantation research, swine have proven valuable because there is no placental transfer of antibodies to the developing pig fetus, so newborn piglets lack maternal antibodies. The skin of the pig is similar to that of a human being in texture, permeability, and thickness. This has made them a valuable animal model for dermal research. Many treatments and medications for skin disease and burns were developed with pigs as part of the overall research. Pigs were also used during development and testing of dermal patches to prevent motion sickness. Swine were also used in the initial development of the computed tomography scan. Swine have been used extensively in nutrition studies. Because they can have gastric ulcers, they are widely used in ulcer research.

> **TECHNICIAN NOTE** The skin of pigs has a texture, permeability, thickness, and repair process similar to that of human skin.

Handling and Restraint

Swine may be restrained with a board to help direct them or hold them in a corner. Hog snares should not be used for capture but can be used to hold the animal in place (Figure 11-17). Avoid overstressing swine because they may develop malignant hyperthermia. Sheep are also susceptible to overheating because they startle easily and have a wool coat.

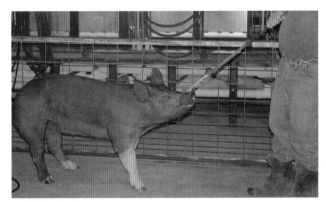

FIGURE 11-17. A hog snare applied to a pig. (From Sirois M: *Principles and practice of veterinary technology*, ed 3, St. Louis, 2011, Mosby.)

CATTLE, SHEEP, AND GOATS

The scientific name for the domestic sheep is *Ovis aries. Capra hircus* is the domestic goat. These animals are ruminants that originated in the Middle East. *Bos taurus* is the European domestic cow; *Bos indicus* is the domestic cow of India, including the Brahma and some miniature cow breeds. Sheep, goats, and cows are social animals and respond well to regular, consistent handling. Sheep and goats have similarities with human beings in cardiovascular and pulmonary anatomy and are used as models in these areas, particularly in the development of surgical procedures. They are also used as models for orthopedic research on diseases and injuries of the bones, joints, and muscles. In fact, sheep have been used to study numerous musculoskeletal conditions, and knowledge about fracture repair, osteoporosis, and osteoarthritis have resulted from research with sheep. Sheep have been used as test subjects for heart valve replacement surgery. Sheep and goats are both used for the production of antiserum, and sheep erythrocytes are harvested for use in some immunologic tests. The earliest work on blood transfusion medicine involved sheep. Pregnant ewes have been used as models for human pregnancy, in part because they give birth to lambs with birth weights similar to those of human babies. This research has led to improved knowledge regarding the hormonal changes that occur in mother and fetus shortly before birth and has improved treatment methods of respiratory distress in premature infants. This work has also contributed to an understanding of the congenital condition patent ductus arteriosus. Sheep were also vital to the research that led to a vaccine for anthrax.

Handling and Restraint

To move animals between enclosures or to capture a single animal for treatment, the animal should be directed to an appropriate location rather than led or pulled. Cattle, sheep, and goats must be acclimated to being moved on a lead. Sheep can be lifted and set up on their rumps if minor procedures must be performed. For more prolonged restraint, a sling may be useful.

Contagious ecthyma is a highly infectious viral disease in sheep and goats. Also referred to by the names contagious pustular dermatitis, contagious pustular stomatitis, orf, and soremouth, the disease is characterized by the development of pustular, scabby lesions on the muzzle and lips (Figure 11-18). The disease occurs primarily in lambs, and lesions around the mouth can prevent nursing or grazing and result in a 15% to 20% mortality rate. In cattle the virus can produce lesions on the teats. The virus is spread to human beings by direct contact with mucous membranes of infected animals or material contaminated by infected animals, including shears, feeding areas, trucks, or clothing.

HORSES

One of the major uses for horses in biomedical research is in harvesting of tissues that can be used in toxicology studies. Horse serum and enzymes from various organs are commonly used for this purpose. Early research into prevention of tetanus and diphtheria in human beings was largely accomplished by using equine animal models. The horse was the first animal in which blood pressure was measured. Research projects aimed at producing a vaccine against West Nile virus use horses. Cloning of horses and donkeys has been performed specifically to provide suitable cells to study prostate cancer

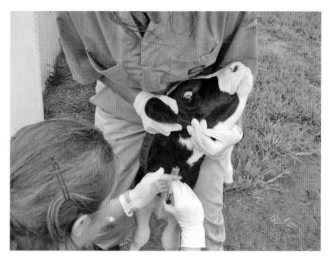

FIGURE 11-18. Ulcerative and proliferative lesions in and around the mouth of this doe are due to contagious ecthyma, or orf. (From Bassert J, Thomas J: *McCurnin's clinical textbook for veterinary technicians*, ed 8, St. Louis, 2014, WB Saunders.)

in human beings. Prostate cancer is essentially nonexistent in stallions, and research into the mechanisms that impart freedom from this disease are being used to develop medications to halt the spread of prostate cancer in human beings.

OPOSSUM

The opossum is the only marsupial that is native to North America. Its scientific name is *Didelphis virginiana*. The opossum is a biomedical model in comparative and developmental biology and medicine. The greatest potential as a research model lies in its semiembryonic state at birth, which presents the only opportunity among North American mammals for direct observation of embryonic development. This semiembryonic state at birth also permits, in the absence of a placental barrier and under minimal maternal metabolic influence, the chemical or physical manipulation of developing embryonic and fetal tissue (Figure 11-19). Laboratory housing of

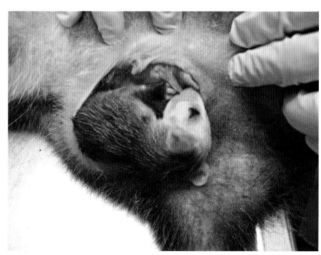

FIGURE 11-19. Young Virginia opossum in marsupium sucking on teat. (From Quesenberry K, Carpenter J: *Ferrets, rabbits, and rodents*, ed 3, St. Louis, 2012, WB Saunders.)

opossums is complicated by the aggressive tendencies and unusual odor of this species. They are prone to a variety of diseases, including tularemia, leptospirosis, and bacterial endocarditis. Infestation with fleas, lice, ticks, and mites as well as a variety of intestinal parasites also occurs. Contrary to popular opinion, they are not especially prone to developing rabies.

BATS

Bats are the only true flying mammals. They are seldom used as experimental animals because they are not well suited to normal methods of animal management. It is difficult and complicated to simulate natural living conditions. However, bats have been used for studies of echolocation and thermoregulation. The thin membrane of the wing is ideal for studies of blood circulation and wound healing.

INVERTEBRATES

A great deal of scientific knowledge has been gained from the study of invertebrates. As with other nontraditional animal models, the use of invertebrates in research has been steadily increasing. In addition to being used as animal models, products from invertebrates are used for medical purposes. Tissue from crabs and sand dollars contains substances that have anticoagulant and antithrombotic activity. Insects are being evaluated as a potential source of pharmaceuticals in much the same way that plants have been for millennia.

Examples of the use of invertebrates in biomedical research include many studies involving the fruit fly. Fruit flies have provided the basis for much of our knowledge of genetics. Studies of the giant squid axon have improved our understanding of ion channel regulation in cells. Marine sea snails have been used in studies of learning and memory and the roles of brain cells and nerve impulses through those cells. The marine sponge has become a useful tool for research of the human immune system and immune-mediated diseases such as rheumatoid arthritis, gout, and lupus erythematosus. Researchers are studying the inflammatory process in the marine sponge and in corals, jellyfish, and sea anemones. Neuropharmacology and neurochemistry have been studied in crabs and mollusks. Research involving retroviruses, such as the human immunodeficiency virus, has been performed with fruit flies. Some fruit flies have been found to have a similar virus. Fruit flies have also been shown to produce a protein similar to the one that triggers expression of the gene that causes Parkinson's disease in human beings. Moths are being used for studies of the olfactory system. Grasshoppers are used in neurology research, and leeches are used in pharmacology research. The list of animal models in the insect world is extensive.

DOGS AND CATS

Although the number of dogs and cats used in biomedical research is extremely small, they have and will likely continue to play a vital role in some research. Because of its ready availability and ease of handling, the dog was one of the first models

when biomedical research was in its infancy in the seventeenth century. The many similarities in anatomy and physiology of dogs, cats, and human beings have made these animals excellent models for some diseases. In particular, the anatomy and biochemistry of the cat brain is very similar to humans. Research with cats as models has provided valuable information in the field of neurophysiology, reflexes and synapse response, and perception of light and sound. Leukemia is a disease shared by human beings and cats, and research with these animals has led to a greater understanding of that disease and its treatment. Cats also develop a viral infection similar to acquired immunodeficiency syndrome infection in human beings. Research on toxoplasmosis, mammary cancer, anesthetics, and techniques for brain surgery has also benefited from the use of cats.

The cardiovascular system of dogs is closely related to that of human beings, and dogs have been used as models for a variety of cardiovascular diseases. Surgical procedures have been developed to prevent stroke and myocardial infarction by opening narrowed arteries in the neck and bypassing diseased or narrowed coronary arteries. The heart-lung machine was developed through research with dogs. Research on dogs also played an essential role in the creation and testing of many artificial devices used to substitute for heart valves and arteries. Artificial hips and joints were initially designed and tested in dogs. Pacemakers and catheters were also developed and evaluated in dogs. Because dogs have a high incidence of kidney disease, they make excellent animal models for this research. The first successful kidney transplant was performed in dogs in the late 1950s. The most common treatment for human cataracts, the intraocular lens, was developed in dogs.

Research with dogs and cats has also had direct benefits for the health of the animals. Improvements in nutrition, diagnostic and surgical procedures, and studies of behavior have led to increased life spans and a better quality of life for pet dogs and cats. Behavioral research with dogs is also being applied to the training of guard dogs and guide dogs.

HOUSING AND HUSBANDRY

Ample references are available that discuss detailed anatomic and physiologic aspects of dog and cat medicine. This section focuses specifically on issues related to keeping dogs and cats in biomedical research facilities.

Dogs and cats used in research are designated as random source, conditioned, or purpose bred depending on how they are acquired. Regardless of their designation, all dogs and cats used for research in the United States must be acquired by a USDA-licensed dealer. The original Animal Welfare Act of 1966 was written specifically to protect stolen pets from becoming research animals. Dealers must provide information to the USDA on the source and eventual disposition of all animals in their care. Random-source animals are those whose health status and medical history are unknown. In some states, animal dealers are permitted to obtain animals that are about to be euthanized in animal shelters. Random-source animals may therefore represent former pets that have either been lost or given up by their owners. In spite of the lower initial costs for purchase of random-source animals, these animals make the least desirable research subjects because they tend to harbor diseases and parasites and must be quarantined for at least several weeks before they can be used.

> **TECHNICIAN NOTE** Dogs and cats used in research are designated as random source, conditioned, or purpose bred depending on how they are acquired.

Animals that are already conditioned for use in research can be purchased from USDA-licensed dealers. These animals may be random-source animals that have been conditioned by the dealer before their sale. The conditioning process is focused on identifying and treating any infectious diseases. The animals are usually immunized and may be spayed or neutered. In addition, some dealers have programs that are designed to acclimatize the animals to the use of the types of caging and food and water devices used in biomedical research. Socialization of the animals may also be performed to ensure the animals will not present a threat to handlers. Purpose-bred animals are the most common type found in biomedical research. These tend to be more expensive, but the animals are accustomed to caging and handling and are known to be free of infectious disease and parasites.

Dogs and cats housed in biomedical research facilities are group housed whenever possible. Group housing of dogs and cats is usually limited to no more than 12 animals in a single enclosure. The Animal Welfare Act contains detailed requirements for space for both individual and group-housed animals. If housed singly, dogs must be provided with exercise, either in a run or by being walked on a leash. Although most dog runs are indoors, outdoor runs are permissible but require special procedures to ensure the animals are safe and conditions are sanitary. Whether housed singly or in groups, cats must be provided with resting shelves above the floor of the cage (Figure 11-20), and there must be a sufficient number of resting shelves, litter boxes, and food and water bowls so that competition doesn't lead to fighting among the animals.

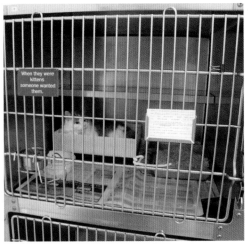

FIGURE 11-20. Cats in cages should be provided with resting boards or boxes elevated above the cage floor. (From August, JR: *Consultations in feline internal medicine*, vol 6, ed 6, St. Louis, 2010, WB Saunders.)

KEY POINTS

- Hedgehogs, chinchillas, and sugar gliders are becoming more popular as exotic pets.
- Exotic animal species that are occasionally used in biomedical research include the chinchilla (*Chinchilla laniger*), the woodchuck (*Marmota monax*), and armadillo (*Dasypus novemcinctus*). Dogs, cats, and a variety of farm animals are used in small numbers in research.
- The large tympanic bullae of the chinchilla make it an excellent animal model for auditory research.
- Woodchucks are used as animal models for malignant hepatoma and hepatocellular adenocarcinoma.
- The armadillo is used in genetic research and for the study of human leprosy.
- Swine have been used in research of the cardiovascular and integumentary systems.
- Sheep and goats are used as models in cardiovascular and pulmonary system research and are often used in the development of surgical procedures related to cardiovascular and orthopedic disease.
- The opossum is a biomedical model in comparative and developmental biology and medicine.
- Bats have been used for studies of echolocation and thermoregulation.

REVIEW QUESTIONS

1. The scientific name for the chinchilla used in biomedical research is _____ _____.

2. The normally low body temperature of the _____ makes it useful as an animal model for leprosy.

3. Improper handling or anything that overexcites the chinchilla can result in a condition that is characterized by epilation, which is referred to as _____ _____.

4. The _____ is used to study embryonic development.

5. Studies of echolocation may use _____ as animal models.

6. The _____ is the gliding membrane that allows the sugar glider to glide through the air.

7. The ideal site for subcutaneous injection in hedgehogs is the haired skin of the _____ or _____.

8. _____ are useful animal models for auditory research.

9. *Marmota monax* is the scientific name for the _____.

10. The common name for the zoonotic disease of sheep that is caused by *Coxiella burnetii* is _____.

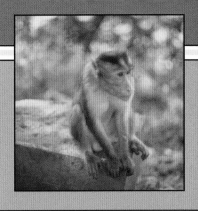

12 Nonhuman Primates

LEARNING OBJECTIVES

After studying this chapter, you will be able to:

- Identify unique anatomic and physiologic characteristics of nonhuman primates.
- Describe breeding systems used for nonhuman primates.
- Identify unique aspects of behavior of nonhuman primates.
- Explain routine procedures for husbandry, housing, and nutrition of nonhuman primates.
- Describe various restraint and handling procedures used on nonhuman primates.
- Describe methods of administering medication and collecting blood samples.
- List and describe common diseases of nonhuman primates.
- Describe appropriate methods of euthanasia that may be used on nonhuman primates.

TAXONOMY

Exact taxonomic classification of the more than 250 species of **primates** is complicated by the fact that many individual variations exist and scientists are not fully in agreement regarding whether some named species truly represent distinct species or simply individual variants. In spite of this, nearly all **simians** share the same general characteristics (Box 12-1).

There are a variety of taxonomic classification schemes for primates. One system groups all primates into two suborders, the Strepsirrhini and the Haplorrhini. Lemurs are members of the Strepsirrhini, and monkeys and apes are classified as Haplorrhini. An alternate system groups nonhuman primates (NHPs) in two orders, the Prosimii and the Anthropoidea. The **prosimians** are the most primitive of the primates. They are all small to medium sized and have a squirrel-like appearance. Examples are lemurs and tree shrews. The anthropoideans, also referred to as simians, include five taxonomic families. The lesser apes, great apes, and human beings represent three of the families. The remaining two are generally referred to as the **New World primates** (NWPs) and **Old World primates** (OWPs). Platyrrhini are NWPs that originate in South and Central America and include the tamarins and marmosets. The catarrhini are OWPs that originate in Asia and Africa and include monkeys. The OWP species

- Arboreal adaptation
- Excellent manual dexterity
- Well-developed sense of sight
- Good hand-eye coordination
- Dependence on learned behavior
- Long infant dependency periods
- Complex social organizations
- Prehensile appendages with opposable thumbs
- Tactile pads and nails on fingers and toes
- Binocular color vision
- Single offspring

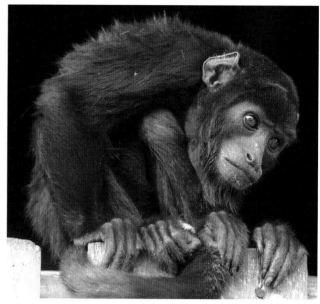

FIGURE 12-3. Pet howler monkey (*Alouatta aloutta*). (From Miller RE, Fowler M: *Fowler's zoo and wild animal medicine current therapy, vol 7,* St. Louis, Saunders, 2012.)

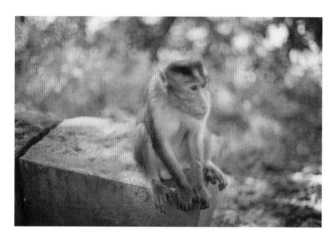

FIGURE 12-1. The rhesus monkey, *Macaca mulatta.* (Image courtesy of CDC/ Dr. Roger Broderson.)

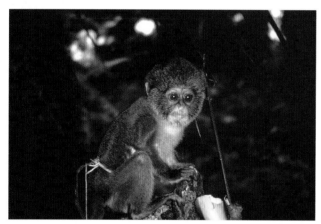

FIGURE 12-2. The African green monkey (*Cercopithecus* spp.) (Image courtesy of CDC/ Brian W.J. Mahy, BSc, MA, PhD, ScD, DSc.)

most widely used in research are *Macaca mulatta* (rhesus monkey) (Figure 12-1), *M. fascicularis* (cynomolgus monkey), *M. nemestrina* (pig-tailed monkey), *Cercopithecus aethiops* (African green monkey) (Figure 12-2), *Papio* species (baboons), and *Erythrocebus patas* (Patas monkey). NWP species used include *Saimiri sciureus* (squirrel monkey), *Aotus trivirgatus* (owl monkey), *Ateles* species (spider monkeys), *Saguinus* species (marmosets), and *Callithrix* species (tamarins, marmosets). *Cebus* species (capuchins) are NWP

species commonly referred to as "organ-grinder monkeys" and are sometimes kept as pets. Howler monkeys (*Alouatta aloutta*) are also kept as pets (Figure 12-3). It is interesting to note that these small primates were originally classified as rodents. Of the great apes, only *Pan troglodytes* (chimpanzee) is used to any extent in biomedical research.

> **TECHNICIAN NOTE** Most primates used in biomedical research are cynomolgus or rhesus monkeys.

UNIQUE ANATOMIC AND PHYSIOLOGIC FEATURES

A detailed discussion of the anatomy and physiology of the various species of NHPs is beyond the scope of this text. A summary of biologic data for some of the more common NHP species is located in Table 12-1. For most species of NHP, anatomy and physiology are strongly correlated to that of human beings. The various simian families do differ significantly in appearance and general characteristics. Specifically, the presence or absence of **prehensile tails**, **cheek pouches**, **ischial callosities**, and distance between the nares can be used to roughly classify a species. Most NWPs have prehensile tails, but this feature is absent in OWPs. The nasal orifices are relatively close together in OWPs and open downward when compared with NWPs. Cheek pouches are present in some OWPs but are always absent in NWPs. Ischial callosities represent hard, keratinized pads on the buttocks and are characteristic of most OWPs and are always absent in NWPs.

> **TECHNICIAN NOTE** Ischial callosities are always absent in NWPs.

TABLE 12-1	Biologic Data for Common NHP Species					
SCIENTIFIC NAME	ADULT MALE WEIGHT (kg)	ADULT FEMALE WEIGHT (kg)	FEMALE PUBERTY (mo)	GESTATION LENGTH (d)	NEONATE WEIGHT (g)	AGE AT WEANING (d)
Aotus trivirgatus	0.813	0.736	30	133	97	75
Ateles fusciceps	8.89	9.16	51.6	226		485
Ateles geoffroyi	7.78	7.29	72	229	512	822
Callithrix jacchus	0.317	0.324	22	148	27	91
Cebus albifrons	3.18	2.29	43.1	155	234	274
Cebus capucinus	3.68	2.54	54	162	230	548
Cercopithecus aethiops	5.023	3.457	54	163.3	314	365
Erythrocebus patas	12.4	6.5	41.2	167.5	504.5	212
Macaca fascicularis	5.36	3.59	51.6	167	345	420
Macaca mulatto	9.355	7.085	42	164	475	316
Macaca nemestrina	9.45	5.7	35	170	472	365
Pan troglodytes	49.567	40.367	126	228	1742	1460
Papio anubis	23.15	12.5	57.5	180	1068	420
Papio cynocephalus	21.8	12.3	66	175	854	365
Saguinus species	0.477	0.517	18	146	43	80
Saimiri sciureus	0.899	0.68	30	160	95.2	51

All NHPs have bony orbits (eye sockets). OWPs have flat skulls with prominent brow ridges, narrow nasal septa, and elongated nares. NWPs have rounded skulls. Brow ridges are absent and the nasal septum is broad with large oval nares. NHPs all have both deciduous and permanent teeth. OWPs have 32 permanent teeth and NWPs have 36. Basic information on the anatomy and physiology of the reproductive systems of commonly encountered NHP species is presented in the section on breeding and reproduction. Additional general anatomic and physiologic data are included in Table 12-1.

ANIMAL MODELS

Primates represent less than 0.025% of all animals used in U.S. biomedical research facilities. The difficulty in procuring animals; their high cost and complicated housing requirements; and concerns regarding injury to workers involved in handling, restraint, and performance of technical procedures are some of the reasons that NHPs are not commonly used research subjects. Despite their infrequent use, however, primates play a vital role in biomedical research. Genetically, NHPs share many similarities with human beings. The chimpanzee and rhesus macaque, in particular, are very closely related to human beings on a molecular level. Primates are also susceptible to many of the same diseases as human beings. Similarities in developmental and behavioral characteristics also exist between human beings and many NHP species. Biomedical research projects involving new treatments, surgeries, and diagnostic techniques use NHPs as the final phase of testing before beginning human trials. This is a particularly important step in cases in which it is illegal or unethical to use human subjects.

TECHNICIAN NOTE Primates represent less than 0.025% of all animals used in U.S. biomedical research facilities.

In an effort to control the use of NHPs in biomedical research, the Interagency Primate Steering Committee, established in 1974, prepared a national plan and recommended research proposal review. Before the use of any NHPs in research, the research is evaluated for the following general criteria.

- Does the research require primates, or can some other species be used?
- Is the species selected for the study appropriate?
- Does the proposal require that only a minimum number be used?
- Will the animals be kept alive and, if not, will tissues be shared with other investigators?

In the United States, national and regional primate research centers coordinate the use of living NHPs as well as any available tissues among scientists throughout the world. This system saves unnecessary use of NHPs for medical research. Research into specific human diseases that currently use NHPs as research subjects is summarized in Table 12-2.

REPRODUCTION

Importation of NHPs into the United States is prohibited except for scientific, educational, and exhibition purposes. Many of the NHP species are listed on the U.S. endangered and threatened species list, and their importation and use are strictly monitored. In addition, many countries with native NHP populations have restricted the exportation of these

TABLE 12-2	NHPs as Animal Models	
DISEASE/ CONDITION	**RATIONALE FOR USE**	**SPECIES MOST OFTEN USED**
HIV/AIDS	Show persistent viremia infected with HIV-1 without signs of disease; can be used to study the infectious properties of the virus	Chimpanzees Gibbons Baboons
Viral hepatitis		Marmoset Chimpanzee
Diabetes mellitus	Spontaneous development of amyloid infiltration into the islet cells of the pancreas	Macaca nigra
Atherosclerosis	Spontaneous development of aortic and coronary atherosclerosis	Squirrel monkeys

HIV/AIDS, Human immunodeficiency virus/acquired immunodeficiency syndrome.

TABLE 12-3	Expected Life Spans of NHPS	
SCIENTIFIC NAME	**COMMON NAME**	**LIFE SPAN (Y)**
Aotus trivirgatus	Northern gray-necked owl monkey	20
Ateles fusciceps	Brown-headed spider monkey	24
Ateles geoffroyi	Black-handed spider monkey	48
Callithrix jacchus	Common marmoset	11.7
Cebus albifrons	White-fronted capuchin	44
Cebus capucinus	White-throated capuchin	46.9
Erythrocebus patas	Patas monkey	21.6
Macaca arctoides	Stump-tailed macaque	30
Macaca fascicularis	Cynomolgus macaque	37.1
Macaca mulatta	Rhesus macaque	29
Macaca nemestrina	Pig-tailed macaque	26.3
Macaca nigra	Celebes or crested black	18
Pan troglodytes	Chimpanzee	53
Papio anubis	Olive baboon	30-45
Papio cynocephalus	Yellow baboon	40
Saguinus species	Tamarins	8-20

species. When importation is possible, it is difficult to obtain healthy animals for use in biomedical research. For these reasons, NHP breeding colonies have been established at the national and regional primate centers. Purpose breeding of NHPs at these centers is aimed at providing animals that are healthy as well as accustomed to life in captivity.

Animals that are acquired from other facilities or are wild caught are subject to quarantine periods before their introduction into the resident colony area. The specific procedures and timing for this quarantine period vary slightly in different facilities. In general, the quarantine period lasts approximately 60 days. During the initial period, the animals are given a detailed physical examination to identify any signs of common diseases. A tuberculosis test is performed, and body fluids and tissue samples are collected for analysis. Fecal examinations and rectal mucosal cultures are usually performed. Radiographs are often taken, particularly of the thorax and abdomen, to identify any diseases or other abnormal conditions that may be present. After this initial quarantine period, the animals are examined every few days and are usually tested again for tuberculosis. In some institutions, a total of five negative tuberculosis tests, performed approximately every 14 days, is required before placing the animal in the resident colony.

BREEDING

Determination of gender in NHP species is usually uncomplicated because of the visible external genitalia. One notable exception is the spider monkey. Females of that species possess an enlarged clitoris that appears similar to the penis of males. Specific reproductive data vary widely among NHPs. Almost all NHPs are polyestrus. Female OWPs and some NWPs exhibit an obvious menstrual cycle, much the same as seen in human beings. In most OWPs the female's cycle lasts approximately 1 month. Menstrual bleeding may be evident in the larger species. In addition, OWP females exhibit a turgescence (swelling) and reddish color change of the external genitalia during estrus. This is commonly referred to as sex skin and is absent in NWPs. Observation of physical and behavioral characteristics can be used in conjunction with examination of vaginal cytology preparations to determine the stage of estrus in NHP species.

> **TECHNICIAN NOTE** Almost all NHPs are polyestrus.

Age at puberty, duration of estrus, and time between estrous cycles vary widely among the groups. Puberty ranges from 3 to 10 years depending on the species, with males maturing a year or so later than females. Additional data for common species of NHPs is given in Table 12-3.

Breeding systems used in NHP facilities include timed mating, paired mating, harem mating, and free-range mating systems. Timed mating programs require that animals be housed individually and the female evaluated daily to determine the optimal breeding time. The female is placed in the cage of the male just before the estimated time of ovulation. This system is useful when exact gestational age must be known, such as for certain postpartum and intrauterine research programs. However, individual caging of animals is expensive. Estimated gestational age can be determined when animals are housed in pairs. With paired mating, the female is observed daily for signs of estrus and subsequent pregnancy. Ultrasound and rectal examination are also used to determine gestational age.

Harem mating involves temporary or permanent housing of one male with a group of females. Animals may also be bred by using free-range systems. This involves housing of a large, mixed-sex group within an enclosure. Both harem and free-range systems are used in production colonies. With paired, harem, or free-range systems, care must be taken to provide adequate space because male NHPs are often aggressive toward females when housed in enclosures that are too small. Artificial insemination of NHPs has been successful in a number of species, including the chimpanzee, rhesus macaque, African green monkey, and patas monkey. This may be accomplished by visually evaluating the females for signs of estrus or by administering hormones to induce estrus before determining the optimal time for insemination. Artificial insemination in NHPs is complicated by the relatively brief potential fertility period of both ova and sperm.

PREGNANCY AND PARTURITION

Methods for determining pregnancy include ultrasound examination and evaluation of physical and behavioral changes. In species that develop turgescence of the sex skin, changes in the degree of color and turgescence can be used to determine whether pregnancy has occurred. In other species, the absence of continual menstrual cycling may be the earliest indication of pregnancy.

Gestation periods vary from approximately 164 days in the rhesus macaque to more than 200 days in some of the smaller NHP species. Pregnancy complications, such as dystocia, endometriosis, and toxemia, can occur. Most female NHPs give birth to a single offspring. Prolonged parenting is the norm for NHPs. The offspring tend to remain with the female parent until weaning age. Weaning occurs between 6 and 8 months, depending on the species. A summary of reproductive data for common NHP species is given in Table 12-3.

BEHAVIOR

Because of the many similarities between behaviors of human beings and NHPs, primate behavior has been extensively studied. A detailed discussion of primate behavior is beyond the scope of this text. Primate behavior is extremely complex and marked by significant species variation. General behavior patterns common to most NHPs include a complex social hierarchy, an inquisitive nature, the need for physical and social interaction with their own species, and a dependence on learned behavior. Many normal primate behaviors are taught to the offspring by the parents, such as identifying and avoiding danger. In addition, NHPs learn by observing others, including their human caretakers.

Studies of primate behavior have provided detailed information on behavior patterns that are characteristic of primates in their natural habitats. Behavior patterns seen in wild NHP species vary somewhat among the species. However, several types of behavior patterns are common to NHP species. These include grooming, foraging for food, and dominant/submissive behaviors characteristic of the development and maintenance of a social hierarchy. Numerous behavior patterns have also been described that serve as communication methods between individuals. This includes a variety of vocalizations; postures; facial expressions; gestures; and displays of jumping, running, and manipulating objects. These behaviors may communicate a variety of information, including dominance; submission; intent to attack; anxiety; and solicitations for mating, grooming, or play. Grooming behaviors, particularly **allogrooming** (grooming of others), serve as a method of communication and may also serve to strengthen the social organization. More submissive members of a group will usually groom those that are more dominant. Captive primates must be given opportunities to develop and express these normal behavior patterns. The lack of attention to this significant aspect of primate care is one of the primary reasons that NHP species raised or kept in isolation usually develop undesirable, abnormal behaviors.

> TECHNICIAN NOTE Grooming behaviors, particularly allogrooming (grooming of others), serve as a method of communication and may also serve to strengthen the social organization.

The Animal Welfare Act requires that research facilities develop and implement plans to promote the psychologic well-being of the NHP species in their care. Methods to meet those requirements have primarily focused on providing environmental stimuli that mimic what would be present in the natural environment of the species. When animals cannot be group housed, cages are often placed so that normal auditory, olfactory, and visual communication among individuals can still occur. Cage "toys" are usually provided to meet the animals' need to manipulate objects and satisfy their natural curiosity. Balls, puzzles, dolls, and foraging devices are common components of primate enclosures. Items typically have a variety of shapes, sizes, and textures and are used on a rotating basis to keep the animals from becoming bored. Foraging devices may be as simple as food hidden inside toys and under cage shelves. Tree feeders are often used for this purpose because most NHP species are arboreal. Visual stimulation may also take the form of colorful cage toys and cage walls painted with bright colors and designs. The presence of a television monitor with moving images is used in some facilities to provide additional visual stimuli. Auditory stimuli can include playing soft music in the primate enclosure area. Preliminary research in this area suggests that this background music can calm agitated animals and reduce aggressive behaviors. Captive NHPs are also usually provided with time to interact with their human caretakers and, in some cases, are given formal training sessions. Captive-reared NHPs respond well to formal training, which also provides an additional enrichment to their environment by allowing greater social contact between the animals and caretakers. NHPs may also be trained to perform essential tasks. For example, a primate that is diabetic can be taught to self-administer required injections of insulin.

> TECHNICIAN NOTE The Animal Welfare Act requires that research facilities develop and implement plans to promote the psychologic well-being of the NHP species in their care.

HUSBANDRY, HOUSING, AND NUTRITION

Specific needs for housing depend somewhat on the species and on the history of the animal. Animals that have been accustomed to group or paired housing usually respond poorly to individual caging. Moving an animal that has been individually caged into group or paired housing can also be difficult and requires special monitoring of the interaction between the individuals. Hand-reared animals may not adapt well to introduction into a primate grouping, especially if the group is composed of individuals reared by their parents.

> *TECHNICIAN NOTE* NHPs are adept at manipulating objects and can easily determine how to open an unlocked cage.

A variety of cages are available for housing NHPs. Most of these are composed of stainless steel and contain slotted or grid floors to allow waste materials to pass through the cage bottom. Cage pans are often present below the cage bottom; these may be designed to allow waste materials from several cages to divert to a central drainage area. The cage usually incorporates an automatic watering system. Cleaning of the cages and cage pans and examining the watering system are usually performed at least once daily. Cages for housing of individual animals often contain built-in squeeze mechanisms to allow restraint of the individual animal. Regardless of the type of cage or cage design, cages must have secure locks because most NHPs are adept at manipulating objects and can easily determine how to open an unlocked cage.

Detailed information on the space requirements for housing of NHPs is contained in the Animal Welfare Act and the Guide for the Care and Use of Laboratory Animals. Specific requirements depend on the species being housed and the type of research being conducted. The Animal Welfare Act groups simian primate species into six groups (Box 12-2). Five of the groups contain species that reach similar adult weights. The sixth group contains the largest of the great ape species and all the brachiating simians. Brachiating simians are anthropoideans that possess anatomic variations of the shoulder region in which the arms are longer than the legs. These animals practice a form of locomotion known as **brachiation**, in which the body is suspended from branches and the animal swings between branches. Some species use their prehensile tails as an additional "limb" when moving in this manner. In addition to the floor space requirement for each of the NHP groupings, the larger NHPs and all brachiating species require enclosures with sufficient height to allow them to make normal postural movements, including brachiation. The requirements listed in the Animal Welfare Act and the Guide for the Care and Use of Laboratory Animals pertain to individually housed animals. When paired or group housing is used, space requirements must consider additional behavioral aspects of primates. Housing of large social groupings or breeding colonies often involves a large indoor cage connected to an outdoor corral. Feeding and

BOX 12-2	Primate Groupings for Determining Space Requirements

Group 1—marmosets, tamarins, and infants (less than 6 months of age) of various species.
Group 2—capuchins, squirrel monkeys and similar size species, and juveniles (6 months to 3 years of age) of various species.
Group 3—macaques and African species.
Group 4—male macaques and large African species.
Group 5—baboons and nonbrachiating species larger than 33.0 lbs (15 kg).
Group 6—great apes over 55.0 lbs (25 kg) and brachiating species.

watering devices are usually located in both the indoor and outdoor areas. Outdoor areas must also contain sufficient shelter to allow protection from extreme weather conditions. Indoor housing is usually maintained at a temperature range of 64° to 84° F and a relative humidity of 30% to 70%.

NUTRITION

Although most NHPs are omnivores, plant material makes up a large percentage of their diet. In their natural habitat, the diet is composed primarily of fruits, leaves, and insects. Commercial diets are readily available and adequate to meet the nutritional needs of NHPs provided that the food is properly stored. Diets formulated for OWPs tend to be slightly lower in protein and fat content than that for NWPs. Pregnant or lactating females and juvenile OWPs are usually given a higher-protein diet than their adult counterparts. In addition, because primates have an absolute dietary requirement for vitamin C, the food must be used within 90 days of milling to ensure adequate levels of this vitamin. NHPs, especially NWPs, are sometimes provided with supplemental feedings of fresh fruits and vegetables. These should be given no more than a few times each week and must be thoroughly washed to avoid transmission of bacterial pathogens to the animals. Pet monkeys are prone to protein deficiency because of overfeeding of fruits and vegetables by their owners. Fresh water must always be available. This is accomplished either through an automatic watering system or hanging water bottles placed outside the cage.

Automatic watering systems must be checked regularly for proper operation. NHP species may refuse food if the watering device is inoperable. In addition, some animals must be taught to use the devices, although they often learn by observing other animals in the colony.

> *TECHNICIAN NOTE* Primates have an absolute dietary requirement for vitamin C.

Primates should be fed a commercial primate diet. Supplemental foods can include moderate amounts of assorted green vegetables, carrots, sweet potatoes, apples, bananas, and oranges, although these should not comprise more than 25% of the diet.

Members of the primate subfamily Colobinae exhibit pregastric fermentation, similar to that in ruminants. In the wild, their diets usually contain a moderately high fiber content. They also spend a significant amount of time foraging. Gastrointestinal problems often develop when captive animals are not provided diets that mimic those consumed in the wild. In addition, some colobus monkeys exhibit sensitivity to gluten and should be fed a gluten-free, high-fiber monkey biscuit. Alfalfa pellets or good-quality alfalfa hay can also be provided.

RESTRAINT AND HANDLING

One of the most significant issues to address in handling and restraint of NHPs is the safety of the handlers. In addition, handlers must be well trained in the procedures needed to minimize stress to the animals. Most NHPs are 4 to 10 times stronger than a human being of the same weight. Bites and scratches from some NHPs can transmit serious and even fatal diseases to the handlers. In many cases, NHP species maintained in biomedical research colonies may have their canine teeth cut to the level of the incisors and capped with dental alloys. Although for most species minimal manual restraint is preferred, for NHP species chemical restraint is usually needed. Some small NHP species can be manually restrained, or a combination of manual and chemical restraint can be used. Regardless of the methods chosen, handlers must always wear protective equipment, including face shields or goggles, protective gloves, and full-length arm covers. Small NHP species (those weighing less than 10 kg) can usually be restrained manually, although chemical restraint is recommended. In most cases, two handlers will be needed. One method of manual restraint is referred to as the collar and catch pole method. This method requires that the animals be housed with a lightweight plastic or aluminum collar. The collar contains two small handles to which a pole can be attached. Two handlers, each with a catch pole, attach the pole to the collar and gently lift the animal from its cage onto a restraint table. The collar is then secured to the table. This method is commonly used in biomedical research facilities. The animals are trained by using positive reinforcement methods to familiarize and acclimatize them to the procedure; most respond quite well.

TECHNICIAN NOTE Handlers must always wear protective equipment, including face shields or goggles, protective gloves, and full-length arm covers, when handling NHPs.

Another manual restraint method that can be used for procedures of short duration in small NHP species involves first immobilizing the animal in a squeeze cage and then grasping the upper arms. The arms are then gently pulled toward the back until the elbows touch. A second handler is usually needed to pry the animal's feet from the cage bars so that it can be removed from the cage. This method represents significant risk of injury both to the handlers and the animal. Many NHP species use their tails for leverage and are capable of reaching the handler with their back feet. The animal must be held out away from the handler's body to minimize this problem.

NHP species may react poorly to restraint. Care must be taken to avoid undue stress on the animals. Restraint must only be performed when absolutely necessary. In some cases, animals become ill or injured after restraint and may need to be temporarily or permanently removed from the colony.

IDENTIFICATION

The methods used for identifying individual NHPs vary depending on the type of housing being used. When maintained in group housing, individuals are usually identified by placing a large identification tag around the neck. An ear tag can also be used, which allows observation of specific individuals from a distance. When housed in single cages, animals can be identified with cage cards. Other methods include implantation of a microchip or tattoos on the thigh or chest. Newly acquired animals can be temporarily identified by applying colored marker or dye to the skin or hair or by shaving a unique pattern in the hair.

CLINICAL PROCEDURES

Administration of medication to NHP species is complicated by the difficulties presented in handling and restraining the animals. Whenever practical, animals that require regular administration of medication should be taught to administer their own medications, or the medication should be placed in a treat or mixed with a favorite food.

INJECTION TECHNIQUES

Parenteral administration of medication can be accomplished by methods similar to those used for other medium to large mammals. Subcutaneous injections are given in the loose skin over the back of the neck. Intramuscular injections are usually given in the triceps, gluteal, or quadriceps muscles. In smaller species, the gluteal and triceps muscle groups have relatively small muscle mass and should be avoided. Intravenous injections can be given in the cephalic or saphenous vein.

When large volumes of medication are needed or the animal requires continual infusion of medications or fluids, a vascular access port is usually placed. The port is surgically implanted in the subcutaneous space along the upper back. The animal can then be trained to present its back for injection or can be connected by a tether system to an infusion pump.

ORAL ADMINISTRATION

Medications that can be given orally are relatively simple to administer to most NHP species. The medication can be placed within a piece of fruit or other treat or covered with peanut butter. Medications can also be crushed and mixed with the food. Some NHPs are adept at picking the medication out or simply eating around it, so animals must be observed to ensure that the medication is actually consumed. For unpalatable medications, an orogastric or nasogastric tube should be placed. The animal should be lightly anesthetized and proper placement of the tube within the stomach verified before administering the medication.

ANESTHESIA

Many restraint techniques, diagnostic procedures, and all surgical procedures require that the animals be anesthetized. For removal of animals from their enclosures, or for procedures of short duration or minimal pain and distress, an intramuscular injection of ketamine is often used. When additional muscle relaxation is needed, the ketamine can be mixed with diazepam, acepromazine, or xylazine. Ketamine, either alone or in combination with other medication, can also be used to preanesthetize animals before placement of an endotracheal tube. An intramuscular injection of atropine is also used before induction of anesthesia to minimize salivation. Other injectable medications used for anesthesia in NHP species include intravenous propofol, tiletamine-zolazepam, and sodium pentobarbital. Injectable medications should not be used as the primary anesthetic regimen when the procedure is expected to take longer than 30 to 45 minutes. One notable exception is propofol. Animals can be maintained at a surgical plane of anesthesia by monitoring anesthetic depth and administering periodic bolus injections of propofol. During anesthesia, the heart rate, respiratory rate and character, and pedal and palpebral reflexes can be used to gauge anesthetic depth in NHPs. During anesthesia and recovery, the animal should be placed on a warm-water blanket or under a heat lamp to prevent hypothermia. Administration of warmed fluids by an indwelling catheter is commonly performed for this reason. Administration of analgesics is an absolute requirement after surgical procedures. For mild pain, acetaminophen or aspirin can be given orally. Injectable analgesics that may also be used include meperidine, butorphanol, and morphine. Animals that have sutures must be maintained in individual cages until the sutures are removed. Normal grooming behaviors of group-housed animals may result in sutures being removed prematurely.

> **TECHNICIAN NOTE** During anesthesia, the heart rate, respiratory rate and character, and pedal and palpebral reflexes can be used to gauge anesthetic depth in NHPs.

COLLECTION OF BLOOD AND URINE SAMPLES

Procedures used to collect blood and urine samples are similar to those used for other large mammal species. Large amounts of blood can be obtained from the femoral vein or artery. This procedure requires that the animal be anesthetized. The venipuncture site must be clipped of hair and surgically prepped. The cephalic and saphenous veins can also be used for blood collection. When repeated sampling is needed, placement of an indwelling catheter or vascular access port is indicated. As with injectable medication administration, animals can be trained to present the catheter site by using positive reinforcement techniques.

Urine samples can be collected either by cystocentesis or a urinary catheter. These techniques are similar to those used for urine collection in dogs and cats; they are relatively simple to perform but require that the animal be anesthetized. Animals can also be housed in a metabolism cage when urine sample collection is required.

DIAGNOSTIC IMAGING

Nonhuman primates must be anesthetized for imaging studies. Standard x-ray equipment and techniques are used as for comparably sized mammals. At least two views of the site of interest must be obtained.

COMMON DISEASES

There are a large number of bacterial, parasitic, and viral diseases that are transmissible between human beings and NHPs. Before beginning work in a primate colony, employees are usually required to undergo a preemployment physical examination and periodic reexaminations. Of particular importance is control of tuberculosis and herpes B infections. Biomedical research facilities have specific procedures that must be followed when a caretaker in the primate facility is bitten or scratched, especially those caretakers who have regular contact with macaques.

INFECTIOUS DISEASES

Although a variety of diseases can be found in NHPs, some are found only in one group of primates. Although a detailed discussion of infectious diseases of NHPs is beyond the scope of this chapter, the more commonly seen conditions in animals maintained in biomedical research and kept as pets are discussed. Particular attention is paid to those diseases that can be transmitted between human beings and NHPs.

Bacterial Disease

The majority of the bacterial pathogens affecting NHPs fall into one of two categories: those that cause respiratory disease and those that cause gastrointestinal disease. In many cases, these pathogens are present in normal animals as latent infection and cause clinical disease only when the animals become stressed. Sources of stress in NHPs include dietary changes, environmental changes (e.g., new cage location, new cagemates), and transportation stress. Mechanisms to minimize stress are vital to prevent serious disease in a primate colony.

Gastroenteritis. Diarrhea is a significant problem in primate colonies. The bacterial agents most commonly associated with gastroenteritis are *Shigella flexneri* and *Campylobacter jejuni*. Other enteric pathogens occasionally isolated include *Yersinia* spp., enterotoxigenic *Escherichia coli*, *Pseudomonas aeruginosa*, and *Aerobacter aerogenes*. Primates (including human beings) may be asymptomatic carriers of these bacteria.

Shigellosis. Animals with active *Shigella* infections are severely ill, dehydrated, and emaciated. When acute colitis occurs there is a foul-smelling liquid stool containing blood, mucus, and necrotic colonic mucosa. Transmission is by the fecal-oral route. Abdominal pain is evident as the disease progresses. Rectal prolapse may occur, and hypokalemia is common. Death may occur within 2 days. Diagnosis is by microbiologic evaluation of rectal swabs. Confirmation of the organism is difficult, and false-negative results are common. Treatment includes fluid therapy and antibiotics.

Campylobacteriosis. Infections with *Campylobacter jejuni* are primarily found in OWPs. Asymptomatic carriers are common. Clinical signs include watery diarrhea and severe dehydration. Diagnosis is by microbiologic evaluation of rectal swabs. The culture must be incubated in a 5% carbon dioxide environment. Confirmation of the organism is difficult. Treatment includes fluid therapy and antibiotics.

Salmonellosis. Although not commonly observed, infections with *Salmonella* species can occur. Clinical signs are similar to those seen with Shigellosis except that vomiting is also present. *Salmonella* infections are usually less severe, although secondary infections such as endocarditis or meningitis have been reported.

Pseudotuberculosis. Pseudotuberculosis can be caused by *Yersinia pseudotuberculosis* (Figure 12-4) or *Y. enterocolitica*. Reservoir hosts include wild rodents and birds. Contamination of feed has been implicated in transmission of infection. Clinical signs include diarrhea and depression. Animals with chronic infections may develop lesions on the liver and lungs that appear similar to those seen with tuberculosis.

Helicobacteriosis. *Helicobacter pylori* organisms have been isolated from the stomach of OWP species, particularly rhesus macaques. Clinical signs may be absent, or occasional vomiting may be present. The organism causes gastric ulcers. Diagnosis requires biopsy and culture of the gastric mucosa. Treatment involves antibiotics to eliminate the organism combined with symptomatic treatments, such as bismuth-subsalicylate therapy.

Respiratory Diseases. A variety of bacterial agents can cause respiratory disease in NHPs. Many of these cause nonspecific clinical signs or may manifest with fever, sneezing, coughing, nasal discharge, lethargy, and anorexia. If treated appropriately, respiratory infections are rarely fatal but many have significant zoonotic potential. *Klebsiella pneumoniae*, *Streptococcus pneumoniae*, *Bordetella bronchiseptica*, *Pasteurella multocida*, and *Haemophilus influenzae* have all been implicated as causative agents of respiratory disease in NHP species. Culture and sensitivity testing is required for diagnosis and as an aid in choosing the most effective antibiotic therapy. Additional supportive therapy may be needed if the animals are anorectic.

The most significant respiratory disease of NHP species is tuberculosis. Tuberculosis can be caused by several strains of *Mycobacterium* (Figure 12-5). The human strain, *Mycobacterium tuberculosis*, is the most common causative agent. Infections with the bovine and avian strains can also occur. Some atypical mycobacteria have also been reported in NHPs, including *M. kansasii* and *M. scrofulaceum*, both of which are potentially hazardous to human beings.

The disease is most commonly seen in OWP species, but all primates are susceptible. Tuberculosis presents a significant zoonotic problem. NHP species can contract the disease from human beings, and infections tend to spread rapidly throughout a primate colony. Transmission is primarily by the aerosol route but can also include bites, scratches, and contact with body fluids. Clinical signs are not remarkable in the early stages of disease. The earliest clinical manifestations are lethargy, weight loss, and general unthriftiness. The disease progresses slowly; later signs

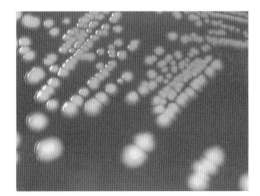

FIGURE 12-4. *Yersinia pseudotuberculosis* bacteria cultured on a sheep blood agar (SBA) medium. (Image courtesy of CDC/ Dr. Todd Parker. Ph.D.; Assoc. Director for Lab. Science/DPEI(Acting) and LRN Training Coordinator.)

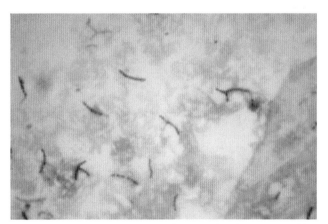

FIGURE 12-5. *Mycobacterium tuberculosis* bacteria using acid-fast Ziehl-Neelsen stain. (Image courtesy of CDC/ Dr. George P. Kubica.)

include respiratory distress, diarrhea, jaundice, and significant lymphadenitis. The disease can take a year to fully develop before obvious signs are present. Definitive diagnosis is difficult and requires a combination of tests, specifically intradermal tuberculin testing and thoracic radiography. The intradermal tuberculin test is usually performed using the skin of the upper eyelid so that the animals do not have to be captured to read the test. The presence of tuberculosis in a primate colony usually requires that the animals be euthanized. Prevention of tuberculosis is therefore a primary focus in biomedical research. Control measures include periodic tuberculin testing and thoracic radiography for animals and caretakers. Medications such as isoniazid are available to prevent tuberculosis infection. However, because development of bacterial resistance is possible, preventive therapy is usually reserved for extremely valuable animals.

Miscellaneous Bacterial Diseases. Melioidosis is caused by the bacterium *Pseudomonas pseudomallei*. It is primarily found in OWPs and apes. Infections may remain latent for many years. Diagnosis involves identifying the typical lesions found in the lungs. *Branhamella catarrhalis* is the causative agent for the disease commonly referred to as bloody nose syndrome. The disease primarily affects cynomolgus macaques, and the most common clinical sign is epistaxis. Tetanus infections can also occur in NHPs. The causative agent is a neurotoxin produced by the bacteria *Clostridium tetani*. All primates are susceptible to this infection. Clinical signs include lockjaw, seizures, and respiratory paralysis. A vaccine is available to prevent infection.

Viral Disease

Primates are susceptible to a large variety of viral agents. Most viral agents have a natural host species and a reservoir host species. The reservoir host usually does not develop clinical infection but remains a source of infection to other species. In some cases, NHPs are reservoir hosts for viral infections that infect human beings. Conversely, human caretakers may be reservoir hosts for viral agents that can cause serious disease in NHPs. Viral agents of concern in NHPs include a number of herpesviruses, poxviruses, hepatitis viruses, and measles.

Herpesviruses. A large number of herpesviruses have been isolated from NHP species. However, most of these are not considered pathogenic to the animals or their caretakers. Herpesviruses of concern include *Herpesvirus hominis* (simplex), *H. tamarinus*, *H. saimiri*, *H. ateles*, and *H. simiae* (B virus).

H. hominis, also known as herpes simplex 1, causes oral lesions (fever blisters) in human beings. In marmosets, gibbons, and owl monkeys, herpes simplex 1 causes a fatal infection characterized by ulceration of the mucous membranes or skin, conjunctivitis, meningitis, or encephalitis. Similar signs are seen with *H. tamarinus* infections in owl monkeys and marmosets. The reservoir hosts for *H. tamarinus* are squirrel, cebus, and spider monkeys. Squirrel monkeys are

natural hosts for *H. saimiri* but infections are rarely symptomatic. In many other NHP species, *H. saimiri* can cause malignant lymphoma and lymphocytic leukemia. The natural hosts for *H. ateles* are spider monkeys. Like *H. saimiri*, this virus can cause lymphocytic leukemia and malignant lymphoma in other NHP species.

> **TECHNICIAN NOTE** Most herpesviruses have been isolated from NHP species and are not considered pathogenic to the animals or their caretakers.

The most significant herpesvirus of concern in NHP colonies is *H. simiae*, also known as herpes B virus. Rhesus and cynomolgus macaques are the natural hosts for this virus. Other members of the genus *Macaca* also carry the virus, and caretakers should always assume that these primates are potential shedders of this virus. Infected animals may be asymptomatic or may develop oral or genital ulcers and conjunctivitis. The disease is transmitted by bites, scratches, and contact with body fluids. Although this is a mild disease in NHP species, human beings develop an encephalomyelitis that is often fatal. Any individual who has come into contact with body fluids from macaques or is bitten or scratched by a macaque should receive immediate medical attention. Primate facilities usually have detailed procedures for the prevention and treatment of herpes B virus infections.

Hepatitis Viruses. Five different hepatitis viruses are capable of infecting human beings and NHP species. The most common of these is the hepatitis A virus, also referred to as infectious hepatitis. Natural hosts for the virus include rhesus and cynomolgus macaques, chimpanzees, and African green monkeys. Transmission is by the fecal-oral route. Infected animals are usually asymptomatic; however, alterations in serum liver enzymes are common and may complicate research results. The disease can be transmitted between human beings and NHPs. Hepatitis B virus, also known as serum hepatitis, is also found in a number of NHP species, particularly chimpanzees. Transmission is by the aerosol route or by contact with body fluids. Most infections are asymptomatic. However, infected human beings serve as carriers for infection and can also develop hepatocellular carcinoma. Caretakers in NHP colonies are usually given a vaccine to prevent infection with hepatitis A and B viruses. Hepatitis C, D, and E viruses are rarely a concern but may be seen in conjunction with hepatitis B infections. Although NHP species can be experimentally infected with these viruses, naturally occurring infections have not been demonstrated.

> **TECHNICIAN NOTE** Caretakers in NHP colonies are usually given a vaccine to prevent infection with hepatitis A and B viruses.

Measles. Measles is caused by a human paramyxovirus also known as rubeola. The disease is generally mild in

NHP species. Macaques and other OWPs seem to be more susceptible than NWPs, and the disease can be fatal in owl monkeys, tamarins, and marmosets. Clinical signs include an exanthematous rash on the chest and lower portions of the body, nasal and ocular discharge, and blepharitis (eyelid inflammation). Respiratory signs are occasionally seen. In some NHPs, particularly marmosets and owl monkeys, the disease can develop into a fatal gastroenteritis when left untreated. Treatment involves supportive therapy. Vaccination of human caretakers is necessary. Caretakers who have come into contact with individuals that have active measles infection should be temporarily prohibited from contact with NHP species. It has been reported that human measles vaccine is effective in preventing the disease in NHPs, and many facilities routinely vaccinate infant macaques with human measles vaccine.

Poxviruses. Poxviruses that are capable of infecting human beings and NHP species include monkeypox, smallpox, benign epidermal monkeypox (tanapox), molluscum contagiosum, and yaba poxvirus. Poxviruses are usually characterized by a maculopapular rash and pustules. The lesions may be highly pruritic, and infected animals are prone to self-mutilation and subsequent secondary infection. Poxvirus infections are usually self-limiting, and recovery imparts immunity. Treatment with steroids, sedatives, and antibiotics is aimed at preventing secondary infection. Vaccinia virus immunization is effective at preventing monkeypox infections in human beings and NHPs.

Simian Hemorrhagic Fever. Simian hemorrhagic fever is caused by a filovirus. This is a highly contagious and fatal viral disease primarily infecting macaques. Asymptomatic carriers include African green monkeys, patas monkeys, and baboons. Clinical signs include fever, facial edema, cyanosis, epistaxis, and dehydration. Multiple cutaneous hemorrhages are present. The mortality rate in macaques is nearly 100%. Transmission to human beings is not known to occur. Another filovirus of NHP species that might be transmissible to human beings has been reported in an outbreak in the Philippines. The virus is related to the Ebola virus, and rodents may serve as reservoir hosts. Clinical signs in monkeys include fever and depression, with rapid progression to coma and death. Although several human beings have been infected with the virus, none developed clinical signs.

Retroviruses. At least six different retroviruses are capable of infecting NHP species. These are often referred to by the collective term simian immunodeficiency viruses. The viruses are in the lentivirus and oncovirus subfamilies. Infected animals may be asymptomatic or may develop any number of disease syndromes and secondary infections, including T-cell leukemia, lymphoma, anemia, atypical mycobacteriosis, intestinal cryptosporidiosis, pneumocystis pneumonia, and candidiasis. There is significant variation in clinical signs and susceptibility from

virus to virus among different NHP species. Transmission between primates usually requires direct or indirect contact with infected blood and other body fluids. Diagnosis can be made by serologic testing or may require viral isolation for definitive diagnosis. Prognosis is poor in clinically affected animals.

Miscellaneous Viral Diseases. Marburg virus caused a disease outbreak in Germany and former Yugoslavia in 1967. Laboratory personnel involved in handling tissues from African green monkeys became infected and died. None of the infected individuals in that outbreak had direct contact with the monkeys. NHP species are also susceptible to rabies infections. Animals housed outdoors are usually vaccinated against rabies. Other viral infections that have been reported in NHP species include chickenpox, lymphocytic choriomeningitis, yellow fever, Epstein-Barr virus, and cytomegalovirus.

Mycotic Disease

Superficial infections with *Microsporum* and *Trichophyton* are known to occur in NHPs. Systemic mycoses include infections with *Candida albicans* and *Pneumocystis carinii*. *Histoplasma capsulatum*, *Nocardia* species, *Coccidioides immitis*, and *Blastomyces dermatitidis* can also infect NHP species but are quite rare. *Candida* is a common saprophyte of the skin, gastrointestinal tract, and reproductive tract. Infections are usually opportunistic in animals that are immunosuppressed or receiving long-term antibiotic therapy. Clinical signs include ulcers or white, raised plaques on the tongue or mouth. Lesions can also be present in skin folds, and the fungus can also attack fingernails. The oral lesions must be differentiated from those seen with monkeypox or herpesvirus infections. Demonstration of the budding hyphae is not diagnostic because the organism is present on the skin of normal animals. *P. carinii* infections are also opportunistic and usually manifest with fever and dyspnea.

Parasitic Disease

Newly imported primates can harbor numerous parasites. Some parasites of NHP species are commensal in NHP species but can cause serious disease in human beings. Some parasites are self-limiting, particularly those whose life cycle requires an intermediate host. Most of these are easily eliminated during the initial quarantine period. Parasites that have direct life cycles tend to be the most dangerous to human caretakers and should be eliminated by pharmacologic treatment.

Blood Parasites. Malaria can be caused by a number of species in the genus *Plasmodium*. Organisms in this genus are protozoal parasites within the phylum commonly referred to as sporozoans. These organisms are obligate intracellular parasites. The most common causative agents seen in NHP species are *P. cynomolgi* and *P. knowlesi*. Diagnosis is based on demonstration of malarial organisms in the erythrocytes (Figure 12-6). The parasite is transmitted

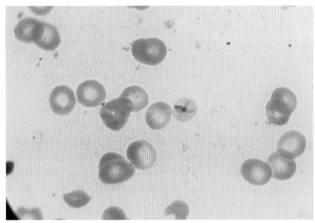

FIGURE 12-6. *Plasmodium falciparum* malarial parasite in a blood sample. (Image courtesy of CDC/ Neva Gleason.)

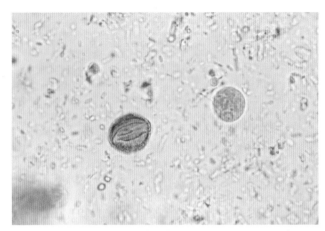

FIGURE 12-7. *Entamoeba histolytica* cysts. (Image courtesy of CDC.)

by a mosquito vector, so it cannot be directly transmitted to human beings. In addition, most *Plasmodium* organisms are species specific and do not infect species other than their definitive hosts.

Toxoplasmosis has been reported in some NHP species. The causative agent is the intracellular sporozoan *Toxoplasma gondii*. Clinical signs of infection are nonspecific and include lethargy and anorexia.

Gastrointestinal Parasites. *Entamoeba histolytica* (Fig 12-7) is a common enteric protozoan, mostly affecting NWPs. NHP species are usually asymptomatic. Transmission is by direct contact with fecal material from infected individuals. Severe infections are characterized by protracted, watery, or bloody diarrhea, constipation, flatulence, abdominal pain, and ulceration of the intestinal mucosa. Diagnosis requires demonstration of the organisms in fresh fecal samples. *Balantidium coli* organisms have been recovered from fecal specimens of NHPs, but this organism is considered commensal to the intestinal tract. Both *E. histolytica* and *B. coli* can infect human beings and cause serious disease.

> **TECHNICIAN NOTE** Both *E. histolytica* and *B. coli* can be transmitted from NHPs to human beings and cause serious disease.

Giardia species are protozoans that inhabit the upper small intestine. Although infections can manifest with diarrhea, giardiasis is often asymptomatic in NHP species. Transmission is by direct contact with fecal material from infected individuals. Proper sanitation prevents transmission of this organism to caretakers. Routine fecal smear examination can demonstrate the presence of the organisms and treatment is not difficult.

Oesophagostomum species are the most common nematode parasites of OWPs (Figure 12-8). Infective larvae penetrate the wall of the large intestine and produce subserosal nodules. Diarrhea is seen when the worm burden is high. The nodules can rupture and cause peritonitis. Other common

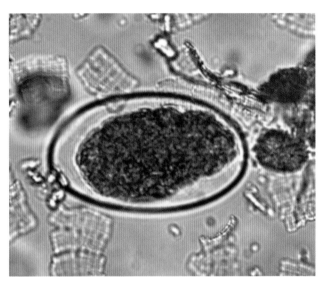

FIGURE 12-8. *Oesophagostomum* spp., egg from a gorilla; this egg was fixed with formalin, and the morula appears somewhat contracted. (From Bowman D: *Georgis' parasitology for veterinarians*, ed 10, St. Louis, Saunders, 2014.)

nematode parasites of NHP species include *Strongyloides* and *Trichostrongylus*. Infection with these organisms is common in many NHP species. The organisms have a direct life cycle and are potentially zoonotic. There are three common species that infect human beings and NHPs: *S. fuelleborni*, *S. cebus*, and *S. stercoralis*. The infective stage of the parasite is a free-living larvae that penetrates the skin or mucosa and migrates to the lungs, alveoli, and trachea. The organisms are then swallowed and cause severe acute enteritis. The initial passage of the organism through the skin can cause pruritus and erythema. Passage through the lungs can cause pulmonary lesions, pneumonia, and possibly death from pericarditis. The affected primate, unless treated and tested frequently, can reinfect itself and may be a continual hazard to human caretakers. Diagnosis involves clinical signs and demonstration of ova or larvae in the feces. Treatment is effective, but proper sanitation is essential in preventing reinfection.

Trichuris organisms are nematode parasites that can also cause pulmonary lesions during migration through the host body. *Prosthenorchis* are nematode parasites found in Central and South American primates. The organisms burrow into the mucosa of the ileocecal junction and can perforate the bowel or cause obstruction when present in large numbers. Cockroaches are intermediate hosts. Elimination of the intermediate host and strict sanitation are essential for control of infection.

Dipetalonema and *Tetrapetalonema* are found in the peritoneal cavity of NWP species; large numbers can be present without apparent harm to the host. *Filaroides* are found in the lungs. The larval form of *Echinococcus granulosus* can cause large, multiple cysts usually found in the abdomen and occasionally in the thoracic cavity. Infection has been reported in wild-caught OWPs.

Ectoparasites. A variety of lice, mites, and fleas are capable of infesting NHPs. Most of these can be transmitted to human beings through direct contact. These organisms are of concern primarily because they are capable of transmitting other infectious agents. *Psorergates* species and *Sarcoptes scabiei* are mange mites that can infest primates and cause sarcoptic mange. *Pediculus humanas* is a sucking louse that is occasionally seen. The flea species, *Tunga penetrans,* and the tick, *Ornithodoros* species, can also infest primates. Diseases caused by these arthropods are usually superficial skin infections characterized by pruritus and scaling. The grooming habits of healthy primates usually prevent severe infestation. Topical treatment of affected primates is effective.

NONINFECTIOUS DISEASES

Because of their relatively long lifespan (Table 12-3) and their similar anatomy and physiology to human beings, NHPs are susceptible to many of the same diseases as human beings. This includes a variety of neoplastic diseases, diabetes, hypothyroidism, arthritis, and cognitive dysfunction. This is one reason why NHPs play such a vital role in the study of human disease.

Neoplasia

A variety of neoplastic diseases have been reported in NHPs. Papillomas and fibromas are fairly common although they usually regress on their own. Fibroma, squamous cell carcinoma, and subcutaneous lipoma have all been reported in NHPs. Renal carcinomas and neoplasia of the digestive tract and larynx have also been reported but are rare.

METABOLIC DISEASES

Some species of NHP are prone to development of goiter. This is seen primarily when a dietary insufficiency of iodine is present. It is also seen in animals with diets high in raw cabbage, kale, or turnips. Affected animals have an enlarged thyroid gland. Clinical signs of hypothyroidism can be present in the offspring of iodine-deficient females.

Diabetes mellitus has also been reported in NHPs. *Macaca nigra,* and *Macaca fascicularis,* particularly those that are obese, have a higher incidence of this disease than other NHP species.

AGE-ASSOCIATED DISEASES

NHPs are susceptible to rheumatoid arthritis, a condition much the same as that seen in human beings. Monkeys can also display cognitive decline with age similar to that seen in some human beings.

HUSBANDRY-RELATED DISEASES

It has been suggested that low humidity predisposes animals to *Branhamella catarrhalis* infection, or "bloody nose syndrome." NHPs housed in outdoor enclosures are also susceptible to heat stroke and hypothermia. Vegetative endocarditis is a common consequence of frostbite.

Dental Disease

Gingivitis, periodontitis, dental caries, and teeth abscess have all been reported in captive NHPs. The anatomic and physiologic characteristics of the oral cavity of NHPs are similar to those seen in human beings and canines. Infant primates may develop gingivitis during eruption of teeth. The gums become tender and swollen and the animal may become febrile. As in human beings, dental caries are related to dietary factors, especially calcium-deficient diets. Cebus and patas monkeys are particularly prone to dental caries.

Nutritional Diseases

Obesity is seen more often than inadequate nutrient intake is. NHPs can rapidly become overweight when excess amounts of a high-quality diet are offered, particularly when activity is limited. Some facilities feed meat to their great apes, but this should be done in moderation because these animals are prone to hypercholesterolemia.

Primates require vitamin D to prevent rickets and osteomalacia. NWPs are particularly susceptible to vitamin D deficiency, especially in animals that are not exposed to daily sunlight. NWPs receiving vitamin D–deficient diets may develop osteodystrophia fibrosa. Vitamin D should be supplemented in these species. Clinical signs of vitamin D deficiency include a reluctance to climb or jump, distortion of limbs and spine, epiphyseal swelling, and spontaneous fractures. Care must be taken to avoid overfeeding of foods high in vitamin D because toxicity can occur, especially in animals housed partly outdoors. Indoor housing may incorporate skylight windows to allow transmission of ultraviolet light into the primate holding areas.

All laboratory primates are susceptible to scurvy, which is caused by vitamin C deficiency. Clinical signs include weight loss, weakness, anemia, gingival bleeding, loss of teeth, and increased susceptibility to infectious disease. Primates with a vitamin C deficiency usually succumb to infectious diseases before clinical signs of the deficiency appear (Figure 12-9).

OTHER PROBLEMS

Acute gastric dilatation, also referred to as bloat, has been reported sporadically in NHP colonies. Although the etiology is not fully understood, theories include improper

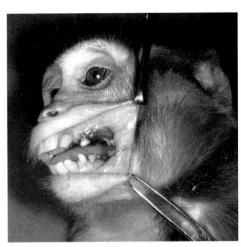

FIGURE 12-9. Ulcerative gingivitis secondary to scurvy (vitamin C deficiency), gingiva, monkey. There is a deep ulcer at the commissure of the mouth and smaller ulcers periodontally. Vitamin C deficiency in primates and guinea pigs can result in gingival erosions and ulcers, and even tooth loss. (From Zachary JF, McGavin MD: *Pathologic basis of veterinary disease*, ed 5, St. Louis, Mosby, 2012.)

husbandry practices and infectious factors. *Clostridium perfringens* has been isolated from the gastric contents of some affected animals. Other suspected causes include accidental overfeeding or overwatering and normal feeding after food restriction. Clinical signs include abdominal distension, shock, and hemorrhage from the nose and mouth. Affected animals may be found dead. Treatment requires relieving the abdominal distension by placing a stomach tube to remove the excess gas and fluid. Antibiotic and fluid therapy are usually prescribed. Control measures include feeding smaller amounts of food more frequently or limiting feeding to the period in which the animals are most active.

Orangutan, baboon, and others have saccular diverticula of the respiratory tract that extend into the subcutis of the neck; in orangutans they are particularly large and reach to the axillae. A wide variety of bacteria, particularly fecal organisms, can cause purulent inflammation of these organs, which clinically results in fluctuant swelling of the neck. In some cases purulent bronchopneumonia results from aspiration of exudate. Treatment for this condition is drainage.

Traumatic injuries, including bite wounds, can occur in any paired or group-housed NHPs. These wounds often become infected with *Staphylococcus, Streptococcus,* or other organisms found in fecal material. Alopecia can be present as a result of self-mutilation or aggression between cagemates. Methods to enhance environmental enrichment should be considered in these cases.

Rhesus monkeys are especially prone to endometriosis, which makes them an excellent animal model for human endometriosis. Although the exact causes are not fully known, the condition is associated with repeated hysterotomies, C-sections, age, and multiple pregnancies; it can also occur without the presence of any of these factors. Clinical signs can be absent, or palpable abdominal masses can occur. Affected animals have uterine enlargement and can develop multiple pelvic adhesions. Eclampsia and preeclampsia, also known as pregnancy toxemia, have been reported in NHPs. The disease is much the same as seen in human women.

EUTHANASIA

Methods of euthanasia vary depending on the species and on whether tissues must be harvested from the animal without contamination from chemical agents. The American Veterinary Medical Association Guidelines for the Euthanasia of Animals discusses only methods and agents for euthanasia supported by data from scientific studies. It emphasizes professional judgment, technical proficiency, and humane handling of the animals. Euthanasia should never be performed in the same room where other animals are housed because this causes unnecessary stress in the remaining animals.

The only acceptable method of euthanasia for NHPs is injectable barbiturate overdose. Conditionally acceptable methods that require approval by the animal care and use committee include inhalant anesthesia overdose and nitrogen, argon, carbon monoxide, or carbon dioxide chamber asphyxiation. In many cases, when postmortem sample collection is not needed, NHPs that are removed from research protocols are sent to primate sanctuaries to live out the rest of their natural lives.

KEY POINTS

- Nonhuman primates are usually grouped into two suborders, the Prosimii and the Anthropoidea.
- Nonhuman primates are used in biomedical research to study acquired immunodeficiency syndrome, viral hepatitis, diabetes mellitus, and atherosclerosis.
- Two common species of nonhuman primates used in biomedical research are the cynomolgus macaque, *Macaca fascicularis,* and the rhesus macaque, *Macaca mulatta.*
- Determination of sex in nonhuman primates species is accomplished by observing the visible external genitalia.
- Several breeding systems are used for nonhuman primates, including timed mating, paired mating, harem mating, and free-range mating systems.
- Facilities that house nonhuman primates must provide programs that promote the psychologic well-being of the animals.
- Housing of nonhuman primates varies for different species and is focused on providing housing mechanisms that allow expression of normal behavior for the species.
- Techniques used for restraint and handling of nonhuman primates species must address the safety of both the handler and the animal.
- There are a large number of bacterial, parasitic, and viral diseases that are transmissible between human beings and nonhuman primates.
- All primates are susceptible to tuberculosis.
- Several herpesviruses can be transmitted between human beings and nonhuman primates.

REVIEW QUESTIONS

1. The scientific name of the rhesus monkey is _____ _____.

2. The scientific name of the chimpanzee is _____ _____.

3. Hard, keratinized pads on the buttocks of most OWPs are referred to as _____ _____.

4. The _____ _____ _____ _____ was created to prepare a national plan for use of NHPs in research and recommendations for review of research proposals.

5. The primate species most often used for studies of atherosclerosis is _____ _____.

6. The Animal Welfare Act classifies simian primates into _____ groups.

7. The bacterial agents most commonly associated with gastroenteritis in NHPs are _____ and _____.

8. The anatomic site typically used for the intradermal tuberculin test in NHPs is _____.

9. The organism that causes oral ulcers in human beings that can cause fatal infections in some NHPs is _____.

10. Contamination of feed has been implicated in the transmission of infection with the organism that causes _____.

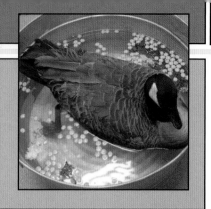

13 Wildlife

LEARNING OBJECTIVES

After studying this chapter, you will be able to:

- Discuss ways to provide nursing care of wildlife.
- Describe regulations and laws concerning wildlife care.
- Describe ways to perform a physical examination.
- Assess the condition of orphaned or injured wild animals.
- Discuss ways to provide supportive care to wild animals.
- Describe methods of sample collection and diagnostic testing for laboratory analysis.
- Identify routes of administration of medication.
- Discuss the ethical treatment and releasability of wild animals.
- Identify potential zoonotic and infectious diseases in common wild animal species.
- Describe the proper use of personal protective equipment.

It is not uncommon for members of the public to find an injured or orphaned native or non-native wild animal on the ground. Generally these individuals are well meaning and want to help the animal get healthy so it can be released back into the wild. If the veterinary hospital decides to take in injured or orphaned wild animals, it must be prepared to not only provide proper housing and diet, it must also provide the animals with experienced staff to safely handle and care for each individual species.

If the veterinary hospital wishes to receive injured or orphaned wildlife from the public or animal control, a specific list of protocols and standard operating procedures (SOPs) need to be written and followed. All clinic members including the front office staff should be aware of the protocols and SOPs. It is very important that all members of the veterinary hospital understand that dealing with injured wildlife can be taxing and emotional. Many animals will have to be euthanized due to injuries that will keep them from returning to the wild. Some wildlife can be placed in permanent wildlife sanctuaries, zoos, or educational centers, but this is rare as many places are already overloaded with common species of wild animals.

The veterinary staff must also be aware of common zoonotic diseases carried by wildlife species. Latex or vinyl exam gloves should be worn while working with wild animals. Proper hygiene as well as keeping the housing facility clean is very important. Wildlife should not be housed with client-owned pets not only because of zoonotic disease potential, but also due to the stress placed on the patients being housed together.

One of the most important services a veterinary hospital can provide is accurate and timely advice over the phone to members of the public. If an adult wild animal can be easily captured and/or picked up by an untrained person, it is very likely that it is sick or injured in some way. Conditions that require immediate medical attention include, but are not limited to, the following:

- Unconsciousness
- Bleeding
- Cold body temperature
- Fractures
- Weakness or inability to stand
- Swelling on head or body
- Seizures
- Eyes closed or matted shut
- Shock
- Puncture wounds
- Maggots present (Figure 13-1)

It is not uncommon for individuals to bring in a healthy, young baby animal that is not necessarily orphaned or injured. Many times people think they are doing the right thing, but in fact they are taking the baby away from the parents when it is not necessary. If the baby is cold, skinny, weak, or if there are dead siblings nearby, the baby is most likely orphaned and needs medical attention. It is important to note that mothers will not abandon their babies simply due to humans touching them. If the baby seems to be warm and strong, it should be returned to where it was found.

If the veterinary hospital is only going to give medical advice over the phone, the staff must provide advice that is medically sound and legal. Some individuals will ask for advice on how to care for the wildlife themselves. It is the responsibility of the veterinary technician or other veterinary staff member to advise the individual that it is illegal and dangerous for nonlicensed personnel to take care of the wild animal.

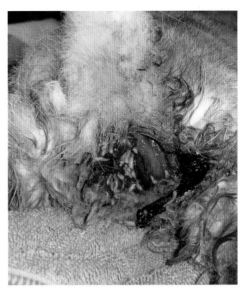

FIGURE 13-1. This rabbit has been infested by maggots. (From Sirois M: *Principles and practice of veterinary technology*, ed 3, St. Louis, Mosby, 2011.)

LEGAL CONCERNS

Native wild animals are protected under a variety of local, state, and federal regulations and laws. It is important for the veterinary hospital to become aware of these regulations and make sure they are followed. Every state has a specific agency responsible for regulating possession of native wildlife. Under many circumstances, a permit is required to work with or possess native wildlife, especially those that are endangered, threatened, or are protected under the Migratory Bird Act. The veterinary practice should develop a relationship with a permitted and licensed rehabilitator or wildlife facility.

> **TECHNICIAN NOTE** The veterinary practice staff must be well versed in the state and local laws related to wildlife that might be seen in your clinic.

INTAKE PROCEDURES AND HISTORY

CAPTURING AND TRANSPORTING WILDLIFE

Capturing a wild animal can sometimes be dangerous. In some cases it may be as easy as simply picking up the animal and placing it in a carrier, but in other instances it may be difficult and require leather gloves, nets, snares, traps, or towels/blankets.

There are a variety of transport cages available to safely transport a wild animal to a veterinary hospital or wildlife center. Anything from a cardboard box to a dog or cat carrier can be used depending on the size and type of the animal being transported. For example, a song bird can be placed in a small box, while a raccoon should be placed in a dog carrier of an appropriate size. When possible, the cage or box should be lined with a towel, indoor/outdoor carpet, or newspaper to help prevent the animal from slipping around

VETERINARY MEDICAL TEACHING HOSPITAL
UNIVERSITY OF CALIFORNIA-DAVIS
WILDLIFE FORM

First name:_____   Home phone:_____

Admission date to VMTH: _____ Time: _____ Date found by Good Samaritan: _____ Time:_____

WNV form received _____ (Initials)

A   Where found:

1   Address, street and city:_____

2   Number of miles from nearest city: _____

3   Description of area or facility found in: (Ex: side of road? In an orchard? Spraying orchard? Barn? A working farm?) _____

4   Was any other wildlife noted in the area at the time? Any interaction with this animal?_____

B   Additional information for stray birds:

1   Species: _____

2   Type of terrain where bird was found: (PLEASE CIRCLE ONE)

Park   Lake   Urban area   Wooded area   Agricultural area   River   Residential area

3   If known-proximity (miles) to sentinel chicken flock:_____

Nearest city or residential area where bird was found:_____

Zip code of bird location: _____County: _____

4   Were any dead birds seen in area where bird was found?   YES   NO

If yes, what species?_____

C   Circumstances of acquisition?

1   What was the animal doing? How was it acting? Attitude?_____

2   How was it caught? _____

D   Was the animal fed?

1   What and how much was offered?_____

2   What and how much did it eat?_____

3   Offered water? _____

4   How much did it drink? _____

E   Any other information or history you can give to help us care for this animal?_____

ACKNOWLEDGMENT

I certify that I do NOT own this animal and understand that the university has sole authority and responsibility for the care and disposition of this animal. I further understand that this animal will NOT be returned to me.

_____
Signature

FIGURE 13-2. Sample intake form. (From Sirois M: *Principles and practice of veterinary technology*, ed 3, St. Louis, Mosby, 2011.)

in the carrier. A towel or blanket can be placed over the carrier to make the environment dark.

The individual capturing the animal should fill out a form giving information about the wild animal (Figure 13-2).

This paperwork should include such information as the address or area where it was found, how it was captured, when the capture occurred, whether the animal was fed, whether any dead wildlife was seen in the area, etc. The wild animal should also have a medical record generated just as if it were a client-owned animal. All physical exam findings, medical procedures, and treatments should be entered into the medical record.

Once the animal has been brought into the hospital or wildlife center, the wild animal should not be handled or looked at in between treatments or feedings. The animal should never be petted, talked to, or played with at any time.

RESTRAINT OF WILDLIFE

Most of the wild animals presented for evaluation are victims of trauma and may have multiple injuries. A complete physical examination is essential. When examining a wild animal, providing supportive care, or obtaining diagnostics, restraint is required for the safety of the patient and the personnel working with the animal. Wild birds have defensive weapons such as beaks and talons and use them when stressed. Many reptiles and mammals can inflict serious bites or scratches. Terry cloth towels, leather welder's gloves, nets, and protective eye wear will be valuable tools to neutralize these weapons.

TECHNICIAN NOTE It is important to properly restrain birds of prey due to their ability to use their beaks and talons for defense. Protective eye wear is a must when working with wading birds such egrets, cranes, and herons.

Capturing a wild animal from a cage needs to be done in a room that can be sealed and has no escape route or hiding places. The door should be locked and the window blinds should be closed. Darkening the room may help reduce the stress of capturing many wild animals. Before capturing any animal, assess how the patient is doing. Some critically ill patients may need time to recover from transport and may need supplemental oxygen prior to restraint. When working with these critically ill patients, it is best to perform your physical exam in stages giving the patient time to recover between those stages. Depending on the species you are working with, general anesthesia may be needed to perform a complete physical examination (Figure 13-3).

RAPTOR CAPTURE AND RESTRAINT

Welder's gloves and a terry cloth towel are often useful when capturing birds of prey. Approach the bird cautiously and place the towel over the patient's head and body. Grasp the bird's body on both sides over the wings and work your hands down to the legs until you have a firm hold on both legs and control of the feet. With the towel remaining over the head and the feet directed away from you, bring the bird to your torso and maintain control of the feet and wings. A stockinette or leather raptor hood can be used to cover the head to reduce stress and restrict vision (Figure 13-4). The legs can be bound together with homemade Velcro® wraps to help retain control of the legs and talons. The use of gloves will reduce the handler's tactile sensation and ability

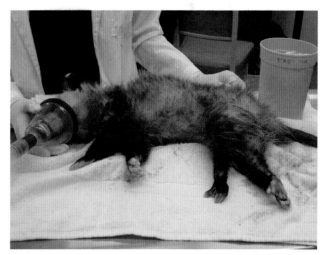

FIGURE 13-3. Wild mammals are generally anesthetized in a chamber or box before physical examination unless they are extremely debilitated. Very sick mammals can be mask-induced, as pictured. (From Sirois M: *Principles and practice of veterinary technology*, ed 3, St. Louis, Mosby, 2011.)

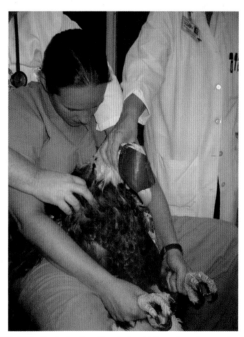

FIGURE 13-4. A leather hood should be placed over the head of the bird to reduce vision and overall stress. (From Sirois M: *Principles and practice of veterinary technology*, ed 3, St. Louis, Mosby, 2011.)

to feel the patients most subtle movements and reactions to the restraint, so once the patient is captured and properly restrained, the leather gloves may be removed.

SMALL WILD BIRD CAPTURE AND RESTRAINT

Small wild birds, such as finches, house sparrows, and scrub jays will frequently present with traumatic injuries after presumably flying into a window or being attacked by a cat. They must be safely and gently restrained for a hands-on physical examination. A small terry cloth or paper towel can be used combined with slow and deliberate movements to minimize stress to the bird. It may be helpful to dim the room lights before proceeding as this calms some birds. To capture, place the towel over the patient, gain control of the head, pin the wings to the body and pick the patient up.

MAMMAL CAPTURE AND RESTRAINT

Capture and restraint of wild mammals will depend on the species you are working with. In many cases, the animal will need to be anesthetized to perform a complete physical examination. If this is the case, the animal is either induced in an anesthetic chamber or in the carrier or cage it is in, or it can be given an intramuscular injection using a syringe pole to sedate or tranquilize it. Once the animal is tranquilized it can be removed from the cage and fully anesthetized. Common wild mammals that need to be anesthetized prior to performing a physical examination include raccoons, canids, most rodents, bats, and any large or potentially aggressive mammal.

> TECHNICIAN NOTE Many wild animals will require anesthesia in order to perform a full examination.

A large towel should be used to help capture wild hares and rabbits. Place the towel on top of the animal and scoop it into your arms while still wrapped in the towel. It is important to note that with improper restraint, rabbits can kick out their hind legs and fracture their backs. In some cases the physical examination can be done with the rabbit covered with the towel. This helps reduce stress to the rabbit. The towel is simply removed from each section of the body as the examination is being performed. In some cases, the rabbit will need to be anesthetized to perform a proper examination. If the rabbit is very sick, young, or calm, all of this may not be needed and the rabbit can be simply restrained by tucking the head between the side of your body and your arm. The other arm should support the rest of the rabbit's body against your own body. Wild hares and rabbits can become very stressed by restraint. Dimmed lights and low voices should be used when possible as this can help reduce stress.

REPTILE CAPTURE AND RESTRAINT

Restraint techniques will vary based on the type of reptile. Exam gloves should be worn when handling these patients because reptiles may shed *Salmonella* spp. bacteria. See Chapter 4 for more details on handling and restraint of reptiles.

Small lizards are generally easy to capture but can be difficult to restrain because they tend to wiggle and squirm while they are being held. Most small lizards can simply be picked up with both hands and taken out of the cage. This is also true of the larger lizard species. If the lizard is aggressive, a towel or blanket along with leather restraint gloves should be used. It is important to remember that lizards can scratch and bite when they are scared or nervous. Wear long sleeves when possible and always keep track of the location of the animal's head. Keeping one hand on the neck, just behind the base of skull, will help prevent getting bitten. Many species of lizards have a natural predatory response to voluntarily "drop" or **autotomize** their tail in an attempt to escape predation. Never capture any species of lizard by their tail.

> TECHNICIAN NOTE Exam gloves should be worn when handling reptiles as they may shed *Salmonella* spp. bacteria.

Most snakes can be easily captured directly out of the carrier or cage they are in. When dealing with nonaggressive snakes, the restrainer can simply pick the animal up and pull it out of the cage. If the snake is aggressive, it may be necessary to use a towel or snake hook along with leather gloves to safely capture it. In these cases, it is easiest to gently toss the towel over the snake and find the head. Once the head has been isolated and restrained, the snake can be safely taken out of the enclosure. If the snake is extremely aggressive or if it is a venomous snake, a snake hook should be used to pin down the head of the snake long enough to safely grasp its head and body. Improper use of the snake hook can cause trauma to the patient; therefore, extreme caution should be taken.

Chelonians are turtles and tortoises. Although chelonians are usually the easiest to capture, they are the often difficult to restrain. Unless working with extremely large tortoises, most chelonians can just be picked up with both hands and placed on the exam table. When examining large tortoises, it is easiest to set up an exam area within the animal's enclosure or on the floor in the hospital's exam area. Because there is so much variation in size and strength, restraint techniques may vary between small and large chelonians. Once the animal's body is under control, it is imperative that the head be properly restrained. Although this is relatively easy when the animal is sick, it can be difficult on strong, healthy chelonians, especially large tortoises and box turtles. There are several ways the restrainer can gain control of the animal's head. Many turtles and tortoises are very curious. If they are set down on the table or the ground, they may just start walking around, allowing the technician to walk up to them and grasp their head with one hand while restraining the body with the other hand. To keep control of the head, it is best to position your thumb on one side of the cranial portion of the neck and position the rest of your fingers (or just the index finger for smaller species) on the other side of the neck just behind the base of the skull. Healthy chelonians are strong, so constant but gentle force may be needed to keep the turtle or tortoise's head out of the shell. Box turtles can be the most challenging chelonians to properly restrain. Because box turtles have a hinge on their **plastron**, many species are able to completely tuck themselves into their shells. The easiest way to extend their head is to gently prop open the cranial portion of the **carapace** (upper shell) and the plastron (lower shell). Extreme care must be taken when trying to prop the shell open. It is suggested that a well-padded object be used when attempting this. This will help avoid traumatizing or fracturing the shell. If initial attempts at capture and restraint are not successful, chemical restraint may be necessary for any reptile, especially large tortoises and box turtles.

PHYSICAL EXAMINATION OF WILDLIFE

As with other exotic species, an initial visual physical examination should be performed prior to the hands-on physical examination. Once the visual examination has been completed, a hands-on physical examination can be completed if indicated. Performing a physical examination on a wild animal is very similar to performing a physical examination on other exotic animals. When performing the physical examination, you should be systematic, proceed in a timely manner, and try to complete the physical portion of the examination quickly. Due to the high stress of many wildlife species, general anesthesia is often required to perform a complete physical examination.

AVIAN

Many wild birds are prey species with survival instincts and frequently alter their behavior when they are in a stressful environment, such as a veterinary hospital. In some cases these birds will mask their symptoms in order to not stand out in their "flock," so they will not be eliminated by a predator or members of their own flock. Covertly evaluate the bird if possible. If the bird does not know it is being watched, it may not be hiding signs of illness. The respiratory rate should be smooth and regular. A healthy bird should show no signs of increased effort. If the bird is exhibiting a tail bob (forward movement of the head or open beak breathing), this could be a sign of respiratory distress and will need immediate attention. Evaluate the **mentation** and stance. If the bird is trying to sleep, not interested in your presence, or laterally recumbent then immediate medical attention is necessary.

> TECHNICIAN NOTE   Birds will often mask symptoms of illness in order to not stand out in their "flock."

MAMMALS

The wild mammal physical examination is performed similarly to other small animals such as dogs and cats. Wild mammals can become easily stressed so it is essential to keep the restraint time to a minimum when necessary. Perform a visual examination then obtain the patient's weight and temperature. Since many of the wild mammal patients are very small, it is best to use a scale that weighs to the nearest gram (Figure 13-5). Many wild mammals will need to be heavily sedated or placed under general anesthesia to perform a complete physical examination.

> TECHNICIAN NOTE   A visual physical examination should be performed prior to performing the hands-on physical examination.

REPTILES

Performing a physical examination on reptiles is similar to performing a physical examination on most mammalian species. Perform a visual precapture and restraint physical examination. During the physical exam, make sure to get an accurate heart rate and respiratory rate. A heart rate is most

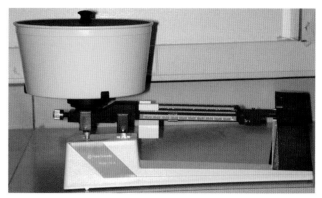

FIGURE 13-5. A gram scale should be used to weigh small wildlife patients. (From Sirois M: *Principles and practice of veterinary technology,* ed 3, St. Louis, Mosby, 2011.)

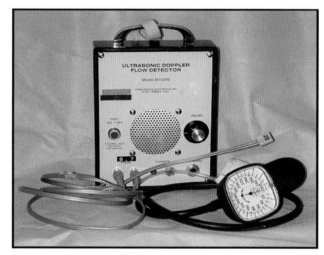

FIGURE 13-6. A Doppler is an essential instrument used to obtain a heart rate in reptilian species. (From Sirois M: *Principles and practice of veterinary technology,* ed 3, St. Louis, Mosby, 2011.)

easily obtained by using a Doppler® (Figure 13-6). Most reptile patients cannot be auscultated with a stethoscope; therefore, a Doppler® is an essential tool to have in your practice. In lizards the Doppler® probe should generally be placed in the same area a stethoscope would be placed on a dog or cat. In chelonians, the Doppler® probe is either placed into the thoracic inlet (on either the left or right side) or on the neck over the carotid artery. In snakes the Doppler® is placed directly over the heart. In most species of snake, the heart is located in the cranial one third of the body. Both the heart and respiratory rates are obtained by simply counting the number of beats and breaths per minute.

SAMPLE COLLECTION AND DIAGNOSTIC TESTING FOR LABORATORY ANALYSIS

Diagnostic procedures that may be needed when working with wildlife include:
- Blood smears
- Fecal flotation and direct smear
- Gram stain
- Tracheal wash

- Cloacal wash
- Nasal flush
- Stomach lavage
- Skin scrape and touch smear
- Dermatologic tape preparation

ADMINISTRATION OF MEDICATIONS AND FLUIDS

BIRDS

The intramuscular and subcutaneous routes are the most common routes for administration of medications. Due to the renal-portal system, injections should only be given cranial to the kidneys. Injections are most often given into the pectoral muscles.

The intravenous route can be used as needed in many species. An indwelling catheter or single injections can be given into the medial metatarsal, cutaneous ulnar, or jugular veins. The oral route is often used to administer medications. Oral medications can be given using a feeding tube or just titrated in with a syringe (Figure 13-7).

MAMMALS

Intramuscular injections are given in the same manner as in dogs and cats. Remember to aspirate the syringe to ensure you are not in a vessel prior to giving the injection. Subcutaneous injections are given in the same manner as in a dog or cat. Larger volumes of fluids can be given in this site. The injection is usually given in the subcutaneous space between the shoulder blades. The patient will need to be held by another technician prior to giving the injection. It is preferred to use a butterfly catheter instead of a regular needle. An 18- to 27-gauge needle can be used based on the size of the patient. The skin should be tented with one hand while the other hand places the needle under the skin and then gives the injection. It is important to aspirate prior to giving the injection to ensure you are in the correct spot. You should not aspirate blood or air. If this happens, start over in a different location.

Intravenous injection of drugs can be difficult in most awake wild mammals. Intraveous injections can be given in the cephalic, saphenous, jugular, or auricular (usually rabbits only) veins. It is important to have the proper syringe and needle size for the injection you are giving. In most cases, a 1.0-ml or insulin syringe with a 27- to 25-gauge needle should be used. Intraveous injections are given in the same manner as in dogs and cats. Intramuscular injections are commonly given in the lumbar or quadriceps muscles. Another technician should properly restrain the patient while the injection is given. Oral medications can be mixed with food or just given orally via a syringe. Putting medications in food is often the best way to medicate wild animals because this causes the least amount of stress.

REPTILES

The intramuscular and subcutaneous routes are the most common routes for administration of medications. Due to

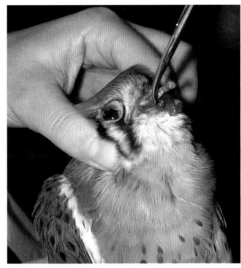

FIGURE 13-7. Wild birds can be fed using a syringe, pipette, forceps (as seen in this picture), or be tube fed using a red rubber feeding tube or metal feeding tube. (From Sirois M: *Principles and practice of veterinary technology*, ed 3, St. Louis, Mosby, 2011.)

the renal-portal system, only the front limbs should be used for intramuscular injections. The intravenous route is rarely used, but administration of fluids and some medications can be given in reptiles. An indwelling catheter can also be placed for continuous fluid therapy replacement, but this can be very difficult.

The intracoelomic route can be used for administration of fluids. The patient should be placed in lateral recumbency with the hind leg extended away from the body. The needle is then placed under the skin and into the coelomic cavity. You must aspirate prior to administering any fluids. If the needle is placed into the wrong spot, fluids could accidentally be given into the bladder or into the lungs both of which are detrimental.

Intraosseous fluids can be given in many lizard species. In lizards, a 25- to 20-gauge spinal needle is placed into the distal portion of the femur or humerus or into the proximal portion of the tibia. A spinal needle is preferred because the stylet will help keep the needle from becoming clogged from a bone core fragment. The catheter is placed using aseptic technique and is sutured to the skin for stability. It is then bandaged to protect the catheter site. This procedure is painful and requires either sedation with analgesia, general anesthesia, or the use of a local anesthetic.

The oral route is often used to administer medications. If the gastrointestinal tract works, feel free to use it! Oral medications can be given using a feeding tube or just titrated in with a syringe.

SUPPORTIVE CARE OF WILD ANIMALS IN THE HOSPITAL

RAPTORS

Raptors receive most of their water intake from the prey they eat; therefore, if they are not readily eating, they can become dehydrated. Fluid therapy and/or force feeding should be considered while in the hospital if the patient is not eating on its own. The most common fluid given to raptors is Lactated Ringer's Solution (LRS) subcutaneously at a dose of 50 to 60 mL/kg/day. Fluids are generally given in the inguinal area. In some cases, IV fluid therapy can be initiated. If the patient is not eating on its own, it needs to be force fed. This can be done either by defrosting and chopping up (if necessary) pieces of mice, rats, fish, or chicks (depends on the species you are working with) or using a manufactured food such as Oxbow Carnivore Care®. Prey is fed by either using tongs to offer the prey or just using your finger to place the prey into the mouth. If a commercial formula is used, it is delivered using a feeding tube. This is done in the same manner as a pet parrot although a rubber feeding tube is generally chosen over the use of the metal tubes usually used with parrots. The mouth is opened and the tube in placed into the distal esophagus. The food should be delivered at a slow pace, watching the back of the mouth to ensure the food is not coming back up the esophagus. If this happens the tube should be pulled out and the bird placed immediately back into the cage. When pulling the tube out of the mouth, the tube should be pinched off so that any residual food is not draped across the glottis causing aspiration. Ideally, babies should be fed using a bird puppet.

> **TECHNICIAN NOTE** Raptors that are not eating on their own will need to be force fed.

Many species of birds only molt new feathers one time per year; therefore, it is extremely important to protect the feathers from being damaged or broken. Multiple missing or broken feathers can prevent the bird from being released back into the wild in timely fashion.

Tail feathers are only replaced about once per year, so it is very important that they are not damaged. Wrapping them with paper packing tape or x-ray film protects them from getting broken.

> **TECHNICIAN NOTE** If the raptor is going to be in the clinic for several days, the tail should be wrapped.

Most metal dog and cat cages can be used for short-term housing of raptors in the veterinary clinic. The cage should be lined with newspaper and most commonly bricks covered with indoor-outdoor carpet are used as perches (Figure 13-8). Bricks are easy to clean, and the indoor-outdoor carpet can be thrown away after the patient has left. The front of the cage should be covered with newspaper as well. This provides a visual barrier between the patient and the rest of the hospital. Adults can be kept at room temperature, but small babies need to be kept much warmer.

NONRAPTORIAL BIRDS

There are many diets and formulas that can be used to provide nutrition to growing songbirds and waterfowl.

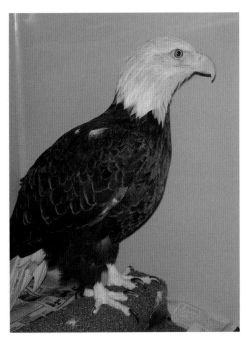

FIGURE 13-8. A common raptor cage setup includes a perch covered in indoor/outdoor carpet. The cage is lined with newspaper. (From Sirois M: *Principles and practice of veterinary technology*, ed 3, St. Louis, Mosby, 2011.)

A maintenance-soaked dog food can be used for short-term feeding in songbirds, but a more nutritional formula should be used for long-term care. Forceps, syringes, pipettes, tongue depressors, and toothpicks can all be used to feed small song birds. Most babies are easy to feed because movement or tapping them on the beak will cause them to gap their mouths open. Care must be taken not to overfeed the bird during each feeding. If the patient is dehydrated, fluids such as LRS should be given at a dose of 50-60 mL/kg/day subcutaneously in the inguinal area. In some cases IV fluid therapy can be initiated.

Song birds should be housed in cages that either have small wire mesh or a dog/cat carrier that they cannot get stuck in or fly through. Perches such as covered bricks, wood branches, or covered PVC pipes can be used. The fronts and sides of the cages should also be covered with newspaper to help keep the stress level down and to provide a visual barrier.

If you are housing water birds such as ducks, geese, and swans you need to provide a swim tank or pool of some sort for them (Figure 13-9).

> **TECHNICIAN NOTE** Water birds must be provided with a place to swim while in the veterinary hospital.

MAMMALS

Mammals can be kept in either a dog/cat carrier (small mammals) or a regular metal dog/cat cage. Again the front and/or sides of the cage should be covered to reduce stress and provide a visual barrier for the animal. Diets will depend on the species you are working with and again there are many diets

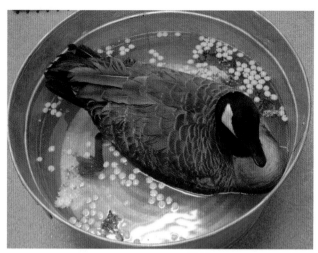

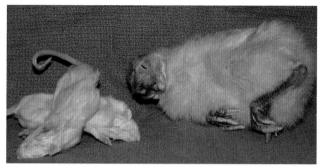

FIGURE 13-10. Prekilled prey items rather than live prey should always be offered to patients such as snakes or carnivorous lizards. (From Sirois M: *Principles and practice of veterinary technology*, ed 3, St. Louis, Mosby, 2011.)

FIGURE 13-9. Waterfowl kept in the hospital should have an area in which to swim on a daily basis. (From Sirois M: *Principles and practice of veterinary technology*, ed 3, St. Louis, Mosby, 2011.)

and formulations available. You will often see that each veterinary hospital and each wildlife center often uses a slightly different formula. It does not really matter what formula is used as long as it is nutritionally sound. It is important for mammalian patients to maintain normal hydration while hospitalized. Assessing dehydration is done in the same manner as in dogs and cats. Fluid therapy should be initiated if the patient is dehydrated. Administering subcutaneous fluids is the most common route used in wild mammals. The fluid rate ranges from 60 to 100 mL/kg/day. LRS is the most commonly administered fluid. Intravenous fluid therapy can be initiated under some circumstances.

REPTILES
Snakes
All snakes are carnivores and feed on whole prey items. The digestive system of snakes has evolved to digest whole prey and defecate the parts of the prey that are not digested such as fur. Ingesting the entire carcass provides added nutrients such as calcium from the bone. Further supplementation is not needed when feeding whole prey. It is never appropriate to feed meat such as chicken breast, hot dogs, or raw beef because this does not provide a complete diet.

It is suggested that prekilled or stunned food be offered to snakes so they will not be harmed by the prey item. Prekilled food can be ordered frozen from several companies. If frozen mice/rats are offered, they must be thawed first (Figure 13-10).

TECHNICIAN NOTE Prekilled or stunned prey should be offered to snakes so they will not be harmed by the prey item.

Lizards
Feeding requirements are based on the type of lizard you are working with. Lizards can be carnivores, herbivores,

insectivores, or omnivores. Herbivores should be fed various types of dark leafy greens and vegetables. Proper leafy greens include, but are not limited to, kale, chard, turnip greens, and escarole. Most insectivores can eat such insects as mealworms, silkworms and crickets. Carnivorous lizards should be fed whole prey. Whole prey includes all the bones, GI contents, muscle, and fur. Whole prey items include mice, rats, rabbits, guinea pigs, and fish (depending on the species you are feeding). Omnivores should be offered a variety of both dark leafy greens and in most cases insects. The quality and variety of food offered is important. Animals should not be fed the same food day after day.

Chelonians
Most aquatic turtles are omnivores, eating fish, invertebrates, algae, leafy greens, etc. Commercial diets are acceptable to feed in moderation, but it is important to make sure they contain essential nutrients needed to maintain good health. Tortoises are herbivores and eat a variety of leaves, grasses, and flowers in the wild. In captivity a healthy diet includes dark, leafy greens, rose petals, hay, and vegetables. Commercial diets can be fed in moderation and should be appropriate for herbivores. Do not feed dog food, tofu, monkey biscuits, or anything that has animal protein in it.

TECHNICIAN NOTE Tortoises are herbivores and eat a variety of leaves, grasses, flowers, etc. in the wild.

If a reptile patient is dehydrated, fluid therapy should be implemented. Assessing dehydration in reptiles is very similar to assessing dehydration in dogs and cats. Evaluate the mucous membranes. Dehydration is indicated when the mucous membranes are dry, pale, and have mucous strands draping from the top to the bottom of the mouth. Note that some reptiles, especially snakes, may have paler mucous membranes then mammals do. Skin elasticity and position of the eyes in the orbits can also be used to assess dehydration. The same techniques used on dogs and cats can be used for most reptiles. If the animal is dehydrated, fluid therapy should be considered and a percentage of dehydration should be estimated for the animal. Accurately estimating percent dehydration for any reptile is based on experience and using the above-mentioned characteristics such as skin tenting, looking at the eyes, and examining the mucous membranes. Fluid therapy routes in reptiles include oral administration, subcutaneous, intracoelomic, intraosseous, and intravenous (although IV fluid therapy can be difficult) fluid administration. Soaking the animal in a tub of warm water (appropriate temperatures will depend on the species) can also be used in conjunction with other fluid therapy routes to help with hydration. Common fluids used in reptiles include LRS and Normosol-R. Maintenance fluid rates in reptiles range from 10 to 30 mL/kg/day.

FOOD PREP

All food should be made just prior to feeding. Even food that sits in the refrigerator long enough can become a heaven for bacterial growth. It is also essential to have proper diets for each species you are working with.

FEEDING FREQUENCY

Baby birds are fed sunup to sundown by the parents. Although it my be hard to feed babies frequently during the day in a busy hospital, it is very important that time is made.

- Hatchlings should be fed every 10-20 minutes
- Nestlings should be fed every 20-30 minutes
- Fledglings should be fed every 45-60 minutes
- Juveniles should be fed every 2 hours
- Birds may not eat at every feeding, but you should still offer food

ETHICAL TREATMENT AND RELEASABILITY OF WILD ANIMALS

The same euthanasia techniques used with other exotic and domestic animals are used on wildlife as well. The animal should be sedated or anesthetized prior to giving the intravenous injection of the barbiturate euthanasia solution. The euthanasia can also be given intraperitoneal (IP) or directly into the heart. Giving the euthanasia solution IP will take longer to become effective. If you are giving the euthanasia solution into the heart, the animal must be anesthetized! It is unethical to give a cardiac injection of euthanasia solution into an animal if it is not anesthetized. If you are working with threatened or endangered species that require euthanasia, you should contact the state fish and wildlife department for permission because there may be rules and regulations regarding euthanasia of these species.

It is unlawful for people to possess bald or golden eagles or their parts. If a bald or golden eagle is euthanized in a veterinary hospital, it should be sent to the national eagle repository for use by federally recognized Native Americans tribes. (National eagle repository: www.fws .gov/mountain-praire/law/eagle/)

If an animal is determined to be non-releasable, it can be placed into a zoo, wildlife education center, or raptor center if they have the proper permits. This can be a daunting task as many facilities already have common species of wild animals.

IMMOBILIZING FRACTURES

Any fracture should be immobilized as soon as possible and pain medications should be provided. The same rules of fracture stabilization used with dogs and cats are used with wild animals as well. The joint above the fracture site and the joint below the fracture site must be stabilized to properly stabilize the fracture. A tape splint can be used to stabilize leg fractures in small song birds. Figure-eight bandages are used in birds that either have a wing fracture or an injury to the wing causing a droop. The figure-eight bandage by itself is used to stabilize a fracture of the radius and/or ulna because the bandage supports the elbow and wrist joints. If the bird has a fracture of the humerus, a body wrap must be placed because the shoulder joint must be stabilized. Stabilization of fractures in mammals and reptiles utilizes techniques similar to those used in dogs and cats.

> **TECHNICIAN NOTE** Figure-eight bandages are used in birds that have a wing fracture.

CHEMICAL RESTRAINT AND ANESTHESIA

It is important to become comfortable with chemical restraint and anesthesia in common wildlife patients that may present to the veterinary clinic. When possible, a premedication should be used to sedate or tranquilize the patient prior to inducing general anesthesia. This will generally produce a smoother induction. Due to the high stress experienced by these patients, the most common way to induce anesthesia is by chamber or box induction. Isoflurane and sevoflurane in oxygen are the two most common inhalation agents used to rapidly and safely induce anesthesia. Mask induction can be used for patients such as birds that can be physically restrained. Many reptile species can be induced using propofol intravenously. Injectable drugs such as ketamine, dexmedetomidine, xylazine, telazol, buprenorphine, butorphanol, and midazolam can be used alone or in combination with each other to sedate or induce anesthesia. The type of species and procedure being performed will determine the appropriate drug combination. A current exotic animal formulary should be consulted prior to giving any anesthetic agent.

Once anesthesia is induced, endotracheal intubation is performed when possible and an intravenous catheter is placed to provide fluid therapy throughout the anesthetic period. Anesthetic maintenance for wild mammals is similar to that for dogs and cats. At minimum the blood pressure (direct or indirect), heart rate, respiratory rate, and temperature should be monitored. Other monitoring techniques include the use of a pulse oximeter, end-tidal CO_2, and electrocardiogram.

Anesthetic recovery can be very stressful for wild animals. Recovery should take place in a dark, warm, and quiet room. The area should be padded to help prevent further injury to the patient. Recovery is generally quick when maintaining on isoflurane or sevoflurane in oxygen. Injectable drugs such as xylazine and dexmedetomidine can be easily reversed. Postoperative pain medications should be administered to provide analgesia in patients recovering from painful procedures. Common postoperative pain medications include butorphanol, buprenorphine, nonsteroidal antiinflammatory drugs, and full mu opioids. Food and water should be offered to the patient once it has recovered from the anesthetic procedure.

STABILIZATION OR LONG-TERM REHABILITATION

Most veterinary hospitals are not set up for long-term rehabilitation, and most places do not have the proper permits to house wild animals for more than a few days. Long-term rehabilitation should take place only if the hospital has a quiet area for the animal to rest, recover, and/or grow. Short-term care (meaning a few days or so) can be provided by many hospitals. Once the animal is brought into the clinic, it should be stabilized and then sent to a licensed wildlife rehabilitation center or rehabilitator as soon as possible. It is very important that the clinic have a clear understanding of the role it is going to play.

ETHICAL TREATMENT AND RELEASABILITY OF WILD ANIMALS

The concept of **releasability** must be considered for every wild animal that is triaged in the veterinary hospital. The overall goal of wildlife medicine and rehabilitation is to release the animal back to the wild so that it can thrive and continue to breed. During the physical examination, one must consider the injuries sustained by the animal and determine whether this animal will be successfully returned to the wild.

> **TECHNICIAN NOTE** The overall goal of wildlife medicine and rehabilitation is to release the animal back to the wild.

It is important to know what types of injuries warrant euthanasia and what types of injuries warrant rehabilitation. Some injuries are much more obvious than others. The patient must be releasable and be able to thrive in the wild. The following common injuries may require euthanasia. Some of them may be more detrimental for certain species (Figure 13-11).

- Compound or open fracture that is more than 24 to 48 hours old
- Complete loss of sight or hearing in any wild animal species
- Impaired vision in one or both eyes
- Nocturnal owls with hearing impairment in one or both ears
- Amputation or partial amputation of a wing or leg

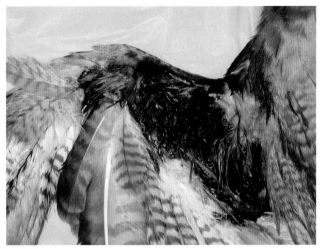

FIGURE 13-11. This red-tailed hawk (*Buteo jamaicensis*) exhibits classic signs of electrocution. Electrocution carries a poor prognosis. (From Sirois M: *Principles and practice of veterinary technology*, ed 3, St. Louis, Mosby, 2011.)

- Any injury to the foot or digits that impairs raptors from hunting and catching prey
- Fractures near a joint such as the elbow or shoulder
- Open fractures with a significant piece of bone missing
- Severe head trauma
- Back injuries that result in loss of limb function
- Animals that have imprinted to humans
- Animals that have an incurable infectious disease
- Mammals with two or more nonfunctional legs
- A rabies vector species from a rabies endemic area
- Rodents or rabbits with a fractured jaw or trauma to the teeth
- Electrocution
- Avian pox virus

DISEASES IN COMMON WILD ANIMALS

Wildlife present to the veterinary clinic for a variety of reasons including various bacterial, fungal, and viral infections; ingesting toxins; trauma including being hit by car, electrocution, being attacked by another animal, gunshot wounds, and fractures. Treatment will vary based on the extent of the injuries and the species you are working with. Listed below are some of the common diseases and presentations of various wildlife species.

Birds of prey commonly present to the veterinary hospital for a variety of different traumatic injuries including gunshot wounds, being hit by a car, flying into a window, being attacked by another animal, and electrocution. Other presentations may include bacterial, viral, fungal, or parasitic infections.

The most common presentation for nonraptorial birds is trauma. Common traumatic injuries include flying into a window, being attacked by a cat or dog, and gunshot wounds. Other common presentations include ingestion of toxic substances. Common presentations for reptiles include trauma such as being hit by a car, being attacked by another animal, fractures, and open wounds. All reptiles can carry *Salmonella* species of bacteria. Contact with reptiles has been directly implicated in human Salmonellosis outbreaks, and the reptiles typically exhibit no signs of illness themselves. Other zoonotic disease potential exists but is not common. Latex or vinyl gloves should be worn at all times when handling reptile species.

Mammals present to the veterinary hospital for a variety of reasons including trauma, bacterial, viral, fungal, and parasitic infections. Common traumatic injuries are caused by being hit by a car, attacked by another animal, and gunshot wounds.

Proper infectious disease precautions should be implemented when allowing a raccoon into your clinic. Raccoons act as a reservoir for rabies in the United States. No parenteral vaccine is approved for use in raccoons, so care must be taken not to be bitten in the clinic.

> **TECHNICIAN NOTE** Raccoons act as a reservoir for rabies in the United States.

Raccoons are carriers of *Balisascaris procyonis*, an intestinal roundworm that is zoonotic to humans. People become infected when they accidentally ingest infected soil, water, or objects contaminated with raccoon feces. Once ingested, the eggs hatch into larvae and travel throughout the body, affecting the organs and muscles. This infection can be fatal.

Raccoons are susceptible to contracting canine and feline distemper. Care should be taken not to carry this disease to your other patients in the hospital. *Trypanosoma cruzi*, *rickettsia rickettsii*, leptospirosis, *Salmonella* spp., are organisms also commonly found in raccoons. Due to the zoonotic potential of many common diseases carried by raccoons, personal protective equipment including gloves, gowns, and goggles should be worn during handling.

Opossums have an impressive immune system and a lower than average body temperature. Because of this, they do not carry many of the standard zoonotic diseases that other animals carry. Although an opossum might carry rabies, it is very unlikely. However, opossums do often carry fleas and other parasites and the potential diseases that go along with those.

Like all animals, squirrels can carry a multitude of parasites. Their droppings are associated with *Leptospirosis* spp. and *Salmonella* spp. Squirrels can also be vectors for the rabies virus; therefore, care must be taken when handling. Bubonic plague is caused by the bacterium *Yersenia pestis* and can be found in rodents. Fleas transmit plague from animal to animal.

One common zoonotic disease found in wild rabbits and hares is tularemia (also known as rabbit fever). Tularemia is a serious infectious disease caused by *Franciella tularensis* spp. This disease is found in lagomorphs in North America and is highly virulent for humans and domestic rabbits. The organism can penetrate intact undamaged skin. In humans

the bacteria rapidly grow in the blood, produce high fever, and can lead to death if the condition goes undiagnosed and untreated.

Bats are the only true flying mammal. Worldwide they are primary predators of a vast number of insect pests and thus help to control insect populations. Bats are actually the most common transmitter of the rabies virus in North America. According to the Centers for Disease Control and Prevention, most of the recent human rabies cases in the United States have been caused by rabies virus from bats.

Armadillos are not really a concern for infectious diseases in people except for one curious note. Many wild armadillos have been known to be infected with *Mycobacterium leprae*, the bacterium that causes leprosy (Hansen's disease). Transmission is through excessive handling or eating the armadillo meat.

Common diseases found in various wild canids include sarcoptic mange, rabies, canine distemper, and parvovirus. Proper precautions should be taken not only to protect yourself against these diseases but to also protect domestic species hospitalized in the clinic.

TOXICOSIS

Heavy Metal Toxicosis

Lead poisoning is common and is caused by ingestion of lead shot used as fisherman's weights or shotgun pellets found in wetlands. Lead shot in other tissues, such as from a gunshot wound, is not a cause of systemic lead toxicosis. Zinc toxicity can occur from ingesting galvanized metal or some coins.

Botulism

The causative agent is *Clostridium botulinum* and is an intoxication rather than an infectious disease. It is contracted by ingestion of the toxin and can be responsible for large die-offs of migrating waterfowl.

Algal Toxins

Freshwaters exposed to warm temperatures can suffer explosive blooms of toxin-producing phytoplankton usually resulting from blue-green algae. Very high concentrations of toxins can occur, which can be neurotoxic and hepatotoxic.

OILED BIRDS

Major oil spills that pollute the sea with crude or heavy fuel (bunker oil) are major environmental problems that affect the surface-swimming and diving birds. Birds that swim into an oil slick can get covered with oil, coating the feather structure and causing loss of waterproofing, insulation, and buoyancy. Birds will vigorously preen their feathers in an attempt to remove the oil and become toxic. The toxicity of different oils varies greatly, and the degree of toxic effect depends on the volume ingested. Hypothermia, dehydration, emaciation, and electrolyte imbalances can occur and need to be treated. Only when the bird is stable can the bathing begin because the process itself is stressful.

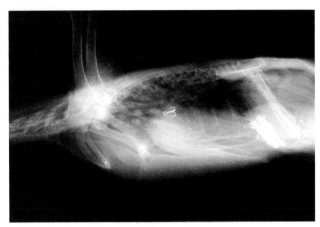

FIGURE 13-12. A treble hook was swallowed by a wild duck. It was later removed using a flexible endoscope. (From Sirois M: *Principles and practice of veterinary technology*, ed 3, St. Louis, Mosby, 2011.)

The recommended detergent used worldwide is Dawn dish soap (Proctor and Gamble) as a 2% solution. A good source for further information is International Bird Rescue Research Center at www.ibrrc.org/.

FISHING TACKLE INJURIES

Birds that present with a fishing line hanging from the mouth should be examined for entanglement externally around the limbs, neck, or beak. Patients should then be radiographed to determine what the bird ingested: hook, weight, or lure (Figure 13-12).

ZOONOTIC AND INFECTIOUS DISEASES IN COMMON WILD ANIMALS SPECIES

Zoonotic diseases are those diseases communicable from animals to humans under natural conditions. Many such diseases are known to exist, and wildlife serves as a reservoir for many of those diseases common to domestic animals and humans (Box 13-1). As professionals in the field of veterinary medicine, we should be alert to the potential for disease transmission from animals. It is important to educate ourselves and the public on this issue. At most you should have no reason to be alarmed or frightened, but should respect the potential for disease transmission and use sound preventive measures. In general, disease is more easily prevented than treated. The diseases discussed below are grouped according to their causative agent or mode of transmission.

RABIES

Rabies is an infectious viral disease that affects the nervous system of humans and other mammals. This virus causes acute encephalitis and eventual death. People get rabies from the bite of an animal with rabies (a rabid animal). Any wild mammal, like a raccoon, skunk, fox, coyote, or bat, can have rabies and transmit it to people. It is also possible, but quite rare, that people may get rabies if infectious material from

---

BOX 13-1   Common Zoonotic Diseases Associated with Wildlife

Bacterial Diseases
- *Chlamydophila psittaci*
- *Salmonella* spp.
- *Campylobacter* spp.
- *Escherichia coli*
- *Staphylococcus aureus*
- *Bacillus anthracis*
- *Streptococcus* spp.
- *Mycobacterium* spp.
- *Leptospira interrogans*
- *Clostridium* spp.
- *Francisella tularensis*
- *Yersinia pestis*
- *Yersinia pseudotuberculosis*
- *Rickettsia rickettsii*
- *Borrelia burgdorferi*

Fungal Diseases
- *Aspergillus* spp.
- *Histoplasma* spp.
- *Blastomyces* spp.

Viral Diseases
- Rabies
- West Nile virus
- Avian influenza
- St. Louis encephalitis
- Eastern equine encephalitis

Parasitic Diseases
- *Giardia* spp.
- *Cryptosporidium parvum*
- *Baylisascaris procyonis*
- *Ancylostoma* spp.
- *Sarcoptes* spp.
- *Encephalitozoon cuniculi*
- *Toxoplasma gondii*

From Sirois M: *Principles and practice of veterinary technology*, ed 3, St. Louis, Mosby, 2011.

a rabid animal, such as saliva, gets directly into their eyes, nose, mouth, or a wound.

SALMONELLOSIS

Salmonellosis is a bacterial disease caused by *Salmonella* spp. bacteria. *Salmonella* spp. exists in virtually all wildlife droppings, and several serotypes are pathogenic to humans and other animals. Salmonellosis can lead to severe cases of gastroenteritis, enteric fever septicemia (blood poisoning), and death. One common means of transmission is through food contaminated by the feces of animals contaminated with the *Salmonella* spp.

CHLAMYDIOSIS

Chlamydiosis is caused by the obligate intracellular bacterium, *Chlamydophila psittaci*. This is a zoonotic intracellular bacterial organism that causes the disease psittacosis in humans and avian chlamydiosis in avian species. The infectious agent is often transmitted by inhaling the organism from dried feces or feather dust from the infected bird.

LEPTOSPIROSIS

Leptospirosis is caused by the bacteria of the genus *Leptospira*. It affects a wide variety of wildlife species, including rodents, skunks, and raccoons. Human cases of leptospirosis usually occur as a result of exposure to urine of infected animals. In some cases, this disease can be very serious and life threatening. Symptoms include fever, headaches, weakness, and vomiting.

HANTAVIRUS PULMONARY SYNDROME (HPS)

Hantavirus pulmonary syndrome, first discovered in 1993, is a deadly disease contracted from rodents caused by the hantavirus. Rodents such as rats and mice are the primary vectors for viruses in this group, and these viruses are found across the United States. Humans can contract the disease by coming into contact with the urine, feces, and saliva of infected rodents. The droppings from infected rodents are believed to be the source of both airborne and direct transmission to other rodents and humans.

BUBONIC PLAGUE

Bubonic plague is best known as the manifestation of the bacterial disease plague caused by the bacterium *Yersenia pestis*. Bubonic plague is an infection of the lymphatic system resulting from a bite of an infected flea. These fleas can be found on wild rodents, most commonly rats. Fleas transmit plague from animal to animal. Early symptoms of bubonic plague include fever, confusion, and fatigue. Untreated bubonic plague has a relatively high fatality rate.

TULAREMIA

Tularemia is caused by *Franciella tularensis* and is a severe bacterial disease carried by rodents that is readily transmissible to humans who come into contact with contaminated food or droppings. The organism can penetrate intact, undamaged skin. In humans the bacteria rapidly grow in the blood, produce high fever, and can lead to death if the condition goes undiagnosed and untreated.

WEST NILE VIRUS

West Nile virus is a virus of the family *Flaviviridae*. This virus is a mosquito-borne disease that infects horses, humans, birds, dogs, cats, bats, chipmunks, skunks, squirrels, and domestic rabbits. It has spread rapidly throughout the United States in the past few years. This can be a serious, life-altering, and even fatal disease. Clinical signs may include depression, anorexia, weakness, recumbency, weight loss, and neurologic signs.

ISOLATION CAGING AREA—PREVENTING THE SPREAD OF DISEASE IN THE CLINIC

Wildlife patients have a high risk of exposure to infectious diseases and can harbor various bacterial, fungal, viral, and parasitic diseases that can be transmitted to domestic pets. It is imperative that you disinfect well between patients. Wildlife suspected of having infectious diseases must be isolated from other patients. Isolation areas must be out of the mainstream of the clinic, where there is minimal foot traffic. Ideally the isolation room should have a ventilation system separate from the main clinic system. Disposable protective shoe covers or foot baths (sodium hypochlorite 10% solution) must be used when exiting this room to prevent the tracking of infectious diseases throughout the hospital. Foot baths should be changed daily or as needed because organic debris can accumulate in the bath and render the foot bath useless.

All veterinary team members who handle animals suspected of having a zoonotic or any infectious disease must wear personal protective equipment not only to protect themselves against infection but also to prevent transmission to others. Personal protective equipment includes disposable outer garments or coveralls, disposable head or hair covers and gloves, safety goggles, and disposable particulate respirators approved by the National Institute for Occupational Safety and Health. Disposable equipment should be considered contaminated and be properly disposed of after use. Nondisposable items such as lab coats and goggles should be cleaned and disinfected between uses. When removing contaminated protective equipment, personnel should remove their outer garments—except for gloves—first and discard them. They should then remove their gloves, wash their hands with soap and water, remove their goggles and particulate respirators, and immediately wash their hands again. If soap and water are not available, an alcohol-based hand gel is sufficient. Washing your hands is the number one way to prevent the spread of disease, so do it between each patient regardless of whether the patient is suspect for carrying infectious diseases. Using these protective measures will help prevent the spread of disease in your clinic and protect those working with the patients.

KEY POINTS

- A specific list of protocols and standard operating procedures (SOPs) need to be written and followed for all wildlife species that the veterinary clinic agrees to treat.
- Latex or vinyl exam gloves should be worn while working with wild animals.
- Native wild animals are protected under a variety of local, state, and federal regulations and laws.
- The individual capturing the animal should fill out an intake form giving information about the wild animal.
- Personal protective equipment is vital when working with wildlife.
- In many cases, wild animals will need to be anesthetized in order to perform the physical examination.
- An initial visual physical examination of wildlife should be performed prior to the hands-on physical examination.
- Birds will often mask symptoms of illness in order to not stand out in their "flock."

- Diagnostic procedures that may be needed when working with wildlife include blood smears, fecal flotation and direct smear, Gram stain, tracheal wash, cloacal wash, nasal flush, stomach lavage, skin scrape, and touch imprint.
- The intramuscular and subcutaneous routes are the most common routes for administration of medications in birds and reptiles.
- Fluid therapy and/or force feeding should be considered for raptor species while in the hospital if the patient is not eating on its own.
- Forceps, syringes, pipettes, tongue depressors, and toothpicks can all be used to feed small song birds.
- Water birds must be provided with a place to swim while in the veterinary hospital. Feed prekilled or stunned food to snakes so they will not be harmed by the prey item.
- The overall goal of wildlife medicine and rehabilitation is to release the animal back to the wild so that it can thrive and continue to breed.
- Wildlife present to the veterinary clinic for a variety of reasons including various bacterial, fungal, and viral infections; ingesting toxins; and trauma including being hit by a car, electrocution, being attacked by another animal, gunshot wounds, and fractures.

REVIEW QUESTIONS

1. If a hospital decides to accept and treat orphaned or injured wildlife, the entire staff must be aware of _____ and _____ in place for care and treatment of wildlife.

2. The veterinary staff must be versed in the _____, _____, and _____ laws in the area regarding wildlife.

3. Upon intake of a wild animal, the hospital must gather what information?

4. _____ _____ _____ must be worn when handling wading birds such as egrets, herons, and cranes.

5. _____, _____, and _____ _____ _____ are often used when capturing birds of prey.

6. Many wild animals require _____ _____ before a veterinarian can perform a thorough physical examination.

7. The heart rate of reptiles is easily obtained using a _____.

8. _____ must be considered in all wild animals during the triage in the veterinary hospital prior to beginning treatment.

9. A wild animal must be able to _____ if released back to the wild.

10. Raccoons are a reservoir for _____ and are carriers of _____ _____, a zoonotic intestinal roundworm.

11. Bubonic plague is caused by the bacterium _____ _____ and can be found in _____.

12. A common zoonotic disease carried by wild rabbits and hares is _____.

13. _____ are the most common transmitter of the rabies virus in North America.

14. _____ _____ _____ is a mosquito-borne virus that can be a serious, life-altering, or fatal disease.

15. Freshwaters exposed to warm temperatures can suffer explosive blooms of toxin-producing phytoplankton usually referred to as _____ _____.

Glossary

A

abscess Localized concentration of pus

acute Sudden onset

ad libitum As much as desired

aerobic Functions in the presence of free oxygen

aerosol Fine particles of liquid suspended in air

afebrile Without fever

aflatoxicosis Disease resulting from ingestion of feed contaminated with toxins (aflatoxins) produced by certain species of *Aspergillus*

Aleutian disease Chronic progressive disorder of ferrets caused by a parvovirus, the Aleutian disease virus

allogrooming Grooming (licking) of others

alopecia Loss of hair

amphibian Organism in the class Amphibia; lives at least part of its life cycle in water

amyloidosis Disease that results from amyloid deposits in the glomeruli of the kidney; common cause of death in aged hamsters

anaerobic Functions in the absence of free oxygen

analgesia Absence of sensitivity to pain

anapsid Describes the skulls of chelonians that have no openings in the temporal region

anesthesia Loss of feeling or sensation

animal models Species used for research of diseases that affect other species

anisodactyl The foot shape of passerines; three toes point forward and one toe points to the rear

anorexia Lack of appetite

anterior Pertaining to the front

antibiotic-associated enterocolitis Colitis associated with antimicrobial therapy that disrupts normal intestinal flora

antibiotic toxicity *See* antibiotic-associated enterocolitis

applied research Involves the use of existing knowledge toward solving a specific biomedical problem; often directed toward detailed objectives, such as development of new vaccines or surgical procedures

apteria Featherless areas of bird skin between feather tracts

arboreal Pertaining to trees; tree-dwelling

aseptic Without microorganisms

ataxia Loss of muscular coordination

athymic Without a thymus gland

audiogenic Produced by sound

auscultate Act of listening

autotomize Breaking away of part of the lizard tail at points of fracture planes of cartilage through the vertebral bodies

axenic Germ free

B

barbering Refers to an action that occurs when a dominant animal chews the fur of a subordinate

barrier-sustained Animals maintained under sterile conditions

basic research Primarily concerned with advancing fundamental knowledge of physical, chemical, and functional mechanisms of life processes and diseases

bicornuate Having two horns

biosafety levels Categories of infectious agents that indicate specific guidelines for handling and management of such agents

blepharedema Edema of the eyelids

blepharitis Inflammation of the eyelid

boar Describes the male of guinea pigs and porcine species

brachiation A form of locomotion in which the body is suspended from branches and the animal swings between branches

brachyodont A type of dentition in which the teeth have short crowns, well-developed roots and a narrow root canal

Bruce effect The manipulation of pregnancy by pheromones; the termination of pregnancy in a recently bred mouse by placing it in a cage with a strange male

bumblefoot Pododermatitis; inflammation of the ball of the foot; usually caused by infection with *Staphylococcus* spp.

buphthalmia Enlargement of the globe due to chronically and notably elevated intraocular pressure

C

cannula Tube

canthus Corner of the eye where upper and lower eyelids meet

carapace The upper or dorsal shell of chelonians

cardiac tamponade Compression of the heart from fluid accumulation in the pericardium

caries Cavities

caudal Pertaining to the tail or posterior end

cavy Common name for a guinea pig

cecotrophs Soft fecal pellets, ingested by animals directly from the anus during the night and early morning

cecotrophy Ingestion of cecotrophs

cere Thickened skin at the base of the nares in birds

cesarean derived Refers to animals delivered surgically by removal of the uterus (hysterectomy) of the mother with delivery of the fetuses in a sterile isolation chamber

cheek pouches Represent evaginations of the lateral buccal wall; an immunologically privileges area in hamsters

chelonian Turtles and tortoises

choana The V-shaped notch in the roof of the mouth in some species that provides communication between the nasal cavity and oropharynx

choke   Common name for the condition that results from the presence of a foreign body in the oropharynx or esophagus

chromatophores   Pigment-containing cells that allow some organisms (e.g. chameleons) to change color

chromodacryorrhea   Refers to increased secretions from the harderian gland; red tears

CITES   The Convention on International Trade in Endangered Species of Wild Flora and Fauna; developed to safeguard species from extinction

clinical research   Live animal research designed to build on the knowledge gained in basic and applied research

cloaca   In birds, reptiles, and amphibians, the terminal end of the urinary, reproductive, and gastrointestinal tracts

coelom   A body cavity; in birds and reptiles, the coelom makes up the thoracic and abdominal cavities

control animal   Animal maintained with an experimental group without receiving the experimental treatment

coprophagia   Ingestion of feces; also called cecotrophy

copulatory plug   Solid mass of coagulated semen and secretions from male accessory sex glands that persists in the female vagina for 12 to 24 hours after mating

corneal reflex   Closing of the eyelid when the cornea is touched

coverts   Smaller feathers that cover the remiges and rectrices of birds. They are for covering the body and play no role in flight

cranial   Pertaining to the head or anterior end

crop   In birds, an outpocketing of the esophagus; the outcropping or dilation of the esophagus located at the base of the neck, just cranial to the thoracic inlet

cyanosis   Bluish discoloration

cytotoxic   Capable of killing cells

D

definitive host   Organism in which an infectious agent develops sexual maturity

dewlap   Loose skin under the throat and neck that may be pendulous in some species or breeds (e.g. rabbits, bloodhounds)

diapsid   Describes the skulls of certain reptiles (lizards, snakes, crocodiles) with two pairs of temporal openings behind each eye

diastema   Space between incisors and premolars

dietary factors   Refers to the quality and quantity of food and water as well as the sanitation of feed and water containers

distal   Furthest from a point of reference

diurnal illumination   Method of providing artificial light for 12 hours each day

dorsal   Pertaining to the back

dosage   Amount of a substance administered per unit of body weight

dose   Amount of a substance administered at one time

E

ectothermic   Refers to species that are unable to generate their own body heat; body temperature is dependent on environmental temperatures

ecydysis   Shedding of the epidermis

elodont   Refers to teeth that are continuously growing with no anatomic roots; tooth that increases in length throughout its life; occur in rabbits, chinchillas, and guinea pigs

emesis   The act of vomiting

enteral   Pertaining to the gastrointestinal tract

epilation   Removal of hair

epiphysis   End of a long bone where new growth occurs

epistaxis   Bleeding from the nose

eructate   Voiding of gas from the stomach via the oral cavity

exophthalmia   Characterized by prominent, bulging eyeballs

exotic pet   Any companion animal other than dogs and cats

experimental group   One that receives a treatment

exsanguination   Loss of blood

extralabel use   Use of a medication in a manner or on a species other than for that which it is approved

extrinsic factors   Involves specific environmental parameters such as temperature, humidity, lighting, noise, and ventilation

F

farrowing   The act of parturition in a sow

febrile   Characterized by fever

fecundity   The ability to produce offspring frequently and in large numbers

flank glands   Sebaceous glands appearing as dark patches on the flank or hip area of hamsters; used for marking territory

focal   Central or localized area

fomite   Nonliving object

fur slip   Loss of patch of fur at a site being grasped; occurs in chinchillas

fusiform   Spindle-shaped; tapering at each end

G

gizzard   Muscular stomach in birds that grinds food into a digestible form

gout   Disease that results from an increase in uric acid in the bloodstream that results in the deposition of the excess uric acid crystals around the joints, in the subcutaneous space, and in the viscera

gnotobiology   The study of gnotobiotic animals

gnotobiote   Animal with known microflora and microfauna

gnotobiotic   Pertaining to gnotobiotes

H

hamster parvovirus   Viral disease of hamsters characterized by incisor abnormalities, testicular atrophy, and domed crania

harderian gland   Accessory lacrimal gland deep in the medial orbit that secretes a porphyrin-rich substance; especially developed in rodents

hemipenes   Paired saclike projections from the posterior cloaca of male snakes and lizards, which together act as a penis and are inserted into the cloaca of the female

heterophil   A leukocyte of avian, reptile, and some fish species containing prominent eosinophilic granules; functionally equivalent to the mammalian neutrophil

hibernation   A deep state of sleep, nearly to the degree of a comatose state. During hibernation, an organism's metabolism and body temperature are in a significantly lowered state

hobs   A male ferret

hoglets   Neonatal hedgehogs

husbandry   Production, housing, and management of animals

hybrid   Animals that are the direct result of mating between two different inbred strains

hyperestrogenism   Condition characterized by and caused by excessive secretion or intake of estrogen; occurs in female ferrets if not mated because they are induced ovulators and remain in estrus for extended periods of time

hyperplasia   Increase in growth

hypothesis   Research supposition

hypsodontic   Teeth with long supragingival surfaces; often grow continuously

hystricomorphs   Rodents in the family Hystricidae; includes cavies and chinchillas

I

icterus   Yellowish discoloration

inbred   Animals resulting from breeding when at least 20 generations of brother-sister or parent-offspring mating have occurred

institutional animal care and use committee   Responsible for all aspects of animal use, education, health, and compliance with all laws and regulations

insulinoma   A tumor of the beta cells of the islets of Langerhans; often malignant; a common tumor in ferrets

intermediate host   Organism in which infectious agents can be maintained

intraorbital   Within the eye

intrinsic factors   Includes such characteristics as species, age, gender, and heredity

in vitro   Outside the living organism

in vivo   Within a living thing

ischial callosities   Thickened, hairless, and often brightly colored skin on the buttocks of some primate species

J

jaundice   Yellowish discoloration

jills   Female ferrets

K

kindling   The act of parturition in rabbits

kurloff cells   Leukocytes characterized by the presence of large, slightly granular cytoplasmic inclusion seen in normal guinea pigs

L

laboratory animal   Any animal used in research or teaching

lacrimal   Pertaining to tears

lacrimation   Production of tears

lagomorph   Organisms in the order lagomorpha. Rabbits and hares

lateral   Away from the midline

lethargy   Condition of weakness or listlessness

lordosis   Postural position with the pelvis elevated

lumpy jaw   Condition caused by a bacterium in the genus *actinomyces* characterized by the presence of a slowly enlarging hard lump

M

macroenvironment   Temperature, humidity, lighting, and ventilation in an area adjacent to a primary enclosure

malocclusion   Improper positioning of teeth

marsupial   Group of mammals whose young are born undeveloped and finish development in a pouch of the female

medial   Toward the midline

mentation   Refers to mental acuity or activity

metabolic bone disease   Refers to condition that is usually the result of long-term dietary deficiency of calcium or vitamin D, a lack of exposure to UV light, and/or a negative dietary calcium-to-phosphorus ratio; common in captive reptiles

microenvironment   Temperature, humidity, lighting, and ventilation within a primary enclosure

mucopurulent   Containing mucus and pus

N

nares   External opening of the nasal cavity

nasal dermatitis   Common condition of juvenile gerbils characterized by inflammation and alopecia around the upper lip and external nares; also referred to by the common names red nose, sore nose, or stress-induced chromodacryorrhea

necrosis   Death

neoplasia   New, abnormal growth

neoteny   Persistence of characteristics of a larval form

New World primate   Primates in the order Platyrrhini; includes squirrel monkeys, owl monkeys, spider monkeys, capuchins, tamarins, and marmosets

O

ocular proptosis   Abnormal forward displacement of the eye

Old World primate   Primates in the order Catarrhini; includes rhesus monkey, cynomologus monkey, and baboons

oncogenic   Capable of causing tumor formation

oviparous   Animals that lay eggs

P

palpate   Examine by touch

palpebral   Pertaining to the eyelid

palpebral reflex   Movement of the eyelids in response to a stimulus

paralytic   Substance that causes immobility

parenteral   Not relating to the gastrointestinal tract

passerines   Bird of the order Passeriformes

patagium   Gliding membrane extending between the body and a limb to form winglike extension that allows an animal to glide through the air

per diem cost   The total costs per day for housing of animals; includes costs of feeding, watering, bedding, cleaning, waste disposal, veterinary care, and other basic animal care requirements, as well as the costs related to operation of the housing facility

per os   By mouth

piloerection   Hair standing on end

pinna   Cartilaginous, projecting portion of the external ear

plastron   Bottom shell of a turtle, crustacean, or arachnid

plexus   Network of nerves or blood vessels

pododermatitis　An inflammation of the ball of the foot of birds, guinea pigs, and other small animals; usually caused by infection with *Staphylococcus* spp

posterior　Pertaining to the rear

potable　Fit to drink

prophylaxis　Preventative

proximal　Nearest to a point of reference

pruritus　Itching

pterylae　The feather tracks on the skin of birds; specific tracts located on the surface of the body where feather follicles are located

ptyalism　Excessive salivation

R

random source　Refers to animals that are not purpose-bred; such animals usually have unknown genetic makeup and health status

reduction　Refers to use of the absolute least number of animals that will achieve the research goals

refinement　Requires that an experimental procedure be chosen that causes the least amount of stress, pain, anxiety, and disturbance of normal life to the animal and still meets the experimental goals. Also requires that those performing procedures are properly trained

relative humidity　Ratio of the amount of moisture in the air at a given temperature to the maximum amount that the air can hold at that temperature

releasability　The ability for a wild animal to be released on recovery based on the injuries sustained

remiges　Contour feathers found on the wing of a bird

replacement　Refers to research that utilizes lower forms of life, computer models, or other artificial means whenever possible

retrobulbar　*See retroorbital*

retroorbital　Behind the eye

righting reflex　A proprioceptive reflex in which an animal is able to right itself after being displaced

S

sacculus rotundus　Unique feature of rabbit gastrointestinal system that forms the terminal end of the ileum

scurvy　The disease caused by a nutritional deficiency of ascorbic acid (vitamin C)

self-anointing behavior　Seen in hedgehogs whereby the animal takes an item such as fish, wool, and various plants into its mouth, mixes it with saliva, and applies the mixture to its spines with its tongue

sentinel animals　Surveillance animals housed for the purpose of identifying abnormal occurrences

septicemia　Presence of bacterial agent in the blood

sexually dimorphic　Refers to species in which the male and female differ in appearance

simian　Member of the suborder Anthropoidea that includes the monkeys and apes

sinus　Air- or fluid-filled cavity

slobbers　Common name for moist dermatitis, especially of the dewlap

snuffles　Upper respiratory tract disease of rabbits caused by bacterial infection, especially *Pasteurella multocida*

sow　Female pig or guinea pig

specific pathogen free　Animals are those that have been demonstrated to be free of certain pathogens

splay leg　Common name for hip dysplasia in rabbits

stock　A type of rat or mouse or other species that has been randomly bred; also refers to a small, square restraining pen with a front and back gate

strain　Type of rat or mouse or other species that has been inbred

straub response　Characterized by erect tail

swim bladder　Structure used for buoyancy allowing the fish to rise or fall within the water by altering the volume of air in this structure

syrinx　Enlargement of the trachea above the sternum. Contains muscles, air sacs, and vibrating membranes that collectively form the voice box of birds

T

tail autonomy　Ability of some species of reptiles to lose their tail when it is grasped by a predator

taxonomy　Science of classifying organisms

thermoneutral zone　Range of temperature for which an animal does not need physical or chemical mechanisms to control heat production or heat loss

tomia　The cutting edge of a beak

torticollis　Head tilt

transgenic　Animals are derived by removing specific DNA sequences from one strain or species and inserting them into an ovum just after fertilization

trichobezoar　Hairball

Tyzzer's disease　Disease caused by the gram-negative, spore-forming, flagellated bacterium *Clostridium piliforme*; reported in nearly all species of rodents and found throughout the world

U

urates　The end product of nitrogenous waste production from the liver; excreted by the kidney as a pasty white to yellow material found in droppings of birds and reptiles

uropygial gland　In the bird, an oil-producing gland, also called the preen gland, used to waterproof feathers; a bilobed gland with one duct opening that empties into a lone papilla, found dorsally at the base of the tail; secretes a lipoid sebaceous material that is spread over feathers during preening to help with waterproofing

V

vagal response　Short-term trancelike state characterized by lethargy and bradycardia that may be induced using digital pressure to the eyes in some species

vasoconstriction　Narrowing of lumen of blood vessels

vasodilation　Enlargement of lumen of blood vessels

vector　Organism capable of transmitting infectious agents

ventral　Pertaining to the abdomen

viremia　Presence of virus in the blood

viviparous　Animals that give birth to live young

W

wheal Raised area or swelling visible on the skin

Whitten effect Synchronization of estrus in female mice through the sudden introduction of a male (or male pheromone)

wolf teeth Small teeth that are present in front of each first molar in rabbits

wry neck Common name for condition characterized by torticollis seen in animals with otitis media or otitis interna

Z

zoonotic Capable of being transmitted between animals to human beings

zoonotic disease Infectious agents that can be transmitted between humans and animals

zygodactyl The foot shape of psittacines; the second and third toes face forward and the first and fourth toes are directed backward

Index

Note: Page numbers followed by "b", "f" and "t" indicate boxes, figures and tables respectively.